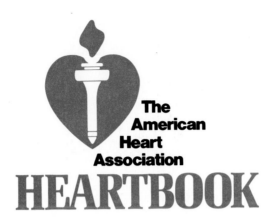

The
American
Heart
Association

HEARTBOOK

A Guide to Prevention and Treatment

of Cardiovascular Diseases

Illustrations by Ilil Arbel

The
American Heart
Association

HEARTBOOK

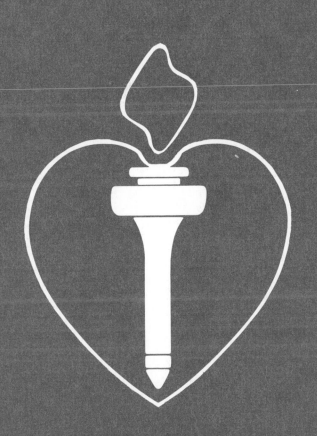

E. P. Dutton   New York

This volume is dedicated to the thousands of scientists whose research over the years has made possible our current understanding of the causes and prevention of cardiovascular disease, and to the millions of Americans in all walks of life who as Heart Association volunteers have raised funds, developed and carried on programs of education and community service—the sum total of whose efforts have dramatically improved the prospect of long life and good health for people everywhere.

ACKNOWLEDG- MENTS

The American Heart Association is indebted to many people who participated in the development of the *Heartbook*. Special recognition is made of the contributions of Mr. William H. White, who developed the concept of this book and gave constructive suggestions throughout its development. The Association owes a very special debt to the authors, who gave generously of their time and talent in writing each chapter. The work of Mr. Gerald M. Astor and Mrs. Viola Roth in editing the chapters into a consistent style was invaluable. The contribution as a consultant of Stephen S. Scheidt, M.D., is gratefully acknowledged.

Special thanks are due to the many people at the American Heart Association, in particular Mrs. Virginia Beckstead. Without them there could not have been a *Heartbook*. We are also indebted to the staff of E. P. Dutton for their special assistance in the final stages of production.

RICHARD HURLEY, M.D.

CONTENTS

Although the importance of the heart has been recognized since ancient times, it was not until 1628, when William Harvey published his treatise *On the Movement of the Heart and Blood in Animals*, that the nature of the circulatory system began to be understood; and it was not until much later, despite the careful experimental methods Harvey had used, that the idea was generally accepted.

Throughout the more than three centuries since the principle of the cardio-vascular system was established, progress in the diagnosis and treatment of diseases of the heart and blood vessels was gradual. A major landmark was the introduction in 1785 of the use of digitalis to formal medicine, after an English physician, William Withering, discovered that the foxglove, a common garden flower, was being used by an old woman to treat the accumulation of fluid known as dropsy. As with many other herbal remedies, the use of extracts from foxglove had been known to folk medicine for many years.

Subsequent pioneers include Augustus Waller, who in 1887 demonstrated the electrical activity of the heart muscle, and William Einthoven, who in 1903 developed the first practical device for measuring that activity—a string gal-vanometer, subsequently refined into the electrocardiogram.

The research in tissue transplantation and anastomoses—the technique of fastening together veins and arteries—by Dr. Alexis Carrel, who won the Nobel prize for medicine in 1912, laid the foundation for the enormous advances in surgery that have begun to revolutionize the treatment of many kinds of cardio-vascular disease.

A major development over the past three decades has been research into the causes and precursors of disease of the heart and blood vessels. Until very recently, coronary attacks and strokes were regarded as manifestations of a degenerative process, the inevitable consequence of aging and genetic makeup, and thus to be fatalistically endured. Beginning in 1948 with the Framingham study, entailing the examination of 5200 men and women at regular intervals, a series of epidemiologic studies have examined how cardiovascular diseases evolve in the general population. After just over thirty years of sustained in-vestigation, a number of major determinants or contributing factors have been identified, some of them modifiable—including high blood pressure (hyperten-sion), elevated levels of cholesterol and sugar in the bloodstream, the cigarette habit, and such living patterns as overeating and too little exercise, which lead to obesity.

During the same period other advances have been made in the diagnosis and treatment of cardiovascular disease. The most notable of these include special intensive-care units for treating patients with heart attack, and the spectacularly improved surgical procedures for dealing with congenital, coro-nary, and valvular heart disease. A variety of drugs for lowering the blood pressure have become available since the first such drugs were introduced in the early 1950s, and have proved more effective than had at first been thought possible.

The mid-1950s saw the development of the heart–lung machine, which takes over the work of a patient's own circulatory system, thus making possible the procedure known as open-heart surgery—as distinguished from other op-erations performed on a beating heart. The heart–lung machine, along with the improved surgical technique, have given back the prospect of health and long life to thousands.

Today through research and the application of new findings lives are being saved; lives of children with inborn heart defects, lives of men and women in their prime. Research to find the causes and prevention of cardiovascular disease must continue, and as answers are found this information must be transmitted expeditiously to the profession and the American public in order to further reduce disability and the unnecessary loss of life.

Since the late 1940s there has been a dramatic drop in the death rate and incidence of rheumatic fever among children. This downward trend has largely been due to better detection and treatment of streptococcal infection, the forerunner of rheumatic fever, thanks to the widespread use of penicillin and other drugs.

For many years, the American Heart Association has been working with the public and medical professions alike to educate them as to the cause, symptoms, and methods of prevention. Another most encouraging development that has occurred in the last thirty years is the downward turn in the cardiovascular death rate, particularly among men from the ages of 45 through 64. Prior to this time, the death rate among men in this age group had been steadily increasing. We believe that important contributing factors to this decline have been reduction in smoking, control of hypertension, and the lowering of cholesterol levels—all of which have been the target of American Heart Association educational programs.

However, all the advances made possible by research and the most carefully planned preventive methods are useless unless the patient and his family are well informed and are willing to put into practice the new knowledge that becomes available to them. The heart education program of the American Heart Association is a dynamic effort to get people to change their behavior in relation to risks which increase the chances of developing cardiovascular diseases, and to accept their responsibility for applying the knowledge they receive.

The public education program of the American Heart Association fulfills the growing demand of the American people to learn more about the progress being made against the nation's leading cause of death. This program allays fears growing out of ignorance, corrects misinformation and misconceptions, and provides a solid base of information upon which the public can act in confidence. It removes barriers that formerly kept many individuals from obtaining the full benefit of medical advances. Dr. Irvine H. Page, one of the earlier presidents of the American Heart Association, once said, "Understand heart disease and you will not fear it." To this I might add, understand heart disease, learn how to prevent it, and you will lead a longer, healthier, and more productive life.

In publishing the *Heartbook*, the American Heart Association has taken another major step in educating the public about the heart and vascular diseases. Hopefully, an educated public will act upon this information and help further reduce the premature mortality and disability from these causes.

To bring the reader the needed expertise to cover the wide spectrum of cardiovascular diseases, the American Heart Association has asked over twenty-five nationally and internationally known authorities to review their areas of specialty. These experts include specialists in pediatric cardiology, adult cardiology, cardiovascular surgery, peripheral vascular disease, exercise physiology, hypertension, cardiac emergencies, stroke, nutrition, behavioral science, preventive medicine, pharmacology, and smoking, to name but a few. Each authority has answered, as clearly as possible, the many questions that are constantly raised by the public in relation to cardiovascular disease. This wealth of knowledge should help to provide a clearer understanding of problems relating to the Heart and Circulatory system and provide valuable assistance to those who have heart disease or who desire to follow a preventive program.

The *Heartbook* is a reference book about the major forms of diseases of the heart and blood vessels. Given its comprehensiveness, it is unlikely that anyone will read it from cover to cover. Rather, an individual who has questions will find most of the answers in the appropriate chapter. The ultimate goal of the *Heartbook* is to provide information which will lead to a healthier heart.

RICHARD E. HURLEY, M.D.
Deputy Vice President
Office of Community
& Medical Program
American Heart Assoc.

LIST OF CONTRIBUTORS

WALTER H. ABELMANN, M.D.
Author of the chapter "Other Forms of Heart Disease," is Professor of Medicine at Harvard Medical School and at Harvard–MIT Division of Health Sciences and Technology, where he also serves as chairman of the Board of Tutors and Advisors. He was Chief of Cardiology at Beth Israel Hospital, Boston, from 1974 to 1978. Author of 150 articles since 1943, he is currently on the editorial boards of *American Heart Journal, American Journal of Cardiology,* and *ACCEL.* He was graduated from Harvard College in 1943 and received an M.D. from the University of Rochester in 1946.

HENRY BLACKBURN, M.D.
Author of the chapter "Risk Factors and Cardiovascular Disease," is Director of the Laboratory of Physiological Hygiene and Chairman of the School of Public Health–Division of Health and Human Behavior, both at the University of Minnesota. His primary interest is in the prevention of heart diseases, concerning which he and his staff are engaged in laboratory and field research around the world. An expert in insurance medicine, he has served since 1956 as chief medical consultant for underwriting for Mutual Service Insurance Companies. Author of 130 publications since 1955, he serves on the editorial boards of *Circulation, Journal of Chronic Diseases, American Journal of Cardiology,* and *American Heart Journal.* He was graduated from University of Miami in 1947 and received an M.D. in 1948 from Tulane University.

ROBERT O. BRANDENBURG, M.D.
Co-author of the chapter "Heart Valve Disease," is Professor of Medicine at the Mayo Medical School in Rochester, Minnesota. A Consultant in Internal Medicine and Cardiovascular Diseases at the Mayo Clinic since 1951, he served as Head of a section of Cardiology from 1960 to 1965 and Chairman of the Division of Cardiovascular Diseases from 1966 to 1974. He was made President-Elect of the American College of Cardiology in 1979 after serving terms as Chairman of the Board of Governors, Vice President, and Secretary. In 1972 he was presented the Award of Merit of the American Heart Association. He was graduated from North Dakota State University in 1940 and received an M.D. from the University of Pennsylvania in 1943.

MICHAEL M. DEHN, M.S.
Co-author of the chapter "Exercise," serves as Program Director and Secretary–Treasurer of the Dallas Cardiac Institute. He is an exercise physiologist at St. Paul Hospital Exercise Laboratory in Dallas and Adjunct Professor at North Texas State University, and Vice Chairman of the American Heart Association Dallas Chapter Exercise Committee. A certified instructor–trainer in cardiopulmonary resuscitation, he received his bachelor's degree from the University of Washington in 1970 and an M.S. in physical education in 1972.

VICTOR G. DE WOLFE, M.D.
Author of the chapter "Peripheral Arterial Disease," is Senior Physician and Director of the Vascular Laboratory, Department of Peripheral Vascular Disease, Cleveland Clinic Foundation. He has been a staff member of the clinic since 1949 and was Head of the Department of Peripheral Vascular Disease from 1961 to 1976. He is a diplomate of the American Board of Internal Medicine, a Fellow of the American College of Physicians, and the author of seventy-four scientific publications. He was graduated from Princeton University in 1940 and was awarded an M.D. from Columbia University in 1943.

HARRIET P. DUSTAN, M.D.
Author of the chapter "Hypertension," is Director of the Cardiovascular Research and Training Center at the University of Alabama Medical Center in Birmingham. She served earlier as Vice Chairman of the Research Division of the Cleveland Clinic. A researcher in high blood pressure for thirty years and the author of more than 150 publications in that field, in 1978 she was chosen the first editor of *Hypertension.* She was President of the American Heart Association from 1976 to 1977. In 1976 *Modern Medicine* presented her with an Award for Distinguished Achievement. Both her undergraduate (1942) and her medical degree (1944) were presented by the University of Vermont.

MARY ALLEN ENGLE, M.D.
Author of the chapter "Congenital Heart Defects," is Director of Pediatric Cardiology at the New York Hospital–Cornell University Medical College where she has just been named the Stavros S. Niarchos Professor of Pediatric Cardiology. At the New York Hospital since 1948, she was Director of Pediatric Electrocardiography for twenty years and Director of Pediatric Phonocardiography for ten years. She has received the Spence–Chapin Award for Outstanding Contribution to Pediatrics, the Cummings Humanitarian Award, the American Heart Association Award of Merit, the Maryland Heart Association's Helen B. Taussig Award, the Citation of the National Board of the Medical College of Pennsylvania and the Woman of Conscience Award of the National Council of Women of U.S. She has served on the editorial boards of *Circulation, American Journal of Cardiology, American Heart Journal,* and *Chest.* She has served on the Board of Directors of the American Heart Association and on the Board of Trustees of the American College of Cardiology. She was graduated from Baylor University in 1942 and received her M.D. from Johns Hopkins University in 1945.

RICHARD I. EVANS, PH.D.
Co-author of the chapter "Hazards of Smoking," is Professor of Psychology at the University of Houston. Film and media editor for *Contemporary Psychology,* he directed or produced thirty-three films, twelve of which are concerned with smoking problems. He serves as a consultant to the National Cancer Institute and the National Science Foundation. He is a member of the editorial board of the *Journal of Behavioral Medicine* and Consulting Editor of the *International Journal of Social Psychiatry* and the *Journal of Dental Research.* He was graduated from the University of Pittsburgh in 1946 and received a Ph.D. from Michigan State University in 1950.

NANCY C. FLOWERS, M.D.
Co-author of the chapter "Arrhythmias," is Professor of Medicine and Director of Cardiovascular Research and Training in the Division of Cardiology at the University of Louisville Department of Medicine. Earlier she was Chief of the Section of Cardiology, Veterans Administration Hospital, Augusta, Georgia. She is President of the Cardiac Electrophysiology Group. Author of over 170 publications and presentations, she has been a member of the editorial boards of *American Heart Journal, Circulation,* and *Geriatrics.* She was graduated from Mississippi State College for Women in 1950 and received an M.D. from the University of Tennessee in 1958.

RICHARD E. HURLEY, M.D.
Author of the Introduction, is Deputy Executive Vice President for Community and Medical Programs of the American Heart Association. He joined AHA in 1960 after several years of research at the Cleveland Clinic and at Case Western Reserve University. In 1979 he was presented the Distinguished Service Award of the American College of Cardiology. He received his bachelor's degree (1951) and his M.D. (1954) from the University of Utah.

C. DAVID JENKINS, PH.D.
Author of the chapter "Behavioral Risk Factors," is Professor of Psychiatry and Director of the Department of Behavioral Epidemiology at Boston University School of Medicine. He was Chairman of the Behavioral Sciences Task Group of the American Heart Association's Risk Reduction Factor Committee and a founding member of the Academy of Behavioral Medicine Research. Author of eighty-seven scientific publications, he has served on the editorial board of *Psychosomatic Medicine* since 1969 and on those of *Journal of Human Stress* and *Journal of Behavioral Medicine* since their inception. He was graduated from the University of Chicago in 1950 and received a Ph.D. in Psychology from the University of North Carolina in 1960.

DONALD F. LEON, M.D.
Author of the chapter "The Annual Checkup," is Vice President for Professional Affairs of the University Health Center of Pittsburgh, as well as Professor of Medicine and Acting Dean of the University of Pittsburgh School of Medicine. He formerly served as Chief of the Division of Cardiology at Magee–Women's Hospital in Pittsburgh and Chief of the Cardiology Section at the USAF Hospital, Scott Air Force Base, Illinois. From 1968 to 1972 he was an American

Heart Association Teaching Scholar in Cardiology. He received an M.D. from Georgetown University in 1957.

DEAN T. MASON, M.D.
Author of the chapter "Congestive Heart Failure," is Professor of Medicine, Professor of Physiology, and Chief of the Section of Cardiovascular Medicine at the University of California School of Medicine at Davis. A member of the editorial boards of fifteen professional journals, he is the author of more than 800 articles and of six textbooks, including Congestive Heart Failure, Advances in Heart Disease, and Cardiac Emergencies. He has also served as President of the American College of Cardiology. His list of honors includes four Cummings Humanitarian Awards. He received both his bachelor's degree (1954) and his M.D. (1958) from Duke University.

FLETCHER H. MC DOWELL, M.D.
Author of the chapter "Stroke," is Medical Director and Chief Executive Officer of Burke Rehabilitation Hospital in White Plains, New York, and Professor of Neurology and Associate Dean of Cornell Medical College. He is also editor of Stroke—A Journal of Cerebral Circulation and Chairman of the Medical Advisory Board of the American Parkinson's Disease Association. He was Chairman of the American Heart Association Council on Stroke from 1972 to 1974. He was graduated from Dartmouth College in 1944 and received an M.D. from Cornell University in 1947.

DWIGHT C. MC GOON, M.D.
Co-author of the chapter "Heart Valve Disease," is Stuart W. Harrington Professor of Surgery at the Mayo Medical School in Rochester, Minnesota, where he has served as a consultant since 1957. He is the former editor of the Journal of Thoracic and Cardiovascular Surgery; he has been a member of the editorial boards of Circulation, Surgery, American Journal of Cardiology, and American Heart Journal. He is a founding member of the Pediatric Cardiac Surgery Club. He received an M.D. from Johns Hopkins University in 1948.

DANIEL E. MC MARTIN, M.D.
Co-author of the chapter "Arrhythmias," is Chief of the Division of Cardiology and Associate Professor of Medicine at the University of Louisville in Louisville, Kentucky. He joined the university as an instructor in 1973 and was an assistant professor for five years before receiving his current posts in 1979. He is a member of the Research Grant Review Committee of the Kentucky Heart Association. He was graduated from Hamilton College in 1961 and received his M.D. from the State University of New York at Buffalo in 1965.

JERE H. MITCHELL, M.D.
Co-author of the chapter "Exercise," is Professor of Medicine and Physiology, University of Texas Southwestern Medical School, and Director of the university's Harry S. Moss Heart Center, both in Dallas. He was an Established Investigator for the American Heart Association from 1962 to 1967, served as Chairman of AHA's Council on Basic Sciences, and currently serves as Chairman of the Association's Exercise Committee. He is a member of the editorial boards of Journal of Applied Physiology, Cardiovascular Research, and Circulation, and author of over 130 publications. A member of the Commission on Cardiovascular Physiology of the International Union of Physiological Sciences, Council on Cardiac Rehabilitation of the International Society and Federation of Cardiology, he was graduated from Virginia Military Institute in 1950 and received an M.D. from Southwestern Medical School in 1954.

RUSSELL M. NELSON, M.D.
Author of the chapter "Cardiovascular Surgery," is Research Professor of Surgery and Director of the Cardiovascular–Thoracic Training Program at the University of Utah. He is a member of the Steering Committee of the American Heart Association and served earlier as Chairman of the AHA Council on Cardiovascular Surgery. He was a Markle Scholar in Medical Science at Utah, served as President of the Utah Heart Association from 1964 to 1965, and was a member of the Board of Directors of the American Board of Thoracic Surgery from 1972 to 1978. He received an M.D. at the University of Utah in 1947 and a Ph.D. in surgery from the University of Minnesota in 1954.

ROBERT A. O'ROURKE, M.D.
Author of the chapter "Symptoms of Cardiovascular Disease," is Charles Conrad and Anna Sahm Brown Professor of Medicine and Director of the Cardiovascular Division at the University of Texas Health Science Center, San Antonio. He is Vice Chairman of the American Heart Association Council on Clinical Cardiology. A member of several editorial boards, he is the author of more than 255 works, including the texts Self-Assessment of Current Knowledge in Cardiovascular Disease and Understanding Diseases of the Heart. He

was graduated from Creighton University in 1957 and received his M.D. there in 1961.

MALCOLM R. PARKER, M.D.
Author of the chapter "Cardiac Emergencies," has been a private physician since 1962. He practices in Los Gatos, California. Currently a Vice President of the American Heart Association, Chairman of its Program Committee, and Chairman of its Task Force on Emergency Cardiac Care at Airports and in Flight, he served earlier as President of the California Heart Association and Chairman of the AHA Committee on Emergency Cardiac Care and Cardiopulmonary Resuscitation. He was graduated from Emory University in 1949 and received an M.D. from the Medical College of Georgia in 1953.

ELLIOT RAPAPORT, M.D.
Author of the chapter "Coronary Artery Disease," is William Watt Kerr Professor of Clinical Medicine at the University of California School of Medicine in San Francisco and Chief of Cardiology at San Francisco General Hospital. He is editor of Circulation, and author of more than a hundred publications. He served as Chairman of the research committees of both the American Heart Association and the California Heart Association and was President of the California and American Heart Association. He was graduated in 1944 from the University of California at Berkeley and received an M.D. from the University of California at San Francisco in 1946.

ROBERT E. SHANK, M.D.
Co-author of the chapter "Diet and Nutrition," is Danforth Professor of Preventive Medicine and Head of the Department of Preventive Medicine at Washington University School of Medicine. Organizations he has served as President include the American Society for Clinical Nutrition, the Association for Study of Liver Diseases, and the Association of Teachers of Preventive Medicine. He has served as a nutrition consultant in Uganda, Zambia, and Sudan and was co-director of nutrition survey teams in Peru and Brazil. A former associate editor of Nutrition Today, he has written 73 articles. He was graduated from Westminster College in 1935 and received an M.D. from Washington University School of Medicine in 1939.

Former chairman of the Nutrition Committee of the American Heart Association, he has served in various capacities of the National Heart, Lung and Blood Institute, the current committee is the Clinical Applications and Prevention Advisory Committee.

LEWIS B. SHEINER, M.D.
Author of the chapter "Cardiovascular Drugs," is a clinical pharmacologist and Associate Professor of the Department of Laboratory Medicine and Department of Medicine at the University of California at San Francisco. He has written over fifty scientific articles and is an editor of Current Topics in Drug Therapeutics. A 1960 graduate of Cornell University, he received an M.D. in 1964 from Albert Einstein College of Medicine.

JOHN T. SHEPHERD, M.D., D.S.C.
Co-author of the chapter "How the Heart Functions," is Dean of Mayo Medical School and Director for Education for the Mayo Foundation. From 1975 to 1976 he was President of the American Heart Association and Chairman of AHA's Research Committee and Council on Circulation. The author of four books, The Physiology of the Circulation in Human Limbs in Health and Disease, Cardiac Function in Health and Disease, Veins and Their Control, and The Human Cardiovascular System: Facts and Concepts, he has served on the editorial boards of American Journal of Physiology, Journal of Applied Physiology, Circulation Research, and other journals. Born in Northern Ireland, he received his medical degree and began his research career at Queen's University in Belfast.

JAY M. SULLIVAN, M.D.
Author of the chapter "Pregnancy and the Cardiovascular System," is Professor of Medicine and Chief of the Division of Cardiovascular Diseases at the University of Tennessee College of Medicine. He served earlier as Physician-in-Chief at Boston Hospital for Women. A Medical Foundation Research Fellow in 1967, he has written over eighty scientific works. He serves on the Medical Advisory Board of the American Heart Association's Council for High Blood Pressure Research. Georgetown University awarded him a B.S. in 1958 and an M.D. in 1962.

J. KEITH THWAITES, M.P.H.
Co-author of the chapter "Hazards of Smoking," is Associate Director of Community and Medical Programs at the American Heart Association National

Center. He joined AHA in 1961 after a decade as Executive Director of the California Heart Association and before assuming his present post was Director of AHA Community Programs. He has served as a member of the board of the National Interagency Council on Smoking and Health and on the advisory committee of Mended Hearts, Inc. He was graduated from George Washington University in 1944 and received an M.P.H. from the University of California at Berkeley in 1951.

LEWIS W. WANNAMAKER, M.D.

Author of the chapter "Rheumatic Fever," is Professor of Pediatrics and Professor of Microbiology at the University of Minnesota. He was Assistant Director of the Streptococcal Disease Laboratory, which was honored by the Lasker Award in 1954 for work on prevention of rheumatic fever. In 1958 he was appointed a lifetime Career Investigator of the American Heart Association. He was Director of the Commission of Streptococcal and Staphylococcal Diseases from 1967 to 1972 and a member of the Rheumatic Fever and Rheumatic Heart Disease Study Group of the Inter-Society Commission for Heart Disease Resources. He has also served on several AHA, NIH and WHO committees and on the editorial boards of a number of clinical and microbiology publications. He received his premedical education from Emory University and an M.D. degree from Duke University in 1946.

NANETTE K. WENGER, M.D.

Author of the chapter "Living With Cardiovascular Disease," is Professor of Medicine (Cardiology) at Emory University School of Medicine. She has served as Vice President of the American Heart Association, Chairman of its Program and Rehabilitation Committees and President of the Georgia Heart Association. She is Co-chairman of the U.S. Department of Health, Education, and Welfare's National Plan for Cardiac Rehabilitation Committee and President-elect of the Rehabilitation Council of the International Society of Cardiology. She has served on the editorial boards of *Cardiac Rehabilitation Quarterly, American Journal of Cardiology, Living, Growing and Dying,* and *Patient Care.* She was graduated from Hunter College in 1951 and received an M.D. from Harvard Medical School in 1954.

STANFORD WESSLER, M.D.

Author of the chapter "Peripheral Venous Disease," is Professor of Medicine at New York University Medical Center and Associate Dean of the NYU Division of Post-Graduate Medical School. A Vice President of the American Heart Association from 1974 to 1975, he has also served AHA as Chairman of the Thrombosis Council, the Council Affairs Committee, and the Publications Committee. A former associate editor of *Circulation* and a former member of the editorial board of *Circulation Research,* he is the author of more than 200 works. He was graduated from Harvard University in 1938 and received an M.D. from New York University in 1942.

MARY WINSTON, ED.D.

Co-author of the chapter "Diet and Nutrition," is Community Program Specialist–Nutritionist for the American Heart Association. Before joining AHA she served as Director of the Dietetics and Nutrition Department at the University of Kentucky Medical Center in Lexington and as Director of the Dietetics Department at Research Hospital in Kansas City. *American Heart Association Cookbook* is among the publications of which she is a co-author. She was graduated from St. Mary College in Leavenworth, Kansas, in 1945 and received both her M.A. (1952) and Ed.D. (1975) from Columbia University.

JOHN J. WITTE, M.D.

Co-author of the chapter "Hazards of Smoking," is Medical Director of the Bureau of Health Education at the Center for Disease Control in Atlanta. He formerly served as Deputy Director of the National Clearinghouse for Smoking and Director of the Immunization Division, both located at the Center. He has been a consultant to British Guiana, Jordan, and Canada and was Executive Secretary of the Public Health Service Advisory Committee on Immunization Practices. In 1972 he received the U.S. Public Health Service Commendation Medal. He was graduated from Hope College in 1954 and received an M.D. from Johns Hopkins University in 1959 and an M.P.H. from Harvard University in 1966.

1

RISK FACTORS AND
CARDIOVASCULAR DISEASE

Henry Blackburn, M.D.

Countries	Average Serum Cholesterol mg. per 100 ml.	Saturated Fatty Acid % Calories
Velika Krsna	157	8.8
Dalmatia	185	9.5
Montegiorgio	196	8.9
Crevalcore	197	9.7
Corfu	198	5.4
Slavonia	198	13.0
Crete	204	8.6
Zrenjanin	208	10.0
Belgrade Faculty	216	10.0
Zutphen	230	19.5
U.S. Railroad	236	17.0
West Finland	254	18.8
East Finland	264	22.2

Of all the recent developments in cardiovascular research, probably none is more important than the clear demonstration that different cultural patterns, life styles, and personal characteristics carry different degrees of risk of eventual heart attack or stroke. The full recognition and implementation of this knowledge could potentially be the most significant measure affecting the collective health of North Americans today.

It has became evident that the "American way" is not an entirely successful experiment as far as health is concerned. People in many other countries have fewer heart attacks and strokes; many have longer life expectancies. If they can maintain a low rate of heart attacks, why can't we? Many facets of day-to-day life are involved. For example, the American eating pattern tends toward overconsumption of meat and dairy products, which are high in saturated fat; a large consumption of sugar and salt; and a decreasing consumption of whole grains, breads, legumes, vegetables, and fruits. In addition, there is the abundance of alcohol, which is readily available, inexpensive, and socially acceptable. There is also the pervasive smoking habit: again, cigarettes are available, cheap, and, for the time being, socially acceptable. Put all this into a motorized, labor-saving, indulgent, and sedentary society that regards physical labor and sweating—except in professional athletics—as largely unrewarding; add commercially determined values and purposeless goals, and the result is an awesome incidence of culturally induced premature disability and death from cardiovascular diseases.

In an effort to pinpoint the causes of coronary heart disease, especially among industrialized societies, major studies of populations throughout the world have been conducted in the last three decades. Evidence concerning the influence of life styles and controllable risk factors is consistent in many of these population studies and is in accordance with clinical observations of patients with premature atherosclerotic heart disease. Laboratory experiments also support the evidence of epidemiological studies. Although controversies persist, understanding is increasing among members of the medical community and the public at large regarding the broad social and economic determinants of heart attacks and strokes and the potential approaches to their prevention.

CONTROLLABLE RISK FACTORS   The major risk factors identified as avoidable, controllable, or correctable in a number of the studies of large population groups include habitual excesses in eating habits, elevated blood fats (lipids), obesity, sedentary life style, high blood pressure (hypertension), cigarette smoking, and personality type. Risk factors over which there is no control are age and aging, sex, race and ethnic origin, country of origin and early environment, and heredity and family history; these are discussed later.

Eating Patterns   The evidence from many sources shows that aspects of diet and eating pattern —that is, food choices, frequency and size of meals—are important to health in general and that a few are strongly related to cardiovascular risk. These include an overconsumption of calories in general and specifically an excess of certain fats, salt, and perhaps sugar in the diet. Indeed, recent research findings put habitual diet and eating pattern in the forefront of personal and public health considerations regarding the risk of coronary heart disease.

How did habitual diet come to be recognized as important in heart disease? How important is an individual's eating pattern to his personal risk of heart attack? As a national problem, how significant is the "American way of eating" in the picture of coronary artery disease and high blood pressure? Why is there still controversy over diet as a controllable risk factor?

One of the first researchers to call attention to the relationship between atherosclerosis and diet was a European pathologist who was studying the relationship between protein intake and kidney disease in rabbits. He noted that rabbits on his high-protein diet had high levels of blood cholesterol and also had fatty accumulations in blood vessels resembling the atherosclerotic deposits he had observed in human arteries during autopsies. Expanding his experiments, he found that the high fat and cholesterol content of the diets, rather than the protein, caused the atherosclerotic arteries. Many years later, in the middle of this century, a number of researchers demonstrated that the levels of fats in the blood could be altered by changes in the diet. They also observed that the most potent factors leading to increased levels of blood cholesterol were consumption of dietary cholesterol and saturated fats, particularly animal fats or industrially "hardened" vegetable fats. Conversely, diets high in unsaturated vegetable fats were shown to lower blood cholesterol levels and neutralize effects of starch and sugar.

Countries	Average Serum Cholesterol mg. per 100 ml.	CHD Deaths, Infarcts per 100
Velika Krsna	156	0.2
Dalmatia	186	1.1
Montegiorgio	196	1.7
Corfu	198	1.3
Slavonia	198	2.0
Crevalcore	200	1.8
Crete	203	0.1
Zrenjanin	208	0.5
Belgrade Faculty	216	0.9
Zutphen	230	3.4
US Railroad	237	3.25
West Finland	253	2.25
East Finland	264	2.4

Then came the systematic observations of a major international study, the Seven Countries Study conducted in the 1950s and 1960s, that cultures characterized by diets relatively high in saturated fats were also characterized by relatively high average levels of blood fats (especially cholesterol) and a relatively high frequency of atherosclerotic diseases. This study, which at its inception involved 12,000 men between the ages of forty and fifty-nine, also showed that communities characterized by low average intake of animal and other saturated fats had low average cholesterol levels and a low incidence of heart disease.

In all, eighteen communities in Finland, Greece, Italy, Japan, the Netherlands, the United States, and Yugoslavia were studied. The men in eastern Finland emerged as having the highest incidence of coronary heart disease, while rates were very low among the men from Corfu and Crete in Greece, from Dalmatia in Yugoslavia, and from Japan. Differences in diet, especially in the types of fat consumed, were considered to be the essential factor. The highest average fat consumption—about 40 percent of the total calories consumed—was found in Zutphen, the Netherlands; Crete; the United States; and eastern Finland. The highest proportion of saturated fats—22 percent—was consumed by the eastern Finns, followed by the Americans with 19 percent. Although the Greeks had an equally high total consumption of fats, only 8 percent was from animal or saturated fats; the rest came from olive oil and other vegetable oils. The Japanese, who had one of the lowest rates of coronary heart disease, consumed the lowest amount of fats, only 9 percent of the total calories and only 3 percent from animal fat.

But what happens when people from countries with a low incidence of heart disease move to another country or area in which there is a higher incidence? Recent studies comparing the incidence of coronary heart disease among Japanese in their homeland with that of those who have relocated in Hawaii and in California show that among those who consume the traditional Japanese diet, which is low in fat and high in complex carbohydrates or starches, there is a pattern of low levels of blood cholesterol and other lipids. But when the Japanese adopt the typical high-fat American diet, which is

Countries	Percent Calories Saturated Fatty Acids	CHD Deaths, Infarcts per 100
Corfu	5.4	1.3
Crete	8.6	0.1
Velika Krsna	8.8	0.2
Montegiorgio	8.9	1.7
Dalmatia	9.5	1.1
Crevalcore	9.7	1.8
Zrenjanin	10.0	0.3
Belgrade Faculty	10.0	0.9
Slavonia	13.0	2.0
U.S. Railroad	17.0	3.2
West Finland	18.8	2.2
Zutphen	19.5	3.4
East Finland	22.2	4.4

A five-year international study, involving a total of 12,000 middle-aged men, showed that communities characterized by a low average intake of animal and other saturated fats also had not only lower levels of serum cholesterol but also a lower incidence of coronary heart disease. The highest incidence was among the men living in eastern Finland and in the United States during the five-year period covered by the survey, compared with the men living in Greece and Yugoslavia. The highest proportion of saturated fat was consumed by the eastern Finns, followed by the Americans. Although the Greeks had an equally high total consumption of fats—about 40 percent of total calories consumed—only 8 percent of their caloric intake was from animal or saturated fats, the difference being made up by the use of olive oil and other vegetable oils.

low in complex carbohydrates and high in simple sugars, the lipid measurements rise, as does the incidence of heart attacks, although these may still be fewer than the average of the adopted country.

More recent experimental studies have shown that monkeys fed American-type diets develop severe atherosclerosis but when their diets are returned to more characteristic monkey fare, the fatty material and the damage to the artery wall decrease. These results and others have led many researchers to conclude that, just as high-fat diets produce fatty arteries in experimental animals, diets high in saturated fat and cholesterol are probably critical factors in the high incidence of heart attacks and strokes among whole communities and cultures. Other associated risk factors may, however, add to the dietary risk to produce the public health problem.

Blood Fats Cholesterol is only one of several lipids found in the blood. In order for the body to transport and use these lipids, they must be combined with another molecule to make them soluble in the blood serum, the fluid portion of blood. This molecule is a protein, which combines with the fats to form lipoproteins, making possible the transport and utilization of fats. Lipoprotein molecules come in various sizes and weights, and the amounts of cholesterol and other lipids they contain vary according to the size and weight.

The heaviest of these molecules is high density lipoprotein (HDL). HDL contains the highest proportion of protein and has recently been shown to be of possible importance in transporting fat away from body cells, thus preventing the accumulation of cholesterol and other fats within the artery walls. There is also evidence that the higher the amount of HDL in the blood, the lower the subsequent risk of fatty artery diseases, heart attacks, and strokes. In general, women tend to have higher levels of HDL than men, and athletes, especially those such as long-distance runners, who engage in very vigorous exercise, also tend to have high HDL. Smokers tend to have lower HDL levels.

Low density lipoprotein (LDL) is lighter than HDL and contains the largest proportion of cholesterol of any of the lipoproteins. There is considerable evidence that a high amount of LDL is a factor in the accumulation of fatty materials in artery walls, and that LDL itself, or LDL cholesterol, is significantly related to future risk of heart attack and stroke. Because LDL level is importantly influenced by diet, it is the measurement which, along with total blood cholesterol, is most related to cultural differences in heart attack rate.

Very low density lipoprotein (VLDL) is lighter still and is the fat-protein molecule in blood which carries the largest amount of triglycerides. VLDL plays an important role in the production of other blood lipoproteins and their transport, but its relationship to fatty artery disease is uncertain. Elevated VLDL may be related to cardiovascular risk directly or related only indirectly because it is a precursor of LDL.

What does this mean to the individual? Evidence is clear that individual risk of a future heart attack, stroke, or other manifestation of fatty artery disease is strongly related to the levels of total blood cholesterol and LDL. The higher the plasma or serum cholesterol level measured during health, the higher the future risk of a cardiac event. The lower the level of cholesterol, the lower the subsequent risk. However, there is no level above which heart attacks are certain or below which they never occur. In general, the frequency of heart attacks is relatively low (by American standards) in persons who have cholesterol levels below 200 milligrams per deciliter (mg/dl) and extremely high in those with cholesterol levels over 300 mg/dl.

The increasing coronary risk according to prior total cholesterol level among 8,000 men followed for ten years in the American Heart Association Pooling Project is shown in the chart:

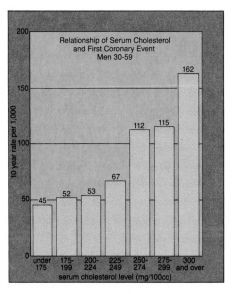

Even in the range of cholesterol levels that most physicians and laboratories in the United States consider normal, there is actually a wide range of risk of heart attack and stroke. Consequently, a clinically normal cholesterol level may not be a true indication of actual risk. There is little controversy among experienced investigators and physicians concerning this evidence. However, there is more to be learned about optimal levels of cholesterol for individual adults, for youth, and for whole countries. For example, in people with high total blood cholesterol levels, it is protective to have higher levels of HDL cholesterol.

Other lipids circulating in the blood which have given rise to a good deal of speculation are the triglycerides, the most ubiquitous form of fat in foods. Triglycerides are so named because they consist of three fatty-acid molecules attached to one molecule of glycerol. They are consumed in the diet and also manufactured in the body and they play a key role in the lipid-carrying function of the blood. Although many patients with coronary heart disease have elevated levels of triglycerides, the evidence that these have any bearing on atherosclerosis is far from complete. One study conducted in Sweden showed that the heart-attack rate among persons with elevated triglycerides is higher than normal, but a number of subsequent studies have found either no relationship or rather tenuous relationships between this lipid and heart disease. One possible exception might be women over the age of fifty—two studies have demonstrated a correlation between elevated triglycerides and future heart attacks in this group.

Another area of concern involves VLDL, the lightest lipoprotein associated with triglycerides. Since it acts as a precursor to LDL, a high level of VLDL may tend to elevate LDL and cholesterol and lower the HDL level.

That there is no conclusive evidence linking elevated triglycerides and VLDL with heart disease does not mean that these elevated levels are of no significance. On the contrary it is known that populations that consume high-sugar diets have elevated triglycerides, as do diabetics, people who drink alcohol regularly, and obese individuals. Women who take birth-control pills also tend to have elevated triglycerides. Preventive physical examinations should therefore include measurement of triglycerides, because this added information helps define more accurately how fats are being handled by the body.

In general, the individual risk of heart attacks rises steadily above a blood cholesterol measurement of 200 mg/dl, and the higher the total blood cholesterol, the greater the risk. The average cholesterol level of Americans is considerably higher than the average in nations that enjoy a lower incidence of heart attacks. The highest levels of blood cholesterol are found in North America, central and northern Europe, New Zealand, and Australia, where the averages range from 220 to 280 mg/dl.

The increasing coronary risk according to prior cholesterol level among 8,000 men followed for ten years in the American Heart Association Pooling Project is shown here. As the cholesterol level increases from less than 175 to 300 milligrams per 100 cubic centimeters and over, the rate of heart attack increases almost fourfold.

Desirable Levels

At the opposite end of the spectrum, populations that are largely vegetarian or those undernourished by Western standards have average blood cholesterol levels ranging from 100 to 140 mg/dl. It should not be assumed, however, that these levels are "ideal" for general health.

In between those two extremes are other population groups which have low cholesterol levels when compared to more affluent Western societies and much lower incidence of heart attacks. These include people in the rural areas of the Mediterranean, Latin America, and the Orient, whose cholesterol levels average 150 to 160 mg/dl. These population groups, which enjoy stable living patterns and diets, are engaged largely in agricultural, pastoral, and fishing pursuits and are particularly free of coronary heart disease. Populations in the more industrialized areas of these regions—Greece, Yugoslavia, Italy, Puerto Rico, and urban Japan—have somewhat higher average cholesterol levels,

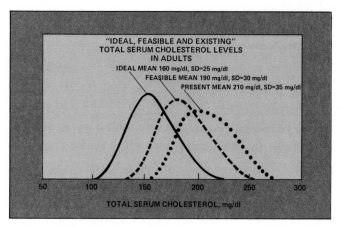

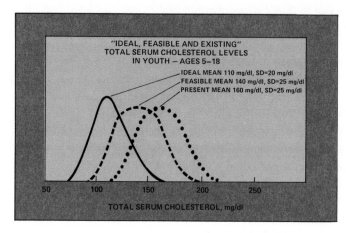

These curves are plots of different cholesterol levels, from lowest to highest. The dotted line curves are the most frequently encountered cholesterol level and represents the present situation for American adults and children. The broken-line curves are those thought desirable and feasible with continuation of present trends in eating patterns. The solid line curves are ideal with respect to population having the fewest heart attacks.

ranging from 180 to 190 mg/dl. Among these groups the incidence of heart attacks is less than half that of the United States and other affluent Western societies.

At a recent international congress on Health Effects of Blood Lipids sponsored by the American Health Foundation, the section on epidemiology concluded that average blood cholesterol levels or 180 to 190 mg/dl may be considered "an upper limit of population averages compatible with substantially reduced risk of fatty arteries, good general health, and low rates of premature mortality."

Another epidemiological aspect emphasized at this meeting was the disparity in the average cholesterol levels among the young in various population groups. A few decades ago, it was assumed that atherosclerosis was a disease of aging. This belief was dispelled by autopsy studies of young men killed in Korea and later in Vietnam, in which it was found that many of these young American men showed evidence of advanced atherosclerosis. Studies around the world have found that the average cholesterol levels of newborns are similar in all population groups—about 65 to 70 mg/dl. But by the ages of five to nine years, wide disparities among populations already exist. In the affluent Western societies the average cholesterol levels in this age group are about 160 to 180 mg/dl, compared to averages of 100 to 120 in populations with lower rates of fatty artery diseases. In reviewing these data at the congress on lipids, the participants caution that "because elevated blood cholesterol levels in childhood tend to track into adult years, it appears desirable and even necessary to have average values of 120 to 140 mg/dl in children to yield adult population values in the desirable range between 150 to 190 mg/dl." Although noting that "genetic factors are very important in determining an individual's amount and types of blood cholesterol," the epidemiologists stressed that "nonhereditary, environmental, cultural, and behavior factors determine much of the *population* differences in blood lipid levels and their associated diseases."

As indicated earlier, high levels of blood cholesterol can be lowered by diet. (In extreme cases, drugs are also used.) According to projections worked out by clinical researchers, an average reduction of 10 percent in total blood cholesterol may be achieved if a new diet provides 30 percent of the calories in fats, no more than 10 percent from saturated fats with dietary cholesterol limited to 200 milligrams a day, and if a higher ratio of polyunsaturated fats is adopted. A further decrease of about 10 percent in total blood cholesterol is possible to achieve if the intake of certain types of fiber, particularly pectins, is increased. Some substitution of vegetable protein for animal protein may produce a further reduction in cholesterol levels.

An additional decrease of about 15 mg/dl may be achieved by moderate reduction in weight. If a regular exercise program is added to this regimen, the payoff may be an increase in HDL—a further potential benefit. Still further reductions may be realized by limiting the total fat intake to between 24 and 27 percent of total calories, with a very low amount of saturated fats. In fact, one Neapolitan community with this type of diet has total cholesterol levels ranging from only 168 to 202 mg/dl and LDL-cholesterol levels of only 97 to 122 mg/dl.

There appears to be sufficient evidence to incriminate metabolic processes associated with excessive blood cholesterol as a cause of coronary heart disease. Examples are:

- The surest and, in fact, the only way to produce fatty arteries in animals is to feed them diets high in cholesterol.
- Cholesterol is predominant in the fat found in the deposits within the artery walls in persons with atherosclerosis.

There is some evidence that lowering cholesterol will help prevent coronary heart disease in people or countries already having much atherosclerosis, but it is not as extensive, as conclusive, or as direct as one would desire. For example:

- Monkeys fed a high-fat diet to increase their levels of blood cholesterol, after returning to their normal low-fat diets, do show evidence of reduction in fatty deposits in their arteries.
- Wartime experiences in Switzerland, Scandinavia, and other European countries during the 1940s suggest that changes in diet, which included reduced consumption of fats and increased consumption of potatoes, beans, and other vegetables, resulted in a lowered incidence of heart attacks in a fairly short time.
- Dietary changes in Europe after World War II, and increased consumption of fats and sugar among immigrants to Israel and the United States, coincided with an increase in blood cholesterol levels and a rapidly increasing frequency of heart attacks.

More evidence is being sought in a number of large-scale studies now underway in the United States and Europe. By the early 1980s, when results of these studies start coming in, there should be firmer evidence as to whether lowering blood cholesterol does, indeed, result in reduced atherosclerosis, as manifested by heart attacks in high risk mid-aged people. Still, this will not indicate the potential for prevention when large numbers of people, beginning in childhood, adopt a more varied eating pattern and reduce other risk factors.

In the meantime, there is much to be gained and, I believe, nothing to be lost from attempting to lower the American level of blood cholesterol by moderate changes in diet. This view is shared by the American Heart Association, whose latest recommendations call for:

- An adjustment in total caloric intake to achieve and maintain ideal body weight.
- A reduction in total fat consumed, to be achieved by a substantial reduction in consumption of animal or saturated fats.
- A substantial reduction in dietary cholesterol.
- A substantial increase in complex carbohydrates and vegetable protein.

High Blood Pressure Many people have the mistaken notion that hypertension (the medical term for high blood pressure) has something to do with "hyper" behavior—that is, the behavior of a tense, nervous, "Type A" sort of person. Although life style and stress may play some role in the disease process, what hypertension actually means is that the pressure at which the blood is being pumped through the arteries is higher than normal. Blood pressure is expressed in two numbers: 110/70, for example. The higher number is the systolic reading, which is the amount of pressure being exerted on the blood vessels during the peak of the heartbeat. The lower, the diastolic reading, is the amount of pressure during the resting state between heartbeats.

While there is no clear definition of where normal ends and high blood pressure begins, most experts agree that a reading of 140/90 is the upper limit of desirable and that blood pressures over this are potential cause for concern because of an increased risk of heart attacks, strokes, and other serious complications. For a person in the "high normal" range, a physician may recommend a reduction in salt intake, weight reduction in some cases, and an exercise program for those who lead sedentary lives. In a small minority of cases of hypertension, a physiological cause, such as kidney disease or a tumor of the adrenal glands, may be responsible for elevated blood pressure; in most patients, however, no cause can be pinpointed, and they are said to have "essential hypertension."

Essential hypertension is clearly a most serious public health problem in the United States today. About 25 million Americans are estimated to have the disease, and thanks to intensified programs to identify cases of hypertension and to bring high blood pressure under control, an increasing number of them are now under treatment. Many experts feel that this improved detection and control is a factor in the declining death rate from both stroke and heart attack in the United States.

The considerable body of evidence linking hypertension and increased cardiovascular risk that has been gathered in recent years includes the following observations:

- The risk of premature cardiovascular disease and death rises sharply with increased systolic or diastolic blood pressures.
- Even within the "statistically normal" level of blood pressure, there are a greater number of heart attacks and strokes among the so-called high normals than in persons with lower blood pressure readings.
- There are indications that the incidence of strokes and heart failure can be reduced in groups of patients whose high blood pressure is lowered by drugs.

Areas that are open to scientific debate or lacking in data include the following:

- Existing evidence is incomplete on the question of whether the benefits outweigh the risks in treating high blood pressure below a diastolic reading of 100.
- The precise benefits of non-drug treatment of borderline hypertension (for example, weight loss, salt restrictions, increased physical activity, and relaxation techniques) are unknown, but promising.
- Sufficient knowledge about the basic mechanisms and causes of high blood pressure is not yet available.

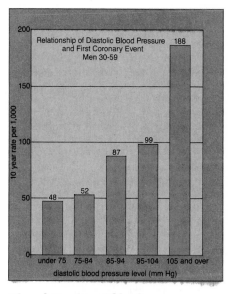

The relationship of blood pressure to the rate of first heart attacks is shown here. As the diastolic blood pressure increases from under 75 mm Hg to 105 mm Hg and over, the rate at which heart attacks occur increases almost fourfold. Figures are from the American Heart Association Pooling Project.

Even though there are unanswered questions regarding the causes and effects of high blood pressure, enough is known to undertake and advise personal and public health programs aimed at controlling hypertension. For example, many Americans, including some physicians, consider increased blood pressure a natural part of aging, but epidemiological studies of other populations have found that this is not necessarily so.

Although the precise physiological cause of high blood pressure is unknown in the majority of cases, a number of studies indicate that there may be an inherited susceptibility to high blood pressure, without which pressures will not be elevated. Since so many Americans have high blood pressure, such inherent vulnerability, if it exists, is probably rather widespread. But an inherited susceptibility is not the entire story; environmental and personal factors, such as increased salt consumption and obesity, appear to play an important role in the development of high blood pressure.

SALT IN THE DIET   There is still considerable research and debate about the role of salt in hypertension, but there is also epidemiological and laboratory evidence to support the thesis that the consumption of salt is a factor. A number of comparative population studies have shown a strong correlation between salt intake and the incidence of adult hypertension and stroke where salt is widely consumed. Moreover, it has been found that severe hypertension may be brought under control by a diet that is nearly salt-free, such as the rice-fruit diet developed some years ago by Dr. Walter Kempner of Duke University, or by drugs that increase the excretion of salt from the body. These drugs are also known to relieve heart failure.

However, many people who consume large amounts of salt have normal blood pressure. Possibly salt brings out an inherent susceptibility to hypertension. In some areas of Japan where large amounts of salt are consumed, the incidence of hypertension is high and stroke is a leading cause of death. In contrast, studies by Dr. Lot Page of Boston and others have shown that people in societies that consume very little salt—such as Middle Eastern nomadic

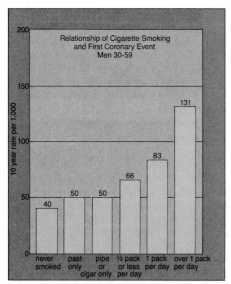

Relationship of Cigarette Smoking
and First Coronary Event
Men 30-59

This chart shows the relationship of cigarette smoking on the rate of first heart attack in a ten-year period. As smoking increases to over one pack/day the rate of heart attack is threefold. (Source: AHA Pooling Project.)

tribes and South Pacific islanders—have virtually no hypertension. The genetic tendency, therefore, may be minimally expressed in a salt-poor surrounding.

How much salt is too much? It has been estimated that if habitual daily salt consumption is less than 1 or 2 grams, or the equivalent of one fourth to one-half teaspoon, there will be little or no hypertension in the population as a whole regardless of genetic susceptibility. As salt consumption increases beyond this amount, however, an increasing frequency of hypertension among adults can be expected, as in the United States and in Japan.

OVERWEIGHT   Obesity is another factor that has been correlated with increased blood pressure. The risk of developing high blood pressure has been shown to be three times as great in overweight persons or those who gain ten or more pounds as the risk for individuals of lower weight. This relationship was brought out in a study in Evans County, Georgia, in which it was found that successful population-wide weight control might reduce the incidence of hypertension by 41 percent.

Because it is not yet possible to identify individuals with inherent susceptibility to hypertension (although research is attempting to provide such means of detection), the two obvious approaches are treatment and prevention. The first entails identifying persons with a persistent diastolic blood pressure of 90 millimeters of mercury or more and providing treatment and adequate follow-up. We possess adequate professional knowledge to achieve this goal; the situation simply requires more efficient means of detecting such persons and encouraging maintenance of the required lifetime drug treatment program. In short, ideal treatment programs exist; it is only necessary for the medical system to extend their use and this is rapidly occurring.

The other approach is a mass hygienic effort toward primary prevention of high blood pressure by changing individual health habits and cultural mores to reduce overeating, lack of exercise, and excessive salt consumption.

Cigarette Smoking   Ever since the first Surgeon General's report on the health effects of smoking, Americans have been well aware of the role of cigarette smoking in the development of lung cancer and chronic pulmonary diseases. But only in the last few years has increasing emphasis been placed on cigarette smoking as a risk factor in the development of coronary heart disease. Evidence linking cigarette smoking and heart attacks includes the following:

• The risk and frequency of heart attacks are greater in persons who smoke and increase according to the number of cigarettes smoked.
• The rate of heart attacks is lower among those who have given up smoking than among current smokers.
• Studies indicate that there are mechanisms linking the components of tobacco smoke with arterial damage and the subsequent development of atherosclerosis. It has also been demonstrated that cigarette smoking decreases the amount of oxygen circulating in the blood and increases the work load of the heart. Smoking also may enhance the susceptibility of the heart to serious rhythm disturbances, an important factor in sudden death. Preliminary evidence from ongoing studies indicates that the cessation of smoking is associated with a reduction in sudden deaths and in deaths occurring after recovery from a heart attack.

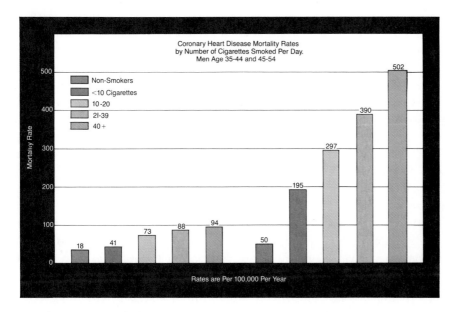

Coronary Heart Disease Mortality Rates
by Number of Cigarettes Smoked Per Day.
Men Age 35-44 and 45-54

Non-Smokers
<10 Cigarettes
10 -20
21-39
40 +

Rates are Per 100,000 Per Year

Actually, there is little controversy over whether cigarette smoking is harmful. The risk of suffering a heart attack may be ten times as great in men aged forty-five to fifty-four who are heavy smokers as in the general population—a difference large enough to indicate that smoking in and of itself may cause a heart attack. Statistical relationships do not establish "experimental proof," but they do provide adequate grounds for recommending that smokers break the habit and nonsmokers do not take it up.

Exercise

The progressive decrease in physical activity and energy expended during work is of the more obvious and profound changes in life style in industrialized societies. Transportation is now rarely under human power. Fewer and fewer tasks require more than very modest effort, and many jobs are completely or partially automated. More and more labor-saving devices clutter households— a second home telephone can reduce the distance traveled by walking by several miles in the course of a year. Many sports activities are vicarious. Even leisure-time activity is often automated and passive, with motor boats and wheels. Add to all this the hours spent in sedentary television viewing, and the total is a markedly reduced output of energy, unaccompanied by any compensating reduction in calorie intake.

There is little question that these changes in mobility and effort have had a marked chronic effect on bodily fitness and on the tendency toward obesity. The amount of body fat has increased at the expense of muscle. The oxygen-carrying function shares in the weakness that comes to any body system that is not regularly exercised. Despite recognition of the important influence of decreased activity on body function, however, twenty-five years of systematic research have not clearly identified any specific role of physical activity in heart attacks or their prevention. In general, the evidence supporting a relationship of sedentary life to coronary heart disease includes the following:

• Men who have sedentary occupations or whose recreational activities involve only minimum physical exercise generally have a somewhat higher heart-attack rate than those who engage regularly in more vigorous physical exertion.

- Physical conditioning with intensive exercise improves the work efficiency of the body; in other words, the same amount of physical work uses less of the reserve work capacity.
- Progressive exercise training can gradually improve work tolerance or rid individual patients of anginal chest pain.
- Experiments with animals have shown that intensive endurance exercise produced increased circulation to the heart muscle.

Job and leisure activity, however, say little about the actual effect of exercise on cardiac risk; for example, high levels of physical activity do not seem to reduce the rate of heart attacks among Finnish lumbermen and farmers, whose traditional diet is one of the highest lipid-raising diets in the world. Even so, comparisons of heart-attack rates in American men according to the energy requirements of their jobs suggest that the more active men experience a somewhat lower incidence of heart attacks. The results, however, have not always shown a gradient of attack rates according to the level of job activity. Moreover, numerous factors tend to concentrate higher-risk persons among the more sedentary occupations; for example, leaving active jobs because of age or illness, and differential retirement and death rates in the more active. Also, individuals who choose physically active jobs may somehow be different from those who choose sedentary jobs, which leads to the question of whether they have a different heart-attack risk from the outset. Efforts to account for such "confounding" factors in the comparison of occupations and to characterize average and peak activities are nevertheless encouraging the idea that activity may have a protective effect.

As for recreational activities, evidence also has been gathered concerning heart-attack rates in men having different leisure-time pursuits. In a systematic survey of British civil servants and of Harvard graduates, those who engaged recently in very vigorous recreational activities were found to have significantly lower heart attack and sudden death rates than those who engaged in very light or moderate exercise.

Still, there are rational explanations for possible protective effects of physical activity on the heart. For example, physical activity is probably the most important factor in over-all control of obesity, which in turn may prevent the development of hypertension. The increased circulatory efficiency resulting from vigorous training enables a person to do physical work with a lower oxygen requirement of the heart. This can be crucial to hearts in which the oxygen supply is adequate for sedentary living but impaired by fatty artery obstructions from delivering blood for more strenuous activity. For example, after the first heavy snowfall each winter, there invariably are a number of reports of sudden death attributed to heart attacks among men shoveling snow. The unusual degree of physical exertion, coupled with the cold, which further increases the heart's work load, may result in a sudden overtaxing of the heart. In contrast, persons who are in good physical condition are not so vulnerable. This does not mean that exercise will prevent heart attacks, only that a heart accustomed to physical exertion is less likely to suffer a coronary event during sudden or unexpected exercise.

Increased diameter of the coronary arteries has also been found in active people, which conceivably could render those arteries less likely to close completely. Increased "collateral," or extra, circulation has been demonstrated in exercised animals, though not in humans. This collateral circulation brings blood to working muscle while bypassing a partially obstructed coronary vessel.

Other benefits of regular exercise include possible anti-diabetic effects, as well as "calming" mechanisms that could render the heart less irritable and thus less susceptible to fatal disturbances in its rhythm.

There are many evidences that the sedentary life style which has accompanied the industrial age is unhealthy. Professional controversy about exercise exists because of the difficulties in relating physical activity habits or physical fitness to any specific risk of heart attack or stroke and will probably continue, since ideal large-scale experiments cannot be carried out among the public to prove beyond a doubt that a sedentary life style may be a factor in coronary heart disease. Since definitive information about exercise is not likely to be forthcoming, professionals can only extrapolate, as in many other aspects of medical judgment, from less than final observations and proceed with direction.

Personality

Most people today recognize that personality, behavior, reactions to stress, and the emotional and spiritual aspects of life have a close relationship with health and physical condition. Adjustments, adaptations, and skills in coping with stress are surely as important to individual (and public) health as physical measurements of risk and other life style characteristics. People can accept, without scientific proof, the fact that inappropriate or inadequate responses to stress can lead to destructive behavior; for example, anxiety may lead to excessive drinking, insecurity to cigarette smoking, depression to sedentary living, rejection to obesity, and so forth. What, however, is the scientific evidence specifically relating these factors to the risk of heart attack or stroke?

Various studies have shown coronary heart disease to be associated with such psychological tendencies as anxiety, neuroticism, depression, aggression, hostility, sense of time urgency, and with such social factors as mobility, status, life events, and dissatisfactions. The problem is that these psychosocial factors are measured by either a subjective questionnaire or an interview, and these are not as testable as physical measurements. There also are no valid external criteria as measures of weight or volume against which to check.

The evidence concerning the relationship of personality and behavior to heart attacks has been obtained mostly in case-control studies; only one major study has been based on long-term follow-up of these characteristics as measured in health and in subsequent disease. In addition, knowledge of behavioral factors is relatively new, and the ability to modify these characteristics has not been established. However, mechanisms exist and are being tested in laboratory experiments in an attempt to relate various behaviors and stress responses to processes affecting blood fats and clotting, blood vessel damage, and susceptibility to heart-rhythm disturbances and sudden death. Further research is required before useful public health recommendations can be made for reducing stress and modifying Type A behavior.

Alcohol

Alcohol consumption has been described as one of the largest health problems in America. The problem is intensified by the wide availability of inexpensive alcoholic beverages and the social acceptability of drinking. Regular alcohol consumption and the early adoption of drinking as a part of life style are characteristic of American society. Indeed, the increase in teenage alcoholism alone is a major public health problem.

Nevertheless, there is little evidence that alcohol consumption plays a *specific* role in the development of heart attacks. This does not mean that there is no correlation; evidence linking alcohol consumption and heart disease includes the following:

- Heavy alcohol consumption is associated with elevated blood pressure.
- Distinctive forms of heart enlargement and heart failure occur in advanced alcoholics, who often tend to be malnourished.
- Alcohol has been shown to impair performance of heart muscle in humans.
- Experimental evidence in animals shows structural and functional derangements of heart muscle cells as an effect of chronic administration of alcohol.

In addition, alcohol contributes indirectly to calorie excess, hypertension, smoking, and sedentary behavior and has powerful subtle effects on the body.

Obesity "Officially," being overweight means being heavier than the average for one's height, age, and sex, based on standard tables of the distribution of weights in the American population. Obesity is officially defined by United States statistical standards as a greater-than-average body content of fatty tissue for weight, age, and sex. But, in fact, obesity is rarely measured except in research studies in which special techniques are used to estimate body fat.

From olden times, when corpulence was equated with good health and prosperity, to the present, when obesity is associated with gluttony, sloth, and social undesirability, both advanced and primitive cultures have smiled or wept, accepted or rejected, admired or decried, and otherwise behaved ambivalently toward obesity. Man's ability to overeat and sore energy as fat undoubtedly had survival value over many eons. But within the period of written history and formal agriculture, this possible evolutionary value has become progressively less necessary. Now, when the energy requirement of work has declined to very low levels, the average life span has lengthened, and food supplies have improved, the ability to store fat for future use would seem to present hazards more often than advantages.

In the United States and other parts of Western industrial society, the diseases of overnutrition and overconsumption are more prevalent than the diseases of undernutrition. The energy demands of active occupations, transportation, and leisure have been reduced drastically. Average per capita calorie intake has also decreased, but not commensurately with the decrease in energy expenditure. Affluence has also led to increased consumption of such foods as fatty meat and dairy products, sugar, and alcohol. The result is a constant and generally losing struggle on the part of large segments of society to maintain stable weight or to attain ideal weight.

As with cigarette smoking, there is now little controversy about the overall medical, social, and personal undesirability of being overweight or obese. Evidence linking obesity and overweight to cardiovascular risk includes the following:

- Insurance experience indicates that the death rate from all causes including cardiovascular ones rises, as relative weight goes from low to above average, and the increase is substantial only in persons whose weight is 30 percent above average.

- Some follow-up studies of United States populations show similar relationships and risks in the upper 10 percent of the population distribution of relative weight.
- Most of the relationship of obesity and overweight to coronary heart disease is with angina pectoris rather than heart attack or coronary death rate.
- Obesity and overweight are widely associated with other risk characteristics thought to have a causal influence in fatty artery disease: specifically, high blood pressure, glucose intolerance and diabetes, and elevated blood uric acid. All these factors can be reduced through weight reduction, as can cholesterol and triglyceride levels.

Scientific controversy over these data persists for several reasons: there are inconsistencies in the evidence. In some regions of the Seven Country Study, those men who were lightest and those who were heaviest had higher death rates than those comfortably in the middle. Furthermore, the treatment of obesity is difficult and very frequently unsuccessful; and a large-scale scientific study to test properly the effect of weight reduction and/or increased physical activity in the primary prevention of cardiovascular diseases is not considered feasible. Thus "proof" of the long-term preventive value of losing weight may not be established. The pragmatic public health view, however, is that such "proof" is not required before recommending prudent and safe preventive measures, for both individuals and society as a whole, to effect the widespread control of obesity.

With respect to personal behavior, every effort should be made beginning with the training of children to establish and maintain controlled eating patterns and regular exercise habits. The social desirability of obese infants should be discouraged. Many adult Americans would have little problem with weight control if they reduced regular alcohol intake and increased exercise to the equivalent of 20 minutes of vigorous walking each day. Most would also have no problem if they followed the American Heart Association's "prudent diet," which calls for reduced consumption of fats, meat, dairy products, and sugar.

FAD DIETS In general, systematic evidence linking fad diets for weight reduction with increased risk of cardiovascular disease is lacking, but there is one major exception—the so-called liquid protein diets. Several deaths from heart attacks have been attributed to these diets, which has prompted the Food and Drug Administration to warn that they should not be used except under the closest medical supervision. Even then, there is a danger to the heart because these diets often result in a loss of lean muscle tissue, which includes the heart. It also should be noted that some fad diets do have the potential of exacerbating the mechanisms of fatty artery disease. A study among hospital employees showed a distinct rise in blood cholesterol levels among short-term users of the low carbohydrate diets, which are really high-fat reducing diets.

Perhaps the greatest harm caused by fad diets comes from the fact that they do not result in long-term changes in eating and activity patterns which are, after all, the basic cause of weight problems. A person will go on a fad diet, succeed in losing the desired twenty-five or thirty pounds, and then quickly regain the weight once he or she goes off the diet. Therefore, fad diets are usually associated with cyclic variations in weight, and many experts consider that these variations probably are not in the best interests of cardiovascular health and, indeed, of health in general. They are accompanied by wide swings in insulin secretion, variation in blood lipids, and the depletion of certain essential nutrients, such as potassium. There is some evidence that coronary heart disease may be triggered or promoted by irregular spurts of lipid accumulation in the blood; it is conceivable that these variations in lipid levels could be related to alternating periods of deprivation and excess calorie consumption and the resulting derangements in blood glucose, insulin, and lipid levels.

Questionable Risk Factors From time to time, reports of other possible cardiovascular risk factors appear. Among those suggested in recent years are coffee, soft water, and excessive intake of vitamin D. In most instances, the evidence behind these implications has not held up.

The soft water theory is a good example. A study of various death statistics found the mortality rate from heart attacks and strokes to be lower in areas that have hard water than in those with soft water. Although the implications are intriguing, the epidemiological evidence is not consistent. There are exceptions to the first reports on the frequency of death in hard-water as opposed to soft-water areas. Laboratory evidence of any specific protective or harmful effect of trace minerals in water is lacking or incomplete. Finally, no research has identified any satisfactory pathological evidence, such as different concentrations of minerals in the body tissue of persons with heart disease as compared to those free of disease, that could point to any particular logical mechanisms which might lead to cardiovascular disease. It is also important to note that the mineral intake in food generally is far greater than the amounts of minerals found in hard water; therefore, any deficiencies in the mineral content of water could be offset by the minerals in food.

UNAVOIDABLE RISK FACTORS So far, I have concentrated on risk factors related to environment or life style. However, there are others that are beyond the individual's control; among these are sex, age, race and ethnic origin, and family history and early environment.

Heredity and Family History Many physicians believe that inherited characteristics are among the most important determinants of eventual heart attacks and strokes. This impression is reinforced by the tragic family histories involving severe lipid metabolic disorders and premature heart attacks. Most of these premature heart attacks can be traced to an inherited disorder known as familial hypercholesterolemia, which is characterized by very high levels of cholesterol in the blood. The pattern of cardiovascular disease in these families is dramatically different from that of the population at large. In many instances, each generation suffers heart attacks and strokes at progressively younger ages. Nothing could be more disturbing than an adolescent's experiencing the chest pains of angina or dropping dead of a heart attack, especially when an older sibling had a similar history and the parents died of heart attacks when relatively young. A few hundred families with exceptionally high susceptibility to heart disease have been identified in recent decades, and in these cases, family history is clearly an unavoidable risk of premature death from coronary heart disease. Although drugs and diet may help forestall early death in some of these persons, there is no known means of preventing the development of fatty artery disease in persons who have inherited this lipid metabolism disorder. Fortunately, the inherited disorder is quite rare; the vast majority of heart attacks in the United States are not related to it.

This fact should not be interpreted to mean that family history is unimportant; if several members of a family have died of heart attacks or strokes at a relatively early age, it should be a signal to pay particular attention to preventive measures. For example, both hypertension and diabetes tend to be inherited, and both are cardiovascular risk factors. Early preventive measures very well can prevent the development of such diseases, even among persons with an inherited susceptibility. However, cardiovascular disease is so common in the United States that it should be considered more a universal trait than a familial one.

Of course, families share more than their genes—familial behavior also is an important factor, especially in the adoption of certain life-style risk factors. Studies show that when both parents smoke, their children are much more likely to smoke cigarettes than are the children of non-smokers. Obesity also tends to run in families, but whether it is a true genetic characteristic or related to family eating habits or a combination of the two has not been shown.

Even so, for most people cultural-environmental influences are more important than inherited tendencies in determining the risk of cardiovascular disease, as can be inferred from population studies evaluating risk-factor levels and heart-attack rates.

As might be expected, the incidence of heart attacks and strokes increases markedly with age; the death rate from these two disorders approximately doubles each decade after the age of thirty. In addition, the mean level of blood pressure, as well as frequency of hypertension, rises significantly with age. In short, the older the person, the greater the likelihood of developing high blood pressure and/or having a heart attack or stroke. Part of this has a very logical explanation: the longer blood vessels are exposed to certain risk factors, such as elevated blood cholesterol levels, the greater the probability that fatty deposits will build up and the rate of their development will accelerate.

But is aging itself a cause of coronary artery disease? It seems doubtful, because even in this society where coronary artery disease is almost a universal characteristic, individuals live to an advanced age without any evidence of atherosclerosis. Moreover, in other parts of the world entire populations live much longer than does the average American and have a very low incidence of heart attacks, strokes, or other manifestations of atherosclerosis. Indeed, there are some cultures in which blood pressure does not rise with age. Therefore, it would seem reasonable to conclude that cardiovascular disease is not an inevitable part of aging, either for individuals or for an entire society.

Statistics show that men are at greater risk than women of developing pre-

PRINCIPLES

1. *Recent research clearly indicates that different cultural patterns, life styles, and personal characteristics carry*

Age and Aging

different degrees of risk of eventual heart attack or stroke. Such controllable or avoidable risk factors as habitual excesses in eating, elevated blood fats, obesity, sedentary life style, high blood pressure (hypertension), cigarette smoking, and coronary-prone personality type behavior have created a great incidence of culturally-induced heart attack and stroke in this country.

2. *Overconsumption of foods, particularly certain fats, salt, and perhaps sugar are significantly related to cardiovascular health and risk. Comparative studies among different nations indicate that cultures with diets relatively high in saturated fats have relatively high average levels of blood fats (especially cholesterol) and*

Sex

relatively high frequency of fatty artery disease. Evidence is clear that individual risk of future heart attack, stroke, and other fatty artery disease is strongly related to the level of blood cholesterol: the higher the level the higher the risk; the lower the level, the lower the risk. High levels of blood cholesterol can be lowered by changes in diet (limiting dietary cholesterol, decreasing the intake of saturated fats, increasing intake of certain types of fiber, substitution of vegetable for animal protein). Moderate reduction in obesity and a regular exercise program, together with a reduction in total fat intake, can further reduce cholesterol levels.

3. *Essential hypertension (high blood pressure not related to a specific physiological cause; such as kidney disease or tumor of the adrenal glands) carries a risk of premature cardiovascular disease, stroke, and heart failure. Although in many cases, the specific physiological cause of hypertension is unknown, there is considerable evidence that salt consumption is a major factor in the cause and progress of the disease. The risk of developing hypertension is three times greater in overweight persons than for those of normal weight.*

4. *Cigarette smoking has only recently been identified as a risk factor in the development of coronary heart disease. Studies have shown that the components of tobacco smoke are linked with arterial damage and the subsequent development of atherosclerosis. Cigarette smoking also decreases the amount of oxygen in the blood and increases the workload of the heart. The risk of suffering a heart attack is greater in men who are heavy smokers.*

5. *Sedentary habits and lack of exercise are also implicated in increased risk of coronary heart disease. Comparison of heart attack rates suggest that more active men have a somewhat smaller incidence of attack. Controversy still surrounds the subject of the relationship between exercise and cardiovascular risk because of the difficulty of conducting large-scale*

mature cardiovascular disease. Evidence implicating sex as a risk factor includes the following:

- At all ages up to about sixty, men have higher death rates from heart attacks and stroke, after that, women tend to catch up.
- Women who have a very early menopause or whose ovaries are surgically removed (surgical menopause) do lose part of their apparent protection and experience a higher incidence of heart attacks.
- Women do not exhibit as high a level of primary risk factors as men.

Even so, it is unlikely that the high incidence of heart disease among middle-aged men can be attributed to their sex alone. But coronary heart disease may take different forms in women. For example, a larger portion of women than men with coronary heart disease experience anginal pains, while sudden death and typical heart attacks are relatively unusual in women.

Some researchers also have pointed to the fact that both men and women appear to be benefiting from the downward trend in heart disease, even though women are acquiring more of the traditional male patterns (holding high-pressure jobs, smoking cigarettes, and leading more sedentary lives). However, this observation may be more apparent than real because of a deficiency in public health surveillance systems. Health behavior and risk factors are simply not monitored adequately enough to make it possible to do more than speculate on any of the trends in cardiovascular disease. For example, although the total death rate from heart disease and strokes is moving down, hospital admissions because of heart attacks may not be decreasing. This leads some to speculate that reduced death rates may be attributed to better medical care of heart-attack victims rather than to an actual decrease in the disease. Others note that larger numbers of Americans, particularly men, have stopped smoking and are undergoing treatment for high blood pressure—factors that also may relate to the reduced death rates. But none of this would explain adequately why women still have lower death rates from heart attacks.

In the past, hormonal differences have been regarded as a possible explanation, primarily because the incidence of heart disease in women does increase after the menopause, when there is a sharply reduced level of female hormones circulating in the body. Whether or not this is correct, the protective forces do not appear to carry over to men. Studies of men who have been given female hormones indicate that, rather than lowering the risk of heart attacks in males, these hormones actually increase the risk. In fact, the studies were cut short when an excessive number of the men in them developed strokes, heart attacks, or blood-clotting problems while taking the estrogens. The same phenomenon has been observed among men who are given female hormones to reduce the growth rate of prostatic cancer. Furthermore, women who have a relative excess of female hormones because they take birth control pills also may have increased risk of heart attacks and other vascular complications. Although the evidence for this tends to be rather mixed, some studies have found that women who both smoke and take oral contraceptives do have a significantly higher incidence of heart attacks and strokes.

In any case, it does appear that being a man entails an increased risk of cardiovascular disease. But women are not automatically free of the risk, and both sexes can improve the odds by concentrating on altering the controllable risk factors.

In North America, several distinct racial differences in cardiovascular diseases have been observed:

- Death rates from stroke are much higher in blacks than in whites.
- The incidence of hypertension is several times as great in blacks as in whites in some areas and substantially higher in the nation as a whole.
- Heart attacks and sudden death from coronary events are more common in whites than in blacks.
- Heart attacks among Orientals in the United States are generally less frequent than in whites but reflect a degree of Western influence in that the rates are higher than in their homelands.

It has not been established whether racial differences such as inherent metabolic differences, cultural influences such as diet, or a combination of the two account for the differences in cardiovascular disease. However, the differences in frequency provide important clues to possible causes and prevention. For example, since blacks suffer a much higher incidence of hypertension and strokes, it makes sense to conduct intensive programs among them to detect, treat, and ultimately prevent high blood pressure. These would include educational campaigns emphasizing the possible roles of obesity and high salt intake in the development of high blood pressure.

Studies show that national origin and early cultural influences are also related to the risk of cardiovascular disease. Evidence implicating these factors includes the following:

- Differences in heart-attack frequency between populations may vary as much as tenfold, as indicated in the Seven Countries Study and other epidemiological studies.
- Migration from countries with a low incidence of cardiovascular disease to countries with a high incidence results within a few years in increased frequency of heart attacks among the immigrants.

A perspective on the role of country of origin and early cultural influences as risk factors in the development of cardiovascular disease is only beginning to develop. For example, it has been widely reported that Yemenite Jews migrating to Israel experience an increase in heart attacks within a decade of migration. However, this group still has a lower overall rate than that of native-born Israelis and Jews of European origin. Similarly, Norwegians who have moved to the United States have an increased risk of heart attacks compared with their counterparts in Norway, but the risk is still lower than that of Norwegian-Americans born in the United States. Another example involves a study of Helsinki policemen—their rate of heart disease is closely correlated with that of their province of origin but often intermediate between that of the province and that of the general population of Helsinki.

The large differences in frequency of heart attacks and strokes among different worldwide populations cannot be reasonably explained by hereditary differences among those populations; rather, life style appears more responsible. Investigators who consider heredity the determining or at least the most important cause of heart attacks and strokes are probably correct for

experiments among the public. Nevertheless, it is certain that physical conditioning with intensive exercise improves the work efficiency of the body and that gradually progressive exercise training can improve work tolerance and rid individual patients of anginal chest pain. Active individuals have increased caliber of coronary arteries, which conceivably could render the arteries less likely to close.

6. *Obesity and overweight are linked to cardiovascular risk and to other risk characteristics thought to have a causal influence in fatty artery disease —high blood pressure, glucose intolerance and diabetes, and elevated blood uric acid. All these associated risks can be reduced through weight reduction, as can cholesterol levels. Weight reduction and control is possible with reduced alcohol intake, increased exercise, and adherence to the American Heart Association's "prudent diet," of reduced consumption of fats, meat, dairy products, and sugar.*

7. *Unavoidable risk factors, those beyond the individual's control, are sex, age, race and ethnic origin, and family history and early environment. Although genetic factors may be critical in certain instances, the influence of family eating patterns and habits, as well as other cultural-environmental influences, are apparently more important than inherited tendencies in determining the risk of cardiovascular disease for the population. Age and aging inevitably increase the risk of cardiovascular problem, but it is doubtful if aging in itself is a cause of coronary artery disease. The same can be said of sex differences: although middle-aged men have a higher incidence of heart disease than women, the higher incidence*

SUMMING UP

cannot be attributed to their sex alone. Both sexes can improve their risks by concentrating on altering the controllable risk factors. It has not

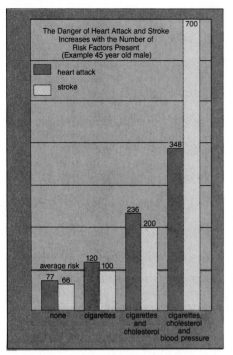

The Danger of Heart Attack and Stroke
Increases with the Number of
Risk Factors Present
(Example 45 year old male)

■ heart attack
□ stroke

The more risk factors are present in one individual, the greater the likelihood of a heart attack or stroke becomes. This chart shows how the risk of heart attack and stroke increases for a 45-year-old man who smokes cigarettes, for one who smokes and has a cholesterol level of 310, and for one in whom the smoking habit is combined with the same cholesterol level plus an abnormally high blood pressure of 180 systolic. Figures are from the Framingham Study.

Prescription for Prevention

been established if racial differences or cultural influences account for the observed racial differences in the occurrences of cardiovascular disease.

8. Worldwide population studies indicate that high blood pressure, elevated blood cholesterol, and fatty artery disease are not necessarily part of the human condition. Changing the cultural and environmental patterns that are high risk factors for cardiovascular disease can do much to reduce this country's rate of premature heart attack and stroke.

the limited numbers of individuals and families with marked metabolic disturbances and an especially high proportion of risks within the United States population. In turn, other investigators are equally correct when they point out that environmental and sociocultural influences, operating in concert with a still unknown and possibly widespread multiple genetic susceptibility, are probably responsible for the mass problem of these diseases and that cultural factors account predominantly for large population differences in frequency of heart attacks.

The more risk factors present, the more likely is possibility of a heart attack or stroke. In fact, each combination of risk factors increases the risk of a heart attack four times above the national average. And the risk factors need not be exaggerated. A person who smokes a pack of cigarettes a day, has a cholesterol level 10 to 15 percent above the average for adults, and has a slight tendency to high blood pressure may have four times the average American risk of suffering a heart attack. Actually, 5 to 25 percent of the population has been found to have modestly elevated multiple risk factors, which puts these people in the same category of risk as a person with extremely high blood pressure or markedly elevated blood lipids.

Of the lessons to be learned from these various studies of cardiovascular risk factors, perhaps the most important is the realization that in the majority of people, modifying the risk factor is not a hopeless task. For example, it is not impossible to effect changes in well-established eating habits. Evidence of this can be drawn from the fact that more and more Americans are cutting their fat consumption by eating fewer eggs and smaller amounts of butter and fatty meats while increasing their intake of low-fat meats and dairy products, vegetarian dishes, and so forth. Americans can break out of their sedentary mold; witness the tremendous increase in the popularity of running, tennis, cross-country skiing, handball, and other vigorous activities. We can detect and control most cases of high blood pressure, as has been indicated by recent studies showing a substantial reduction in the number of untreated hypertensive patients. And many experts believe that these various measures are beginning to pay off; witness the downturn in cardiovascular mortality in the last ten years.

The lessons from population studies worldwide indicate that high blood pressure, elevated blood cholesterol, and fatty artery disease are not necessary parts of the human condition. If the lessons from other countries and from research in the United States were applied at a national level—for example, increasing physical activity to avoid weight gain, halving salt intake by not adding any at the table and avoiding salted foods, halving the intake of saturated fats by reducing the amount of fatty meats and dairy products consumed and increasing the amount of lean meat, cereals, and vegetables, and eliminating the smoking habit—a very large reduction of the nation's burden of premature heart attacks and strokes is predicted, and eventually their virtual disappearance as major causes of disability and death is not unthinkable.

2

HAZARDS OF SMOKING

Richard I. Evans, Ph.D.,
J. Keith Thwaites, M.P.H.,
John J. Witte, M.D.

Cigarette smoking is the most significant preventable cause of premature death and disability in the United States today. Among the health problems attributed to cigarette smoking are coronary heart disease; cancer of the lung, oral cavity, larynx, pharynx, and urinary bladder; chronic bronchitis; emphysema; complications of pregnancy, infant health, and obstructive pulmonary disease. Medical science has produced substantial evidence to support this statement, including the fact that male and female cigarette smokers report more acute and chronic conditions such as chronic bronchitis and emphysema, chronic sinusitis, peptic ulcer disease, and arteriosclerotic heart disease than persons who never smoked.

When one smokes cigarettes, the chances of getting a serious disease are far greater than if one does not smoke. However, the most encouraging thing about giving up the habit is that when individuals who have smoked for a long time choose to stop, their overall mortality ratios after fifteen years are similar to those who never smoked. Nevertheless, while the greater percent of individuals understand and recognize the dangers of smoking, it has been estimated that more than fifty million people still continue to use cigarettes in the United States today.

The single most important effect on health due to cigarette smoking is the development of heart attacks. In 1975, approximately 25 percent of the 650,000 deaths from coronary heart disease (CHD) were attributed to cigarette smoking. This is equivalent to more than 160,000 preventable deaths per year, or a needless loss of life every three minutes. Other deaths attributed to smoking in that same year include 64,000 for lung cancer, 20,000 for cancers of other sites, and approximately 22,000 from chronic obstructive pulmonary diseases. It is significant that when an individual who smokes cigarettes has such risk factors as hypertension, high blood cholesterol, or diabetes, the risk of acquiring CHD is greatly increased.

The risk of developing lung cancer is ten times greater for cigarette smokers than for non-smokers. Lung cancer risks increase directly with the number of cigarettes smoked per day, level of carcinogenic substances, total lifetime number of cigarettes smoked, number of years of smoking, age at initiation of smoking, and depth of inhalation. When a cigarette smoker also drinks alcohol, the risk increases so that the combined effect is greater than each factor acting independently.

Cigarette smoking has also been found to reduce exercise performance. For example, as few as ten cigarettes a day can adversely affect endurance and cardiorespiratory fitness. At any given age life expectancy for cigarette smokers is greatly shortened. Prospective studies have shown that a thirty-to-thirty-five-year-old who smokes two packs of cigarettes a day has a reduced life expectancy of from eight to nine years as compared to a non-smoker of the same age.

It has been demonstrated that the danger to one's health increases according to the number of cigarettes smoked. Although the smoker can reduce the health risks by smoking a smaller number of cigarettes, switching to cigarettes featuring low tar and nicotine, taking fewer puffs and not inhaling, the only sure way to enhance one's health and increase longevity is to abstain from smoking entirely. Switching to cigars or pipes is not a satisfactory substitute as many smokers of these tend to inhale. (See Other Forms of Smoking.)

The 1979 *Report of the Surgeon General on Smoking and Health* identifies smoking as causally related to coronary heart disease for both men and women in the United States, and cigarette smoking as a major independent risk factor for the development of fatal and non-fatal myocardial infarction. The report also indicates that cigarette smoking appears to be a risk factor for a second heart attack and diminishes survival following a heart attack for those who continue to smoke. The amount smoked is indicated as being directly related to the degree of risk. Smokers who quit reduce their risk of dying from coronary heart disease; the reduction approaches that for the non-smoker following a total abstinence of ten years. Although smoking low tar and nicotine cigarettes reduces risk, it by no means reduces that risk to the level of the non-smoker.

HOW SMOKING AFFECTS THE HEART AND CIRCULATORY SYSTEM

Atherosclerosis is manifested by the deposit on the inner walls of the arteries of atherosclerotic plaques which distort and narrow their diameter. This in turn reduces the flow of blood through them and creates a condition called ischemia. When ischemia becomes severe any organ or tissue which cannot get an adequate blood supply is no longer able to function effectively. As a result, a clinical disease such as coronary heart disease, stroke, or peripheral vascular disease develops.

It has also been shown that cigarette smoking is associated with more severe atherosclerosis of the aorta and coronary arteries than has been found in non-smokers. Smoking is also reported as being responsible for increased deaths from arteriosclerotic aneurysm of the aorta (a ballooning effect that can lead to its rupturing).

The mechanisms by which cigarette smoking is associated with higher rates of coronary heart disease are not yet fully understood. Recent research would indicate that carbon monoxide may be one of the factors in the cigarette smoke that lead to the development of atherosclerosis, resulting in angina pectoris and heart attacks.

Carbon monoxide (CO), one of the most poisonous by-products of cigarette smoking, is a colorless, odorless gas which makes up anywhere from about 1 to 5 percent of cigarette smoke. Because it has an extremely strong affinity for hemoglobin (which carries oxygen to the tissues), any inhaled CO quickly displaces the oxygen in the blood, forming carboxyhemoglobin (COHB). Carbon monoxide may cause damage by injuring the walls of the arteries, enhancing the deposition of cholesterol in the development of atherosclerosis, which narrows the arteries, diminishing the supply of oxygen and other nutrients. In addition, carbon monoxide is the principle contributor to diseases of the respiratory system and sudden death from coronary heart disease.

Nicotine is generally understood to be the addictive element in tobacco that acts on the adrenal glands and on certain heart tissues to release powerful stimulants called catecholamines. The catecholamines raise the blood pressure and the heart rate, causing the heart to work harder, thus requiring a greater amount of oxygen. But as smokers take in nicotine, they are also inhaling carbon monoxide, which decreases the amount of oxygen in their blood. Thus, nicotine in combination with carbon monoxide may be the predisposing factor in the development of heart disease and heart attacks.

In addition to speeding up the heart rate and causing a rise in the blood pressure, nicotine also causes a constriction of the blood vessels. Smoking even one or two cigarettes will cause an increase in the heart rate of fifteen to twenty-five beats per minute and will raise the systolic blood pressure by as much as 15 percent. The constriction of blood vessels additionally leads to a decrease in blood flow to the fingers and toes and aggravates or initiates such peripheral vascular conditions as Buerger's disease and Raynaud's phenomenon. For smokers, the risk of acquiring peripheral vascular disease in diabetes mellitus is also increased. Cessation of smoking benefits the prognosis of peripheral vascular disease and is an important factor in its surgical treatment.

More than four thousand components of tobacco smoke have been identified. Many of these (some of which are trade secrets) are potentially harmful, and several have been implicated in the development of specific diseases, including coronary heart disease. Ninety percent or more of cigarette smoke is comprised of about a dozen gases that have been identified as being hazardous to health. The remainder consists of particulate matter, the best known constituents being nicotine and tar.

It is significant to note that if an individual is subject to several risk factors, the total effect of any combined risks is greater than the sum of risks taken singly. In other words, if each of the four risk factors mentioned above had an independent rating of 1, they would add up to 4. However, by interaction, the combined effect would now result in a total of 6 or more. Many researchers report that the reduction in smoking, particularly among men, has been an important factor in the lowering of mortality rates. The decline in mortality from cardiovascular disease is probably due to many factors including control of cholesterol, high blood pressure, and weight, as well as of smoking. It is also recognized that improved acute medical care of heart attack victims has had some impact in reducing death rates.

SMOKING AND CEREBRAL VASCULAR ACCIDENTS (STROKE) There is conflicting evidence as to whether there is an increased risk of cerebral vascular disease (stroke) due to smoking. Cigarette smoking may well be a risk factor for stroke at all ages. However, other causes of stroke become proportionately so important in later years that the risk attributed to smoking is masked by the large number of cerebral vascular accidents due to other causes.

OTHER FORMS OF SMOKING Those individuals who smoke pipes and cigars usually do not inhale very much smoke. This apparently lowers risk that they will develop lung cancer. Nevertheless, that risk is still greater than that for non-smokers. Both pipe and cigar smoking are associated with increased mortality ratios for cancer of the upper respiratory tract, including cancer of the oral cavity, the larynx, and the esophagus. For pipe or cigar smokers who inhale the smoke, the risk of developing lung cancer is at least equal to or greater than for those who smoke cigarettes. It is significant to note, however, that while the lungs of cigar and pipe smokers are exposed to less smoke than the lungs of cigarette smokers, the smoke exposure which occurs in the upper respiratory tract approximates that as for all smokers. The amount of smoke in the larynx and the oral cavity is about the same for pipe and cigar smokers as for cigarette smokers. There is also evidence that pipe smoking is directly related to cancers of the oral cavity, including lip cancer. With alcohol and smoking having an increased risk due to their interaction, the risk is further heightened. The degree of risk for cigar smokers is directly proportional to the number of cigars that are smoked each day.

Finally, it must be pointed out that pipe and cigar smokers are at an increased risk compared to non-smokers of developing chronic obstructive pulmonary disease. As compared to cigarette smokers, however, the mortality rates are somewhat lower.

Any switch from cigarettes to marijuana may be likened to jumping from the frying pan into the fire. Since marijuana contains greater amounts of tar than tobacco and possibly other harmful substances, the risk, instead of decreasing, may increase. Also, the long-term effects have not yet been determined. In addition, the marijuana smoker tends to inhale deeper and to hold the smoke in the lungs longer to gain a greater effect, resulting in a higher absorption of any harmful substances. There is also clinical evidence that marijuana smokers have an increased incidence of bronchitis, and research on animals indicates the strong possibility of an increase in lung cancer, emphysema, and other respiratory diseases.

OCCUPATIONAL HAZARDS RELATED TO SMOKING

Certain occupational exposures are associated with an increased risk of dying from lung cancer. Cigarette smoking interacts with the carcinogens in question to produce a much greater risk of developing lung cancer than from occupational exposure alone. Workers in the uranium and the asbestos industries who do not smoke have only slightly increased lung cancer rates as compared with the rest of the population, but for cigarette smokers the rates are dramatically elevated. Asbestos workers who smoke have 92 times the risk of developing lung cancer than non-smoking workers, and uranium miners who smoke have 10 times the risk of non-smoking uranium miners. Industrial workers who smoke and are exposed to rubber fumes, coal dust, or chlorine are also subject to an increase in lung damage.

SMOKING HABITS OF HEALTH PROFESSIONALS AND TEACHERS

A majority of smokers and non-smokers are of the opinion that doctors, other health professionals, and teachers should set a good example by not smoking. A report issued in 1977 by the Center for Disease Control of the Public Service indicates that physicians, dentists, and pharmacists are indeed leading the downward trend. A national survey among health professionals conducted in 1975 and again in 1978 confirms this decrease. Those health professionals who are still continuing to smoke are not only smoking fewer cigarettes, but are also more likely to smoke lower tar cigarettes than smokers in the general population. Nurses, on the other hand, have shown an increase in smoking. A survey of nurses in 1969 showed 37 percent to be current smokers. A similar survey in 1975 showed 39 percent of the nurses smoked cigarettes. Thus, the percentage of nurses who smoked actually increased during this interval. This may be partly due to the same reasons accounting for the increase among all females.

Contrary to popular belief, a study released in 1967 showed that only 28 percent of female teachers and 18 percent of male teachers actually smoked.

The decline in smoking among health professionals is indicative of their growing concern on the hazards of smoking to health, and enhances their credibility and role as examplars in persuading smokers to quit. It is perhaps ironical that most smokers say they have never been advised by a doctor to quit smoking or cut down on cigarettes, despite figures showing that more than 70 percent of smokers who smoke a pack or more a day have said that they would give up cigarettes if urged to do so by a physician.

Doctors in growing numbers are posting "No Smoking" signs in their offices and clinics, with instructions to staff to remove ashtrays and enforce the rules. The utilization of literature on the hazards of smoking cessation techniques by health professionals and teachers is also on the increase, and helps to reinforce patient counsel and classroom instruction. There is also a growing interest in eliminating cigarette machines in hospitals, including gift shops and other health facilities.

ADULT SMOKING The proportion of adults in the United States who regularly smoke cigarettes began a steady decline about the time of the release of the *Surgeon General's Report on Smoking and Health* in 1964, which widely publicized the health hazards of smoking. Of interest is the reduction in the death rate from CHD in the subsequent years following this report.

In 1965, the Public Health Service conducted a national survey on smoking habits of persons 20 years of age and older. Forty-two percent of the individuals surveyed admitted to being current cigarette smokers (53 percent of the men and 32 percent of the women). A similar survey in 1975 showed a sharp reduction to 34 percent of the proportion of individuals who smoked (39 percent of the men and 29 percent of the women).

This cannot help but reflect the increasing concern of adults in relation to the hazards of smoking. In addition, the survey showed that a very high percentage of individuals who continued to smoke would like to quit if there were an easy way for them to do so. While there continue to be more men than women who smoke, the comparative decline in smokers over the past ten years shows that men are quitting at a faster rate than the opposite sex. This may be indicative that women have more difficulty than men in giving up the habit.

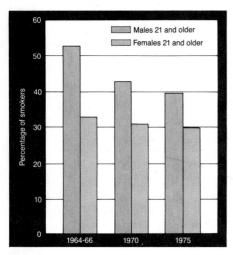

Of interest is the fact that the number of cigarettes consumed per person in the United States has declined from 4,345 in 1963 to 3,965 in 1978. The per capita cigarette consumption in 1978 was the lowest in twenty years. This reduction is no doubt due to the combined efforts of voluntary and public health agencies in informing the public on the hazards of smoking.

Changing percentages of the total adult population, male and female, who smoke cigarettes.

Although the percentage of smokers in the population continues to decline, the tobacco industry reports that sales of its products are increasing. The reason for this apparent conflict is a population growth that exceeds the decline in the percentage of individuals who smoke. For example, between 1970 and 1975, the adult population grew by some eleven million people, increasing the number of adult smokers by approximately one million. There are indications that with the lowering of tar and nicotine in cigarettes, some smokers feel less satisfied, with the result that they increase the number of cigarettes they smoke, and thus the possibility of an even greater risk.

Also, since 1970 women are smoking an average of two additional cigarettes a day. To this must be added the increased number of teenage girls who have taken up smoking. The total increase in the amount smoked in 1975 as compared to 1970 comes to approximately 15 billion cigarettes, thus accounting for the record sales reported by the tobacco industry. Most of today's smokers know that cigarette smoking causes disease and premature

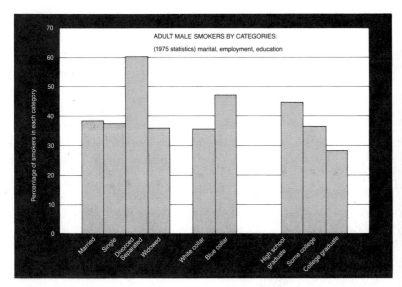

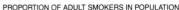

PROPORTION OF ADULT SMOKERS IN POPULATION

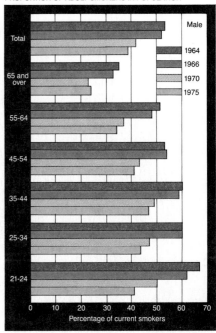

death and are concerned about the possible effects of smoking on their health. Some of the reasons given for smoking are:

CRAVING OR PSYCHOLOGICAL ADDICTION   There is growing evidence that heavy smokers may become addicted to nicotine, which sets in motion a craving that can only be assuaged by another cigarette. In other persons, there may not be so much a physiological addiction as a psychological one, such that over a period of time they have convinced themselves that they could not cope with life situations without indulging in cigarettes.

A SENSE OF INCREASED ENERGY OR STIMULATION   Many smokers feel a cigarette gives them a needed lift at a time when they are feeling low. They report it helps them to wake up in the morning and to start out the day with a positive attitude.

A survey by the U.S. Public Health Service in 1975 showed a reduction in the number of persons 20 years of age and older who smoked since a similar survey made ten years before. Although there are still more male than female cigarette smokers in the United States, men appear to be quitting at a faster rate than women.

PROPORTION OF ADULT SMOKERS IN POPULATION

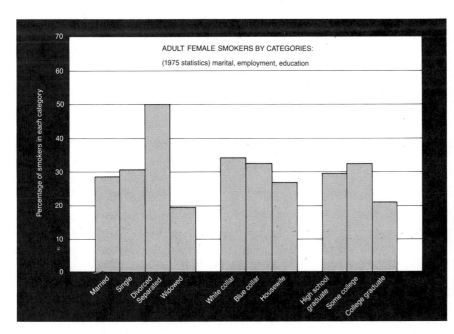

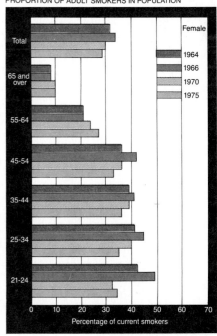

THE SATISFACTION OF HANDLING OR MANIPULATING THINGS   A cigarette, some smokers say, gives them something to do with their hands and provides a mild form of distraction, a feeling of security. This phenomenon frequently occurs in dealing with others.

THE ACCENTUATION OF PLEASURE AND RELAXATION   A large number of smokers feel that smoking is a form of pure enjoyment which provides psychological enhancement and puts them at ease with the world. Often this is the situation when one has a cup of coffee or indulges in alcoholic beverages.

THE REDUCTION OF NEGATIVE FEELINGS SUCH AS ANXIETY OR ANGER   When under tension or in adverse or strange situations, a cigarette is often said to provide a feeling of calm, a pacifier in situations that are difficult to deal with. These situations include meeting new people, dealing with others, and being in a tense situation with one's superiors. Such smokers also say it makes it easier for them to cope with day-to-day problems and irritations.

HABIT   Other smokers have just adopted a bad habit, possibly emulating a parent, a sibling, a close friend, or someone they admire. Often these people may not enjoy cigarettes but continue to smoke out of pure custom. They are not fully conscious of what they are doing when they automatically pick up and light a cigarette.

Those who continue to smoke cigarettes, many of whom have tried to cut down or quit, do so even though there is a rising concern from their families and friends and an increased hostility from non-smokers.

Helping people to stop usually requires a variety of appeals and cessation techniques as the smoker is motivated by highly personal reasons and rationalizations. Cessation methods are discussed more fully later in this chapter.

SMOKING-RELATED HEALTH PROBLEMS UNIQUE TO WOMEN   Researchers have concluded that women could conceivably reduce by 75 percent their chances of a heart attack by not taking up the habit or by quitting. Studies also show that young women smokers between the ages of eighteen and thirty-five tend to be outgoing, somewhat rebellious against authority, and strongly influenced by peer pressure. They are more likely than non-smokers to have boyfriends, husbands, and friends who smoke; generally they come from families in which one or both parents smoke. A majority of young women smokers believe that smoking could harm an unborn child and either reduce the number of cigarettes smoked or quit during pregnancy. Unfortunately, most women resume the smoking habit after their babies are born. (See the section on Effects of Second-hand Smoking on Infants.)

Smoking was first recognized as a health problem for men in the 1930s, when a sharp increase in lung cancer rates for men was noted, but for several reasons no similar increase at that time was noted for women. As a group, women started smoking later than men, primarily because the habit was socially unacceptable for women during this period. Consequently, it was not until the last decade that sufficient numbers of women had smoked long enough to provide the data necessary for meaningful research. Recent national surveys indicate that in the last twenty years, women are not only taking up smoking in larger numbers but are also beginning to smoke at an earlier age. (See Teenage Smoking.)

The same health risks as for men who smoke are now being documented for women smokers, Heart attack, lung cancer, cancer of other specific sites, bronchitis, and emphysema are diseases that occur among women smokers at rates far greater than among non-smoking women. Women's lung cancer rates have tripled since 1964, the Surgeon General has reported, and if present rates continue, by 1985 it will overtake breast cancer as the leading cause of death among women. Additionally, it has been found that women smokers incur unique risks for themselves and for their offspring. (See Smoking During Pregnancy.)

SMOKING DURING PREGNANCY

Risks associated with cigarette smoking during pregnancy include spontaneous abortions, infants with lower birth weight, and increased fetal or infant death near the time of delivery. Women who are heavy smokers also have a greater risk of complications of pregnancy. These effects are reported as being reversible, provided the pregnant woman stops smoking by the fourth month. However, many pregnant women do not fully understand the increase in risk as a result of their smoking. There are unique health hazards both to the woman who smokes and to the developing fetus. Smoking mothers show an increase in the risk of premature separation of the placenta, which can lead to fetal and maternal death, and also of placenta praevea. There is also an increased incidence of congenital malformations and crib death (sudden infant death syndrome) in infants whose mothers smoke during pregnancy. With these facts in mind, women who smoke should make every effort to quit, particularly during the period of gestation.

SMOKING AND ITS EFFECTS ON CARDIOVASCULAR DISEASE AMONG WOMEN TAKING ORAL CONTRACEPTIVES

Women thirty years of age or older who smoke and utilize estrogen-containing oral contraceptives subject themselves to a ten-fold risk of having a heart attack compared to women who do not smoke. This higher risk of heart attack occurs in all age groups and is a problem of increasing severity. Many women are terminating the use of oral contraceptives rather than attempting to stop smoking. The point often misunderstood is that cigarette smoking is the main cause of the increased health hazard, and that this can be reduced by giving up cigarettes.

EFFECTS OF SECOND-HAND SMOKING ON INFANTS

Children under one year of age who are exposed to smoke have a higher frequency of admissions to hospitals for respiratory illness as compared to children of non-smoking parents. This increased risk for children of getting pneumonia, bronchitis, and tonsillitis suggests that the smoke generated by parents in the home is responsible for the higher incidence of these diseases. Smoke may act by increasing the infant's susceptibility to infectious agents, thus leading to these respiratory problems. The relationship between parental smoking and pneumonia, bronchitis, and tonsillitis in children should be a concern of smoking parents if they wish to improve their children's chances of remaining healthy. To this must be added their role as exemplars, for it has been convincingly proven that the children of smoking parents are more likely to take up the habit.

TEENAGE SMOKING

The effects of smoking on health develop over many years, with mortality rates from all causes significantly higher for smokers who start the habit in their prime. Studies in humans and animals have clearly demonstrated that cigarette smoking is responsible for lung damage and dysfunction at a very young age. Atherosclerosis, which often leads to heart attacks and strokes, is also a smoking-related disease that can have its genesis early in life. Unfortunately, the long-term effect of smoking on health is a problem that too many youngsters ignore.

National surveys of teenage smoking habits reveal that the frequency of smoking is increasing among young girls in this group. Among males twelve to eighteen years of age, approximately 16 percent regularly smoke cigarettes, and this rate has been stable for several years. In contrast, the proportion of females who smoke has increased steadily, from 8 percent in 1968 to 15 percent in 1974, at which time the number of teenage female smokers almost equaled the number of male smokers. Since 1968 alone, the percentage of girls aged twelve to fourteen who smoke has increased eightfold. Among the group between the ages of thirteen and nineteen, there are now six million regular smokers, and the number of regular smokers under the age of thirteen has reached 100,000.

One reason why this trend may continue is because of the large expenditure for tobacco advertisng (over half a billion dollars per year), which portrays smoking as being chic and sophisticated and is clearly intended to lure young people to take up the habit. However, the relationship between exposure to the mass media and the initiation of smoking is difficult to separate from the other influences to which the teenager is exposed, including such factors as whether or not the parents or siblings smoke and peer pressure. Also, one cannot discount the changing status of women in this country, providing greater freedom for females to pursue many activities that were once predominantly male-oriented. The cigarette industry has made a point of exploiting this changing status by directing much of its advertising at this lucrative target group.

The nature of the family and the smoking habits of parents and siblings is of prime importance in determining whether children take up cigarette smoking. For instance, teenagers in families with both parents present are less likely to smoke than those in single-parent families. In families where one or both parents smoke, the children are more likely to use cigarettes. Where there is an older brother or sister who smokes, the youngster is three times as likely to be a smoker and is four times as likely to smoke as one who has a no-smoking exemplar in the family. The influence of peer pressure is particularly important: almost nine out of ten teenage smokers report that at least one of their four best friends is a regular smoker, while only one in three non-smoking teenagers says that a regular smoker is one of his or her four best frends. This exemplar/peer role is one that needs much more research to determine how peer pressure can most effectively be combated.

Cigarette smoking among teenage girls seems to be connected with rebelliousness, whose manifestations include smoking marijuana and drinking excessively. Cigarette smokers also tend to have a greater dislike for school, are poorer students, and are less prone to continue their education beyond high school.

Among young women most likely to quit smoking are those who are younger or more athletic, those active in clubs, and those who are employed.

Because of the concern over the rapid increase in teenage girl smokers, more research data is available for this group than on teenage boys.

Despite all that has been said about teenagers and smoking, 92 percent of teenagers surveyed believe that smoking is harmful to their health, and 85 percent say that they do not plan to be smokers five years from now.

COPING WITH THE TEENAGE SMOKING PROBLEM

Increased emphasis needs to be placed on prevention of smoking among children and adolescents. Parents who smoke should recognize that their example is important, as is their understanding of the other forces, such as peer pressure, that cause their offspring to take up the habit. One approach parents can take is to provide assistance to their offspring in understanding the hazards of smoking, to emphasize the positive aspects of not smoking, and to give support to those children who do smoke in their efforts to quit. Information and facts are not enough. There is also evidence that the excessive use of fear can have the opposite effect. Efforts should be made to train the child to resist social pressures from their peers. Youngsters who have learned to say "No thank you, I don't smoke" when offered cigarettes by their peers are better able to handle the situation when it arises. Additionally, parents can help by supporting legislation aimed against misleading and glamorous advertising. With the immediate and positive effects of being a non-smoker on one's future health, this information is particularly important for those children who are athletically inclined.

Several programs are underway in many institutions around the country to discourage and, if possible, prevent smoking among children and adolescents. Undoubtedly, special efforts will be placed on school programs that try to train the child to resist social pressures to begin smoking. Parents can also help by supporting efforts to prohibit the use of vending machines for tobacco products to which children and adolescents have access. Legislation to make it illegal to sell or offer tobacco products to children should also be encouraged.

INVOLUNTARY SMOKING

Involuntary smoking, where there is public exposure to air pollution resulting from tobacco smoke, is sometimes referred to as passive or secondary smoking. The chemical constituents found in smoke-filled atmospheres are derived from two sources, mainstream and sidestream smoke. Mainstream smoke comes from the cigarette that is puffed on by smokers and exhaled into the air. Sidestream smoke, which comes from a smoldering cigarette that is held in the hand or has been placed in an ashtray and continues to burn there, has a higher concentration of carbon monoxide.

Although over four thousand individual constituents of cigarette smoke have been identified, most research has focused on carbon monoxide, nicotine, benzopyrene, and acrolein. Tobacco smoke also contains glyco protein, a highly allergenic substance to which approximately one-third of the population are sensitive. This material can also activate blood clotting pathways. Carbon monoxide (CO) has been linked with the development of atherosclerosis, a condition which can lead to heart attacks and strokes. Of the other twelve hundred substances which as yet have not been adequately researched, it can be assumed that many of them may be harmful to man.

The carbon monoxide level in the air of an enclosed room is determined by the number of cigarettes being smoked at any one given time, rather than the cumulative number of cigarettes that have been smoked. Studies of enclosed public places, including taverns, nightclubs, sports arenas, etc., can show high concentrations of carbon monoxide well above the ambient air quality standard (9 ppm).

Smokers carry levels of carboxyhemoglobin (COHB) three to four times greater than non-smokers. An important study has shown, however, that even low levels of COHB can lead to critically low levels of oxygen (hypoxia) in diseased areas of the myocardium, thus leading to fatal episodes of ventricular fibrillation.

Special populations at risk from involuntary smoking include children under one year of age, who have an increased chance of developing respiratory illness when their parents smoke. Other groups include individuals with chronic diseases, especially cardiovascular disease. Persons with chronic bronchitis and emphysema have been shown to have increased mortality under conditions of severe outside air pollution, which are only accentuated if inside areas are contaminated by tobacco smoke. The impact of short-term exposure on such individuals has not yet been adequately evaluated.

The nuisance effect of tobacco smoke is receiving increased recognition. It has been conclusively shown that smoking is related to irritations of the eye, nose, and throat involving a substantial percentage of the population. As a result, there is an increase in legislation to ban smoking in public places and in the setting aside of special smoking areas in airplanes, trains, and restaurants. There are also a growing number of offices and industrial sites that provide smoke-free areas for workers.

Interpretations of current data on the health effects of exposure to tobacco smoke do not demonstrate a definitive cause-and-effect relationship between involuntary smoking and specific disease conditions. However, medical decisions are rarely based on the results of controlled studies. In this context, the evidence for the deleterious effect of tobacco smoke on the body is stronger than that for many other risk factors of disease.

THE HIGH COST OF CIGARETTES In 1976, Americans smoked 620 billion cigarettes at a cost of over $14 billion. The next year, Americans spent $16 billion on cigarettes. The following chart provides a clear indication of the direct cost of smoking to the consumer.

COSTS TO THE SMOKER BASED ON NUMBER OF
PACKS OF CIGARETTES SMOKED PER YEAR

	COST PER YEAR BASED ON 65 CENTS PER PACK		COST OVER 30 YEARS FOR 1 PERSON
NUMBER OF PACKS PER DAY	1 SMOKER IN THE FAMILY	2 SMOKERS IN THE FAMILY	
3	$713.75	$1427.50	$21,412.50
2	$472.50	$ 944.00	$14,175.00
1	$236.25	$ 472.50	$ 7,087.50

Included in the purchase price of cigarettes are the excessive costs of cigarette advertising, which in 1977 alone came to over $500 million.

It has been estimated that $17 billion is lost to this country each year as a result of smoking-related illness, medical care, accidents, absenteeism, and lost work output. The National Center for Health Statistics Report estimated in

1965 that smoking-related illness each year cost the United States 77 million work days lost, 88 million days spent ill in bed, and 306 million days of restricted activity. Data from 1974 have indicated more than 145,000,000 excess days of bed disability for the U.S. population in one year. Overall, it has been estimated that more than 10 percent of all hospital and medical expenses in the United States are tobacco-related, resulting in an increase in the overall cost of health and life insurance and taxpayer-supported health programs.

The careless use of cigarettes also accounts for a large number of home and forest fires that occur each year. In the United States during 1976, it was reported that residential fires claimed more than 6,200 lives and caused $1.4 billion in property damage. The National Fire Protection Association reported that more than a fourth of all residential fires and 56 percent of all fatal residential fires are ignited by smoking materials. The property loss in smoking-related non-residential fires, and in medical expenses and wage losses of people injured or killed in smoking-caused fires, pushes the indirect toll of smoking even higher. A controversial issue with smoking and non-smoking taxpayers alike is the Department of Agriculture's subsidy of the tobacco growers, which in 1977 amounted to some $60 million.

Much of the cost resulting from cigarette smoking must be shared by the non-smoker who becomes the victim of increased taxes and insurance rates. There is some hope for the non-smoker, however, in the growing numbers of insurance companies that are lowering their rates for the cigarette abstainer, reflecting lower costs for policies covering life, auto, home-owners', and health insurance.

RIGHTS OF THE NON-SMOKER

There has been a growing conviction that non-smokers have the right to breathe air free from cigarette smoke. Nearly two-thirds of the population are reported to find it annoying to be near a person who is smoking, with more than a third of the smokers also feeling this way. In 1964 and 1966 only 52 percent of the population agreed that smoking should be restricted to fewer places. But in 1975 the percentage jumped to 70 percent. Over half the smokers would currently like to see smoking in fewer places despite growing restrictions on smoking. Three-fourths of the adult population surveyed felt that management should have the right to restrict smoking in offices and factories whether or not it posed a safety hazard. In the last year or so there has been increased pressure to restrict smoking at sporting events that are held in enclosed areas, particularly where the ventilation is inadequate. There has also been a successful suit in the law courts in behalf of the worker's right to a smoke-free environment at his place of employment.

CIGARETTE ADVERTISING

In 1977, the amount spent on cigarette advertising by tobacco companies came to some $500 million. The six major tobacco companies, each marketing several leading brands, manufacture 99.9 percent of all the cigarettes purchased in the United States today. The top twenty brands alone account for approximately 93 percent of all cigarette sales, with the top four assuming 40 percent of all advertising costs.

Since the ban on cigarette advertising on television in January, 1971, the tobacco companies have been concentrating their efforts in magazines and newspapers, on billboards, posters, and areas frequented by the general populace, especially public transportation. Following the ban on television commercials, concentration on media of this type has dramatically increased. A particular target is young women; several brands have made a point of focusing their attention on this growing market, with some success.

A review of current advertising practices indicates that many companies concentrate on special audiences or interest groups, despite the claim of the tobacco companies that the prime objective of advertising is to get smokers to switch brands.

The themes that are used fall into several basic categories: satisfying taste and smoking enjoyment, low tar and nicotine content, identification with an attractive personal image in settings that imply social recognition, as well as the unique attributes of the cigarette itself, such as style, filter, length, and packaging. Often the advertising is associated with clean air and healthful outdoor surroundings. There is a growing public concern in regard to the tactics employed by cigarette manufacturers in their efforts to attract new smokers, particularly those who are younger.

In 1964 only 36 percent of the population favored a ban on cigarette advertising, but by 1970 60 percent of the population supported its elimination. It is interesting to note that by 1975, over half of the smokers surveyed themselves supported a total ban, feeling perhaps that cigarette advertising made it difficult for them to quit. Another reason frequently cited was that smokers do not wish to see others take up the habit.

Cigarette advertising apparently not only attracts new recruits to the habit, but additionally has its impact in maintaining a large clientele that continues to make the cigarette manufacturing business a most profitable one.

FEDERAL AGENCY REGULATIONS A government study of transportation practices shows that 60 percent of nonsmoking passengers and 38 percent of all passengers are bothered by cigarette smoke.

The Interstate Commerce Commission (ICC) regulates smoking on buses and passenger trains, and permits smoking only in the rear 30 percent of the seating on interstate buses, such as Greyhound and Continental Trailways. Bus drivers are not permitted to smoke inside these vehicles. On intercity and interstate trains, smoking is permitted in designated smoking cars, lounge and snack cars, but not in dining cars. The Civil Aeronautics Board (CAB) has promulgated and made effective official rules requiring that *all* air passengers who so desire must be seated in sections of the aircraft in which smoking is prohibited and that such restrictions *must* be enforced by all airline personnel. These rules require "each carrier to insure that smoking is not permitted in 'no-smoking' areas and to enforce its rules with respect to the segregation of passengers in 'smoking' and 'no-smoking' areas."

Should problems persist in obtaining compliance, a formal complaint should be lodged with the Civil Aeronautics Board in Washington, D.C. Although the CAB has a formal complaint procedure for smoking violations, only the carrier can be fined—as is true of trains and buses. However, since airlines are subject to fines up to $1,000 for each violation, they have an incentive to see that smoking rules are enforced.

LOW TAR AND NICOTINE CIGARETTES It has been demonstrated that individuals who smoke low-tar, low-nicotine cigarettes tend to inhale more deeply and to hold the smoke in their lungs longer. This, in effect, means that they expose themselves to the same hazards inherent in smoking high-tar and high-nicotine cigarettes.

In an earlier study of more than a million men and women, the consequences for health of smoking high tar and nicotine cigarettes were compared with the effects of smoking brands low in tar and nicotine. Although total death rates were lower for smokers of low tar and nicotine brands than for smokers of high tar and nicotine brands, these death rates were still considerably higher than for non-smokers. The study established tar as a major contributor to deaths from cigarette smoking and presents an argument refuting the claim that low tar and nicotine cigarettes are safe. The addictive properties of cigarettes would likely drop with a decrease in nicotine yield, and smokers might find it easier to take the final step into cessation. In the meantime, the widespread health problems associated with tobacco usage might be reduced. There is also a belief that widespread use of a so-called "safer cigarette" would actually reduce risk, but this would require two questionable assumptions: first, that there would be no increase in the number of cigarettes a smoker consumes and secondly, that smoking did not begin at an earlier age.

The main purpose of cigarette filters is to reduce the level of tar and alkaloids, including nicotine, and trace elements in tobacco smoke. Actually, the risks of lung cancer are reduced when smokers switch from non-filter to filter cigarettes, primarily as a result of the reduction in tar levels. In regard to coronary heart disease, however, one study suggests that the risk may increase when a smoker switches from non-filter to filter cigarettes, primarily for the reason that there could be a higher carbon monoxide level from inhaling the smoke of filter cigarettes, particularly if more of them are smoked to offset the decrease in the nicotine effect.

FILTER CIGARETTES

Of the 29 million Americans who stopped smoking between 1964 and 1975, it is estimated that 95 percent of them quit on their own, and that only about 2 percent of those who wanted to quit attended formal smoking cessation programs.

Nine out of ten smokers interviewed in 1975 said that they had either tried to stop smoking or would if there was an easy method of doing so. Men appeared to be more successful at quitting than women, and lighter smokers and persons concerned about their health were also more likely to succeed. Unfortunately, there is no way to ascertain accurately why people stop smoking. Some statements reflect a last-straw situation rather than the underlying motives for quitting. Reasons most often cited as the incentive to stop smoking are "mastery of my own life," "disease prevention" or "setting an example for my children." Several studies reveal that successful ex-smokers have usually tried to stop smoking several times and are more apt to stop for reasons of health than for any other. The longer one smokes, there is not only an increased likelihood of developing a related disease, but also more difficulty in giving up the habit.

One of the more commonly used techniques to get people to stop smoking has been to arouse fear of the consequences, which are often portrayed in vivid detail. This approach all too often has backfired, however, as the individual who has been so affronted often smokes even more in order to relieve his or her anxiety.

There are no gimmicks, gadgets, techniques, or approaches that are universally successful in helping a smoker to quit. Tapering off may not facilitate

SMOKING CESSATION PROGRAMS

the quitting process for many habituated smokers. The smoker should have a personal commitment to stop and must set a date for doing so. Stopping "cold turkey" can be difficult, but many smokers use this technique successfully, finding the tapering-off method impractical. Many smokers who try to taper off instead of quitting cold turkey may actually prolong the agony of withdrawal, thereby increasing the possibility of remaining habituated. In effect, smokers utilizing this technique remain in a constant or chronic state of withdrawal. The process may actually reinforce their smoking behavior, leading to a relapse and return to smoking. Withdrawal symptoms usually last anywhere from four weeks to as many as twelve—but several former smokers have reported a desire to smoke that lasted as long as five years.

Encouragement and reinforcement are helpful in the first few days and weeks after quitting. Such support should come from the smoker's family and friends, as well as the physician and members of the office staff. During the early days and weeks after quitting, it is helpful to provide an environment free from smoke and smokers, and to reduce other situations where the temptation to start again may be difficult to resist.

GROUP PROGRAMS   Those people not able to quit on their own need outside help, and can be referred for free help to smoking cessation clinics run by the major voluntary agencies, or to commercial groups that conduct cessation programs for an established fee. The effectiveness of these groups varies, but on the average they have a success rate of from 30 percent to 46 percent, as measured by persons who are not smoking one year later.

National voluntary health agencies such as the American Heart Association, the American Cancer Society, and the American Lung Association have educational materials such as pamphlets, posters, films concerning smoking; some have sponsored group cessation programs for a number of years through their local chapters. Such programs are usually based on a national model provided by the parent organization and utilize the volunteer services of physicians, trained psychotherapists, counselors, and ex-smokers. Positive reinforcement and group interaction are stressed, with avoidance of scare tactics and aversion therapy (punishment) approaches. A typical program would consist of a group of eight to twenty persons who meet with a therapist or non-medical person for two hours twice a week over a period lasting four to six weeks. Participants learn why they smoke, identify ways to quit, and are motivated and supported by the leader and other group members. Most cessation clinics largely rely on group dynamics, on helpful tips from successful quitters, and on a mutual desire to stop smoking. The important aspect of this type of approach is the presence of continuing support. Other institutions and foundations also offer smoking-withdrawal methods. In recent years, several profit-making corporations have entered the field of group therapy smoking cessation programs. Perhaps the best known organization is "Smoke Enders," which began in 1969 and now has chapters in thirty cities around the country. Participants attend nine weekly meetings of two hours each. At the conclusion of the course, reunion meetings are organized for purposes of reinforcement. The importance of such reinforcement and follow-up programs is a key factor in getting smokers to reach a point of continuing total abstinence.

Many organizations offer five-day group therapy smoking cessation programs. Generally, groups vary from fifteen to several hundred persons, and the program consists of five consecutive day or evening meetings lasting one and a half to two hours each. The program usually includes lectures, inspirational messages, films and group interaction aimed at behavior modification. Other methods involving behavior modification include techniques where an unpleasant reaction is emphasized, such as being subjected to the ill effects of rapid smoking or of an electric shock.

It must be pointed out that the absence of uniform reporting data among organizations conducting cessation programs makes it difficult to compare their rates of success. It is suspected that many commercial smoking programs are often not aware of their failures since people who fail to stop smoking very likely feel guilty and don't go back.

Because of the widespread use of aversion therapy, a further explanation of the technique warrants attention. When this method is used, the smoker is made to feel uncomfortable on the premise that if smoking is connected with something unpleasant, he or she will be less likely to continue the habit. Positive reinforcement in the form of something pleasant is often provided when the person doesn't smoke. The extremes of such techniques are employed by various types of anti-smoking programs. The rapid-smoking technique has also been used. Here the individual is required to inhale smoke every six seconds until he or she becomes dizzy or nauseated. The carbon monoxide thus enters the body at such a rapid rate that it becomes extremely unpleasant. However, this technique is not without dangers and is strongly discouraged for individuals with heart and lung conditions. Other aversive methods include electric shock and blowing smoke in the face of the smoker. One relatively harmless self-help technique is for the smoker to wear an elastic band on the wrist and when the urge to smoke becomes too strong, to snap it smartly so that it hurts.

Another method calls for a substitute such as chewing gum or providing a small reward that ordinarily would be denied. One other approach to the control of smoking has been the Water Pik one-step-at-a-time method. This technique involves the progressive reduction of nicotine content in the cigarette smoke by utilizing a series of filters. Still another approach to control smoking has been the use of Tabmint, an anti-smoking chewing gum. When this gum is chewed at the same time as tobacco smoke is inhaled, the result is an unpleasant taste. Other newer methods being experimented with include hypnosis and acupuncture. Further research on these is needed, however, before any definite conclusions can be reached.

The use of drugs as a tobacco substitute has often been tried. One such drug is laboline. The use of a placebo (an innocuous medication) has been found to be equally effective.

The most important thing about any of these programs is that from the start the individual must realize that the decision to stop smoking must be his or hers, and that no one else can take the first step toward managing one's own behavior.

One of the big problems with all methods is that of backsliding. Studies have shown that from 70 to 80 percent of addicted smokers who have stopped start again after anywhere from six months to a year. The importance of constant vigilance needs stressing. Indulgence in just one cigarette can restart the habit. Avoidance as far as possible of situations where one could be tempted to smoke continues to be a wise precaution. None of the methods described

PRINCIPLES

1. *A person who smokes cigarettes has a far greater chance of getting a serious disease than a non-smoker. In addition to coronary heart disease, cigarette smoking has been*

indisputably linked with cancer of the lung, oral cavity, larynx, pharynx, and urinary bladder; chronic bronchitis, emphysema; obstructive pulmonary disease; and complications of pregnancy and infant health. Although cigarette smoking is the most serious controllable risk factor for many diseases, a smoker can reduce the risk to the level of one who has never smoked, simply by giving up the habit. Reducing the amount smoked, or using low-tar brands, and not inhaling are no substitutes for giving up the habit entirely.

WEIGHT CONTROL IN SMOKING CESSATION

2. *The 1979* Report of the Surgeon General on Smoking and Health *presents evidence from over 30,000 scientific studies linking smoking to coronary heart disease among both men and women. The presence of carbon monoxide in cigarette smoke may be one of the factors that leads to the development of atherosclerosis and ultimately to a heart attack. Nicotine, the addictive element in tobacco, combines with carbon monoxide to act on the adrenal glands and certain heart tissues. As a result, the heart rate speeds up, the heart is forced to work harder, blood pressure rises, and blood vessels constrict. In addition to nicotine, many more of the over 4,000 components of tobacco smoke have been implicated in the development of coronary heart disease and other diseases.*

3. *Cigarette smoking may also be a risk factor for stroke at all ages, but evidence for this is not as conclusive as for cardiovascular disease.*

4. *Cigarette smoking also interacts with carcinogenic materials in many industries, placing smokers who work in such industries at still greater risk.*

5. *The percentage of smokers in the population is declining, although actual sales of cigarettes has increased. This seeming contradiction indicates a shift in the*

is a substitute for self-management. Smoking is a personal problem that has to be handled by the smoker and no one else.

Almost all adults now believe smoking is hazardous to one's health. Belief in the dangers of smoking, however, seems to be far from sufficient to make the individual stop and remain an abstainer. Smoking control programs must therefore do much more than supply information. The focus should be on modifying the specifics of smoking behavior of any given individual.

Likewise, there is a belief that a change in attitude toward smoking would lead to its control. Rarely can we depend on this approach. In fact, it is more likely that by first changing smoking behavior, there will be a change in attitude toward smoking. Despite some of the discouraging results from several of the methods described, it must be remembered that with virtually all approaches, many smokers have been successful in breaking the habit. The process begins with individual motivation.

The decision to quit smoking is often accompanied by the mistaken notion that weight gain is inevitable. Although such gains may occur, usually they can be prevented through careful planning and awareness. The gain is primarily due to an increase in appetite and food intake. Most smokers report that their sense of taste has improved; this is also a factor in the greater consumption of high-calorie and tasty foods. The gain is usually not permanent; in time most ex-smokers revert to their former weight. Possible solutions to the problems that often arise while trying to stop smoking include the following:

LENGTHENED MEAL TIMES   The smoker who has previously hurried through dinner for a cigarette now finishes ahead of others, consumes second helpings, and replaces the after-dinner cigarettes with a rich dessert. To avoid this situation, each meal should be carefully portioned. Extra food should be put away so that seconds are not readily available. Among the strategies that might be employed are to slow down eating by cutting food into smaller pieces; to put the fork down between mouthfuls and swallow all the food from each bite before refilling the fork; to sip ice water frequently during the meal; gradually to extend the time between bites; to eat only what is on the plate—no seconds; to use small plates so there seems to be more food; and to get up from the table immediately after the meal is finished. If possible, there should be some activity to avoid the temptation to eat more. Beverages should be served in another setting. If necessary, the dessert and the beverage can be saved for a late-evening snack, low-calorie fruits, plain cake or cookies being substituted for the rich dessert. Another food idea is to brush one's teeth immediately after the meal as a signal that eating has ceased.

ORAL CRAVING   The individual who wants something in the mouth to substitute for a cigarette often resorts to frequent nibbling. Possible solutions to this problem include carrying sugarless gum or artificially sweetened mints. Only one piece of candy should be eaten at a time, giving it time to melt so that it lasts much longer. Finding things to do with the hands such as creative crafts, home repairs, and gardening, will often keep one from nibbling. While at home, one might also choose to nibble on food that requires some work, such as unshelled nuts or seeds that must be cracked, or foods that must be peeled, thus requiring the use of both hands and the mouth.

THE EVENING SNACK   Ex-smokers often have a strong desire to nibble in relaxed situations such as watching television. To combat this tendancy, low-calorie foods should be substituted for those high in calories. It might be helpful to have a variety of raw vegetables prepared and available when needed, such as raw carrots, celery sticks, green pepper strips, fresh mushrooms, tomato wedges or cherry tomatoes, cauliflower buds, or cucumbers. These can be served plain or marinated with a low-calorie cottage cheese dip. Munching on plain crackers, rye crisps, breadsticks, pretzels, unbuttered popcorn, or dry cereal snacks can also be helpful, provided that the amount eaten is kept to a minimum. Control of the environment is also important. Tempting foods high in calories should be kept out of sight or, better still, not be available in the house. Food should be removed from the living area so as not to be accessible when the impulse to snack develops. It is also helpful to place suitable snacks where they are clearly visible and easily reached. Other methods include substituting another activity when the urge to eat occurs; portioning the snack by never taking more than one serving at a time; and by changing the meal schedules. Sometimes moving the dinner meal to a later time may lesson the desire for evening snacks.

ENVIRONMENT   Certain activities or social situations lead to eating, drinking, and a cigarette. Coffee breaks, cocktail parties, poker games, and sporting events are all smoking-associated activities. Every effort should be made to avoid such situations whenever possible, particularly during the early stages of smoking cessation. Some helpful activities include taking a walk, choosing a sport or activity in which one can participate. Every effort must be made to break the association between the food and smoking, so that food does not replace the cigarette. One should have skim milk, fruit and vegetable juices, tea, low-calorie carbonated drinks, or bouillon during coffee breaks. Fruit can be found in vending machines or cafeterias or brought from home to serve as a snack. Alcoholic beverages should also be controlled, since drinking contributes to calories and may also reduce defenses against the temptation to eat or smoke. One way of reducing intake is to decrease the alcohol by having just one drink followed by refills consisting of a low-calorie mixer or plain water.

Not all of these ideas will be appropriate for any one individual. However, an awareness that eating is an established pattern which can be altered through a number of techniques may awaken individuals to evaluate their habits, define their problems, and develop plans to cope with these situations when and if they arise.

Smokers who wish to stop must start with the conviction that they really want to quit and can do so if they put their minds to it. Having arrived at this point, it is important to outline in writing the motives and reasons for giving up smoking. The reasons must be very personal ones and a list of them should be reread several times a day, particularly in the early stages of quitting, as constant reinforcement is critical. The positive conviction that one can master the habit and that the will-power exists to control one's life and future destiny are very critical. The plan for stopping should include as a target a definite date when cigarettes will be discarded. As part of this resolution, in order to improve one's overall health, the smoker should

type of cigarettes being smoked and in the age and sex of smokers. More low-tar cigarettes are being sold and more women and teenage girls are taking up the habit.

6. *Women smokers are now running the same health risks as their male counterparts: they have far greater rates of heart attack, lung cancer, other cancers, bronchitis and emphysema than women who don't smoke. Special risks are incurred by women in pregnancy. These include spontaneous abortion, lower birth weight for infants, greater risk of complications during pregnancy, and increased fetal or infant death near the time of delivery. These effects are reversible if the woman stops by the fourth month of pregnancy. Taking oral contraceptives increases the risk of heart attack tenfold for the woman who smokes. In addition to these risks to herself, the smoking mother can expose her infant and young child to increased risk of acquiring pneumonia, bronchitis, and tonsillitis from "second-hand" or passive smoking.*

7. *Since 1968 there has been an eightfold increase in the percentage of teenage girls who smoke. This can be contrasted with the stable rate of smokers found among teenage males. Research indicates that peer pressure and home and parental smoking habits are strong influences on teenagers who decide to smoke. Parents have a heavy responsibility to guide their teenage children in the matter of smoking, particularly in the face of well-financed tobacco industry advertising campaigns and the easy access to cigarettes in stores and vending machines.*

INDIVIDUAL PROGRAMS TO STOP SMOKING

8. *Cigarette-smoking-related illness, medical care, accidents, absenteeism and lost work output is estimated at $17 billion a year. Data from 1974 shows that more than 145,000,000 days of disability were incurred by the population in that one year as a result of cigarette-smoking problems.*

9. *The tobacco industry's efforts to convince the smoking public that low-tar, low-nicotine cigarettes are "safe" is deceptive. Smokers tend to inhale these cigarettes more deeply, retaining the smoke in their lungs for longer periods. The smoker also tends to smoke more cigarettes to satisfy his craving for nicotine. Other forms of smoking—cigars, pipes, marijuana—also expose the smoker to excessive risk of the same diseases as does cigarette smoking. Although marijuana users insist the weed is harmless and safe, marijuana actually contains even greater amounts of tar than cigarettes, may also contain other harmful substances, is inhaled more deeply than cigarettes, and its smoke is retained in the lungs for longer periods.*

10. *The rights of nonsmokers are now protected by city, state, and federal government regulations in transportation and in many public places. In 1975 over 70 percent of the population agreed that smoking should be restricted in public places.*

11. *It is possible to stop smoking, and 29 million Americans did so, without benefit of formal and expensive courses or behavior-modification programs. A strong personal commitment to stopping, and a firm date for stopping, are necessary steps, along with a frank admission of the difficulties of accepting a long period of withdrawal symptoms. Positive reinforcement and support from family and colleagues can reduce the temptation to begin again. The misconception that weight gain is inevitable is one of the greatest stumbling blocks to stopping. The person trying to stop should recognize that food should not be used to fill the gap usually occupied by the after-dinner cigarette or the cigarette break during the day. Leaving the table immediately after eating, keeping a supply of low-calorie snacks, and avoiding places and occasions associated with cigarette smoking are some ways of coping with the desire to substitute food for cigarettes.*

get a general physical checkup including a determination of blood pressure and, if necessary, dietary counsel to offset the possibility of gaining weight. One may also find benefit from engaging in supervised physical activity. The positive feedback from such action will reinforce the determination to give up smoking as well as enhance one's sense of well-being. Some successful methods that have helped many smokers to quit include the following:

Listing the reasons for giving up smoking, those that are personal and meaningful. A written outline of the reasons for smoking and the situations where it takes place serves a useful purpose in that it enables the smoker to understand more clearly why, when, and where he is smoking and to develop strategies for most effectively coping with the problem. Teaming up with a partner who is also interested in a smoking withdrawal program, to compare notes and provide mutual reinforcement, can be helpful. To join with several smokers in maintaining a record of their smoking patterns can also be useful. Across the top on an 8½-x-11-inch sheet of paper, the following headings can be listed:

Time	Occasion	Feeling	Value
7:00 a.m.	Rising	Depressed	1

The value on a scale of 1 to 5 will give highest rating to 1 and lowest to 5. Record every cigarette that is smoked on this sheet. Fold the sheet lengthwise, wrap it around a cigarette pack, and secure it with two or three rubber bands. Carry it with you at all times. Every time a cigarette is needed, unwrap the tally sheet, fill in the appropriate information, and rewrap the package. In due course, start eliminating the least valued cigarettes, leading finally to the most important.

Other effective advice includes the following:

Carry cigarettes in a different place each day, making it more difficult to reach the pack; never buy a carton of cigarettes and only buy one pack at a time; switch brands at least twice during the week; do not carry matches or a lighter; gradually reduce the number of cigarettes smoked each day; record each morning the number of cigarettes to be smoked that day, and record at night how many were actually smoked; walk, exercise or take a shower in place of a cigarette; avoid situations and associations that might make it tempting to smoke, e.g., television, coffee, alcohol, parties or get-togethers where there may be considerable smoking; constantly reinforce the desire to quit by reading the reasons and motives for quitting. "If you don't succeed, try again."

Should the self-help method prove too difficult, one of the group programs outlined earlier in the chapter can be tried. If the motives and reasons for quitting are strong enough, eventually the smoker must win the battle. The rewards are too important to settle for less.

Although the smoker may be able to reduce the health risks of smoking by using fewer cigarettes, switching to filtered low tar and nicotine cigarettes, taking fewer puffs and by not inhaling, the only sure way to better health is to abstain from smoking entirely.

3

DIET AND NUTRITION

Robert E. Shank, M.D.,
Mary Winston, ED.D.

Among the controllable factors that have been linked to cardiovascular disease (see chapter 1), there is now clear evidence that diet and nutrition are of paramount importance. Habitual excesses in eating habits (especially of fats, salt, and possibly sugar), often resulting in obesity, are high on the list. Thus, knowing something about the nutrients in foods, the roles they play, and how to properly choose foods are important steps toward a healthy heart and good health in general. It is also important to understand that the nutritional needs of each age group—infancy, childhood, adolescence, adulthood, and old age—are distinct, and vary from stage to stage.

NUTRIENTS IN FOOD Over fifty nutrients are known to man. It is suspected that as scientists learn more, they will discover that there are others essential to human nutrition.

The macronutrients—so called because the body uses them in large amounts—are fats, carbohydrates, and proteins. They are the only important sources of energy and the body's main chemical building materials. Alcohol, when consumed in quantity, could conceivably be called a macronutrient because it constitutes a source of fuel, and it must be taken into nutritional account since it replaces other foods. The second group of nutrients are those called micronutrients, because the body uses them in such small amounts. These are vitamins and minerals.

Water is an important nutrient because it constitutes the largest component of our food. It does not supply energy, but it plays a crucial role in body chemistry.

The body itself cannot manufacture or synthesize all of these substances; many of them must come from an external source.

The processes of digestion and absorption, by which the foods we eat are made available to the body, begin in the mouth, where the first step in the digestion of starches is initiated. The process continues in the stomach, where fats and proteins are broken down, and in the small intestine, from which the nutrients are released into the bloodstream. The energy also made available from the fats, carbohydrates, and proteins is measured in units known as calories—defined as the amount of energy required to bring up the temperature of one cubic centimeter of water by one degree Celsius. The measure used in studying human nutrition is actually a kilo-calorie, or the scientist's calorie multiplied by one thousand (in other words, the amount of heat needed to raise the temperature of one liter, or approximately one quart of water by one degree Celsius). As it is somewhat confusing for the layman, the kilo-calorie is generally referred to as a calorie in discussions of nutrition.

FATS Fats in foods most commonly take the chemical form of triglycerides, which are made up of carbon, hydrogen, and oxygen, and include a three-carbon compound, glycerol, to which are attached three molecules of fatty acids. Triglycerides are not soluble in water. Those that are solid at room temperature are called fats; if a fat is liquid, it is considered an oil. Triglycerides are the form in which fat exists in meats, cheese, fish, nuts, vegetable oils, and the greasy layer on the surface of soup stocks or in a pan in which bacon has been fried. Vegetable fats are generally liquid; the corn oil and cottonseed oil used in cooking are examples. The difference in consistency reflects the difference in chemical structure betwen animal and vegetable triglycerides.

The fatty acids from animal sources are predominantly saturated, whereas those from vegetable oils owe their fluidity to being relatively "unsaturated" —that is, they contain fewer associated hydrogen atoms. They are known as polyunsaturated fats. The human body is limited in its capacity to manufacture fatty acids of the latter kind, and thus must obtain them from the food it consumes. The proportion of these polyunsaturates essential to its functioning is very small—about one percent of the total calories consumed.

FATS AND THE CHEMISTRY OF DIGESTION   An important component of the digestion and transport of fat is the process of emulsification—in other words, the distributing of small globules of fat in an aqueous medium, such as takes place when vinegar (a watery substance) is combined with vegetable oil to make a salad dressing.

The triglycerides and other lipids in foods are emulsified in the stomach and intestine through the churning action caused by contraction of these organs following a meal. The secretions of the liver and gall bladder provide bile acids that assist in stabilizing these emulsions. As triglycerides are distributed in small globules within the intestine, enzymes (known as lipases) secreted by the stomach and the pancreas act to split each molecule of triglyceride into two molecules of fatty acid and one of glycerol, with a remaining third fatty acid still attached. These compounds, held in even smaller globules (micelles), are brought to the surface of the intestinal cell, where they are absorbed and reassembled, and from which they are released into the lymphatic system and eventually into the bloodstream in the form of tiny droplets called chylomicrons. These droplets have on their surface a compound made up of protein plus fat, known as a lipoprotein. They also contain, along with fat-soluble vitamins and other nutrients released by the intestinal cell, the soapy, waxy substance known as cholesterol (from the Greek words *khole*, "bile," and *stereos*, "solid"—so called because it was first discovered in gallstones).

In a healthy person, the triglycerides and other fatty substances normally move into the liver and into storage cells known as adipocytes to provide energy for later use. Fat in certain quantities is important in maintaining the body's structure; because of the physical characteristic of not being soluble in water, it is an essential part of the membranes of cells, and provides insulation for conserving body heat. If fat were water-soluble, it could not serve any of these functions, since the aqueous fluids of blood and tissue would dissolve and wash it away. This is discussed below, in the section on reducing cholesterol.

CARBOHYDRATES

Of the caloric total in the average American diet, it is estimated that 44 percent is derived from carbohydrates, as compared with 42 percent from fat and 14 percent from protein.

SUGARS   During the digestive process, all carbohydrates are eventually broken down into simple sugars or monosaccharides, mainly glucose, fructose, and galactose, each of which contains six carbon atoms. Grains, vegetables, fruits, and honey, along with cane and beet sugars, molasses, and maple syrup, are all sources of glucose; fruits, honey, and sugars also provide fructose. Milk products are the main source of galactose, as well as providing glucose. Table sugar or sucrose is a disaccharide, formed by the linking of one molecule of glucose and one of fructose. The average annual consumption of sucrose in the United States is approximately 110 pounds (50 kilograms) per person—more than 500 calories a day, or roughly half the entire intake of carbohydrates. Milk sugar or lactose, the disaccharide found in milk products, contains one molecule of galactose and one of glucose. During the process of digestion, galactose and glucose enter the bloodstream at a rapid rate, whereas fructose and other simple sugars are absorbed much more slowly.

Glucose, the chief sugar in human metabolism, is utilized by all tissues. Some organs, such as the brain, use it almost exclusively for energy; others, such as skeletal and cardiac muscle, use the fat in cells primarily to meet the need for energy. In the cells of the liver and muscle tissue, many molecules of glucose may be linked together to form glycogen, an animal starch or polymer, to be released when necessary to maintain normal levels in the blood. But the quantity of glucose that can be stored in this way is relatively small (about 150 grams or 600 calories at one time), so that when a larger quantity is consumed, the excess glucose is converted to fat and stored in adipose tissues. In this way, overindulgence in carbohydrates (but especially the chemically simpler sugars) contributes to obesity, thus adding to the risk of cardiovascular disease.

STARCHES Consisting of many molecules of monosaccharides, starches are important components of such vegetable foods as potatoes, sweet potatoes, beans, and cereals. As compared to sugars, they are relatively insoluble and need cooking to break them down and permit the digestive process to begin. The stalks and leaves of vegetables, including such kinds as lettuce, spinach, and celery, and the outer coverings of seeds, contain cellulose, a polymer like glycogen, consisting of many glucose molecules linked in a straight chain. Unlike glycogen, cellulose is almost resistant to the digestive process and is thus not available as a source of energy. It is a very important factor in the diet, however, because the fiber and bulk it provides help maintain tone and movement in the bowel during the process of digestion.

ALCOHOL Currently, about 4 percent of the average caloric intake by adult Americans is in the form of alcohol, made by the fermentation of grains or fruits. Most alcoholic drinks contain few nutrients other than calories. When they are included in a meal, they merely add calories and, eventually, un- wanted pounds. It should be obvious why most therapeutic or weight-reduc- tion diets begin by placing alcohol under a strict embargo, or at most, permit a glass of white wine, the alcoholic drink with the fewest calories. Aside from other, well-documented dangers, the excessive consumption of alcohol fre- quently replaces other foods of greater nutritional value, further endangering the whole body. Alcoholic beverages in small quantities do enhance appetites and add to the pleasure of eating, but they must be recognized as potent contributors to obesity.

PROTEINS Proteins consist of large molecules made up of smaller units called amino acids. They differ from both fats and carbohydrates, the chief sources of energy in human nutrition, in that besides the common elements of all three—carbon, oxygen, and hydrogen—the amino acids contain nitrogen, a necessary component of the diet. In addition, nearly all proteins contain sulfur, and some incorporate molecules of phosphorus, iron, zinc, and copper as well. The protein in the human diet is important in maintaining and repairing tissue proteins, which do not exist for a lifetime but are constantly being broken down and resynthesized. The same is true of the hormones that control body processes, the enzymes that are required for metabolism, and the antibodies that ward off infection. The hemoglobin that is an essential component of the blood is itself a protein.

The need for protein food is greatest during periods of most rapid growth. By adulthood the requirement has been stabilized—except during pregnancy and breast-feeding, when greater amounts of protein food should be eaten. Most people in the United States consume far more protein than they need. The recommended quantity for an adult under ordinary circumstances is no more than 0.8 grams of protein for each kilogram (2.2 pounds) of body weight, or about 56 grams for a man of average size and about 46 grams for a woman of average size.

Food proteins vary in their usefulness as sources of nitrogen and essential amino acids. Of the twenty-two amino acids commonly found in animal proteins, eight (isoleucine, leucine, lysine, methionine, phenylalanine, threonine, tryptophan, and valine) are required by adults and must be derived from the diet; they cannot be synthesized within the body. Infants require an additional amino acid, histidine. Whenever one or more of these essential amino acids are not present in sufficient quantity during the synthesis of a body protein, this synthesis is limited quantitatively by the availability of the essential amino acid lowest in supply. Generally speaking, proteins from animal sources—such as dairy products, beef, poultry, pork, and fish—provide somewhat larger quantities of the essential amino acids, in proportions that make them more readily utilizable by the human organism, than do vegetable proteins. Zein, the protein in wheat flour, may be improved in its biologic value by the addition of the essential amino acid lysine, or if it is consumed at the same time as another protein (e.g., from a legume such as dried beans, or a milk product) that provides the lysine in which wheat flour is lacking. Similarly, the proteins of beans and rice, eaten separately, are not comparable in biologic value to those found in meats; but consumed together they are significantly more nutritious because the deficits in essential amino acid content of one are partially met by another.

PROTEINS FOR A VEGETARIAN DIET   Vegetable foods provide protein without significant fat, and are cheaper than those from animal sources. On the other hand, vegetables must be eaten in greater bulk to obtain comparable calories. All the essential amino acids are available from eggs and low-fat dairy products, which are thus excellent supplements to a vegetarian diet—except for the high cholesterol content of egg yolk. It should be remembered, however, that egg white does not contain cholesterol, and that the white contains the protein.

As a source of protein, fat-free dairy products are especially recommended. Skim milk, low-fat milk, evaporated skim milk, nonfat dry milk and buttermilk made from skim milk, yogurt made from skim milk, fruit ice, imitation diet ice milk (made with skim milk), and sherbet are all valuable foods. Cheeses made from skim milk are low in fat and high in protein. These include dry cottage cheese, farmer's cheese and pot cheese, and ricotta (if made from skim milk), imitation cheese made with skim milk and corn oil, and sapsago cheese.

Any vegetarian who eats no animal products must be especially careful in choosing vegetables so that all the needed amino acids are supplied at a single meal. The following table offers a guide to planning vegetarian meals with these requirements in mind.

FOR QUALITY PROTEIN * FROM VEGETABLE SOURCES, USE ANY FOOD FROM COLUMN I IN COMBINATION WITH A FOOD FROM COLUMN II

	COLUMN I	COLUMN II
Legumes	Beans: Aduki, Black, Cranberry, Fava, Kidney, Limas, Pinto, Marrow, Mung, Navy, Pea, Soy (Tofu) (Sprouts)	Low-fat dairy products
	Peas: Black-eyed, Chick, Cow, Field, Split	Grains
	Lentils	Nuts & seeds
Grains	Whole Grains: Barley; Corn (Cornbread) (Grits) Oats; Rice; Rye; Wheat (Bulgur, Wheat Germ) Sprouts	Low-fat dairy products
		Legumes
Nuts & seeds	Nuts: Almonds, Beechnuts, Brazil nuts, Cashews, Filberts, Pecans, Pine nuts (Pignolia), Walnuts	Low-fat dairy products
	Seeds: Pumpkin, Sunflower	Legumes

* Low-fat dairy products (milk, yogurt, cheese, eggs, cottage cheese), in addition to being used as a supplement to the above, may be used alone as quality protein.

PROTEINS AND THE CHEMISTRY OF DIGESTION Digestion of food protein begins in the stomach. The secretions here provide acids and an enzyme, pepsin, which initiates the process of fracturing the long chain of amino acids into somewhat smaller chains called polypeptides. When the stomach discharges its contents ino the duodenum, pancreatic secretions provide alkaline solutions to neutralize the acids of the stomach, along with a variety of additional enzymes. These secretions break down the polypeptides and undigested protein into very small units, known as dipeptides and tripeptides, and finally into the constituent amino acids. After being absorbed by the upper portion of the intestine, the amino acids enter the bloodstream and are carried to the liver and other tissues.

When the body's needs for amino acids have been met after a meal, the remaining amino acids are freed of their nitrogen and enter into systems of energy metabolism that draw at the same time upon carbohydrates and fat. Since the source of all but a very small proportion of the nitrogen in foods is protein, the total quantity of nitrogen in food protein can be compared with nitrogen losses from the body to ascertain whether enough protein is being taken in—an assessment known as nitrogen balance. When the balance is negative—i.e., when the nitrogen lost in the urine and feces exceeds that in the food that is consumed—more food sources of protein are called for. If, on the other hand, the balance is positive, the body's needs for protein synthesis and replacement are being met, and some of the amino acids are being utilized along with carbohydrates and fat to meet the body's need for energy. A negative nitrogen balance that continues for more than a few days will bring about loss of body weight. The first stage in the process consists of a loss of water, which is reflected in a lowered weight on the scales. During the second stage, the body begins to draw upon its stored fat in order to maintain its normal processes—as is desirable in one who is overweight. The third state of starvation begins to draw upon the body's store of protein, and thus to break down the tissue needed to sustain life. In children, this means a cessation of growth. A continued negative nitrogen balance reduces the protein content of the blood; fluid or edema collects in and under the skin of the feet and ankles; there is damage to the liver and a thinning of the mucosa or absorptive surface lining the intestine.

To maintain a positive nitrogen balance, the intake of food must provide sufficient fat and carbohydrate to meet the body's energy needs and to spare the protein from depletion. It is for this reason that calories as well as protein must be available in the needed amounts. For a person who is underweight, it should be remembered that pounds can be added simply by consuming more food. The extra calories—no matter whether they are derived from carbohydrate, fat, or protein—are likely to be deposited largely as fat if one is relatively inactive. If one is physically active on a regular basis, the formation of new tissue, particularly muscle, from the protein and carbohyrate consumed will be favored, and less fat will be deposited.

CALCIUM AND PHOSPHORUS Among the minerals that are needed to build and repair bone and the skeletal framework of the body, calcium and phosphorus are the most important. They are found primarily in milk and dairy products. Of the 0.8 grams each of calcium and phosphorus that are the approximate daily requirement for an adult, a cup of fluid milk provides about 0.3 grams of calcium and 0.25 grams of phosphorus. The mineral content of milk is the same whether it is whole, low-fat, or skimmed. An ounce of most kinds of cheese will afford about the same quantity as a cup of milk. Other relatively good sources of calcium and phosphorus are contained in such vegetables as spinach, greens, and beans of all varieties.

MINERALS

The body of an average-sized man will contain about 1,200 grams of calcium, amounting to about one-sixtieth of the total body weight. Of this, 99 percent is deposited in bone as a phosphorus-containing compound. The calcium and phosphate molecules in the bone are not there for a lifetime, but are periodically removed and replaced by new molecules. It has been estimated that about 0.7 grams of calcium in the bones of an adult is turned over in this manner daily.

The small quantity of calcium in the body which is not a constituent of the bones—about 10 grams or two teaspoonsful—has very important functions. It is involved in the contraction of skeletal and heart muscles, in the coagulation of blood, and in the structure of cell membranes.

Phosphorus also has many functions to fulfill in the chemistry of the body besides its contribution, along with calcium, to the structure of the bones. In the form of phosphate, it is involved in many reactions important to the transfer of energy within cells and in the blood.

SODIUM AND POTASSIUM   The major source of sodium in the current American diet is table salt (sodium chloride). It is estimated that on an average, adults consume from 6 to 18 grams of sodium chloride daily—a quantity that adds up to as much as fifteen pounds a year. Of this amount, the sodium content is approximately 40 percent, or from 2.4 to 6 grams daily. The actual nutritional requirement is probably somewhere between one-half and one gram a day. There is reason to believe that the excessive consumption of salt is a contributor to hypertension or high blood pressure, which in turn adds to the risk of heart attack.

Sodium is a metallic element found in the blood and other body fluids, and present naturally in many foods. Its concentration in body fluids is precisely controlled by hormones that are secreted in response to an increase or decrease in the amount of sodium present, and that cause the kidneys to eliminate or retain it accordingly.

Potassium is found in a higher concentration than sodium within the body cells, and is effective in determining many of the functions of enzymes. Like sodium, potassium is found in a variety of foods, but is not added to by the use of the salt cellar. When diuretic drugs are being taken because of an excess of water and salt, deficiencies of potassium (and also of sodium) may occur, and must be checked.

IRON   Iron, another mineral, is an essential component of hemoglobin, the pigment in blood that is responsible for carrying oxygen extracted from inhaled air to the various tissues of the body. It is also needed for the formation of myoglobin, a muscle pigment, and for the activity of a number of important enzymes. The quantity of iron taken in daily must be sufficient to replace what is lost from the body or is needed to build new tissues in the growth of infants and children, or during pregnancy. Unlike other minerals, iron is not excreted through the kidneys but is lost from the body primarily as the outer cell layers are shed by skin or living membranes. In women during the reproductive years, there is an additional loss of iron by way of the hemoglobin contained in menstrual blood. The iron requirement for women is therefore greater than for men. The usual diet of most Americans provides iron in many forms and from a wide variety of sources, adding up to an average content of about 6 milligrams of iron for each 1,000 calories. Liver, meats, chicken, green and yellow vegetables, and enriched breads are all rich in iron. From about 1.0 to 1.5 milligrams of iron are needed daily—an amount that is usually absorbed by the body from a daily intake of from 9 to 18 milligrams present in the diet. During pregnancy, particularly the latter half, the requirement for iron increases markedly. Since the usual diet is unlikely to provide the needed amount, it is best to take iron pills or medicinal iron to prevent anemia—that is, a deficiency in the oxygen-carrying capacity of the blood—in the mother and infant.

OTHER ESSENTIAL MINERALS OR CHEMICAL ELEMENTS   MAGNESIUM   Like potassium, magnesium is an important component of most cells and contributes to the activity of enzymes. It has a role in conduction of nerve impulses as well. Stores of magnesium are found in bone. When a deficiency occurs in the human body, manifestations include rapid beating of the heart, and abnormalities will appear in the electrocardiograph. Many foods provide magnesium, particularly those of vegetable origin. So long as a variety of foods is eaten, the usual American diet affords about 120 milligrams of magnesium per 1,000 calories. Dietary deficiencies occur rarely, but have been observed in children suffering from a shortage of protein calories, and in adults who drink alcohol to excess.

ZINC This is another mineral required by the human body. Foods that contain zinc in significant amounts include meats, liver, eggs, oysters, milk, and cereal grains. The average daily intake is on the order of from 10 to 15 milligrams. For adults, the recommended amount is 15 milligrams. There seems, however, to be no evidence of a deficiency in the United States.

TRACE ELEMENTS A number of other chemical elements must be provided, though in minute quantities, if normal growth is to occur in childhood and if health is to be sustained during adulthood. Among them are copper, selenium, cobalt, manganese, iodine, and fluorine. Each trace element has its own very specific function to perform, and if it is not available to the body, problems will arise. Too little iodine causes an enlargement of the thyroid gland, and a goiter is the result. Too little fluorine leaves the teeth susceptible to decay. A deficiency in copper leads to a defect in the walls of the blood vessels in experimental animals, and the result is hemorrhage.

VITAMINS

During the process of digestion and metabolism, new chemical compounds are continually being formed by the uniting of atoms from several elements, or by the splitting of larger molecules (see the discussion of fats, carbohydrates, and proteins in this chapter). Other chemical compounds, which cannot be newly formed or synthesized by the body, are nevertheless required in very small amounts for physiological processes. These are the vitamins, and they come largely from the food we consume. (One of them, Vitamin K, may be produced by bacteria that are normally present in the intestines.) The entire concept of vitamins is relatively new. The first vitamin was recognized in 1914. Up until that time, diseases that were later found to be caused by vitamin deficiency had been common, in the United States as well as elsewhere—among them scurvy, rickets, pellagra, beri-beri, and pernicious anemia.

The discovery and isolation of vitamins, and the determination of their mode of action, ushered in a whole new era in the science of biochemistry. Many were eventually discovered to be co-enzymes, determining the direction and rates of specific chemical reactions. Once it had become feasible to manufacture them in relatively large quantities, the addition of fat-soluble vitamins to milk and other dairy products, and the enrichment of white flour and bread with water-soluble vitamins, became customary. In addition, vitamins in pill or capsule form can be taken as supplements to the diet. As has been emphasized, however, they are not a food substitute, or an alternative to overeating.

FAT-SOLUBLE VITAMINS Those vitamins that are not readily soluble in water, and that accompany fats in foods and in the body, include Vitamins A, D, E, and K.

Vitamin A, known chemically as retinol, is required in visual processes in the retina and particularly for vision in dim light; for growth of bones; and for maintaining normal skin and lining membranes of the body. The vitamin is stored in relatively large quantities in the liver. The chief food sources of Vitamin A are in animal products, including liver, eggs, kidneys, whole milk or low-fat skimmed milk with the vitamin added, butter, fortified margarine, and fish liver oils. About one-half of our Vitamin A is consumed in these forms. The remainder derives from plant foods, notably the dark green and yellow vegetables and fruits. Yellow vegetables contain minerals called carotenes, which are converted to Vitamin A after ingestion in food.

Vitamin D functions in the control of absorption of calcium and phosphorus from foods in the intestine, and in the metabolism and deposition of these minerals in bone. A deficiency produces the disorder known as rickets. Vitamin D is produced in the body by the action of ultraviolet light of the sun on ergosterol in the skin. Food sources include milk irradiated with ultraviolet light, fortified margarines, milks and butter, eggs, and fish.

Vitamin E, chemically identified as alpha-tocopheral, is an antioxidant which protects Vitamin A, fats and other components of the body from oxidation. In addition, it has a role in preserving the structure of red blood cells. A deficiency state in humans has not been recognized. Vitamin E is widely distributed in foods; the richest sources are wheat germ, vegetable oils, lettuce, and whole grain cereals.

Vitamin K, known chemically as menadione, has an important role in controlling blood coagulation, and is involved in synthesis by the liver of a number of factors or chemical compounds essential for the coagulation process. A deficiency is accompanied by hemorrhage. Green and leafy vegetables are a good source of Vitamin K. Since the bacteria in the intestine ordinarily produce it in sufficient quantities to meet the body's needs, however, a deliberate effort to provide this vitamin is needed only under very unusual circumstances—e.g., the taking of an antibiotic that has reduced the bacterial content of the intestines.

WATER-SOLUBLE VITAMINS *Thiamine,* also called B_1, forms, along with phosphate, a co-enzyme that is important in energy metabolism. Thiamine is required for normal function of many tissues, most notably of the heart and nervous systems. Diets deficient in thiamine cause the disease known as beriberi. Food sources of thiamine include enriched flour and bread, whole grain cereals, pork, poultry, beef, milk, and eggs.

Riboflavin, known also as Vitamin B_2, functions in the body in two co-enzymes important for cell respiration, utilization of protein, and growth. A deficiency in man is associated with skin lesions on the face and at the angles of the mouth. Rich sources of riboflavin include milk, cheese, organ meats, fish, poultry, eggs, green and yellow vegetables, and enriched breads and cereals.

Niacin (nicotinic acid) is converted in the body to two co-enzymes which are involved in cell respiration and in the metabolism of fat and carbohydrate. A niacin deficiency produces the disorder known as pellagra, which is accompanied by skin lesions, diarrhea, and mental dysfunction. Niacin derives from the following food sources: liver, enriched and whole grain cereals or breads, lean meats, poultry, fish, peanuts, milk, and potatoes. In addition, an essential amino acid, tryptophan, is converted in the body to niacin in a ratio of one part niacin from each 60 parts of tryptophan.

Vitamin B₆ represents three related chemical compounds in food, namely pyridoxine, pyridoxal, and pyridoxamine. As a co-enzyme, it is importantly involved in the metabolism of protein and amino acids. Vitamin B_6 has important roles in the function of the central nervous system and in the synthesis of hemoglobin. Deficiency causes anemia. Meats, liver, whole grain cereals, and vegetables are food sources for Vitamin B_6.

Folacin has the chemical name of pteroylglutamic acid. Like most other B vitamins, it functions as a co-enzyme important to formation of red blood cells and to synthesis of nucleic acids. Deficiency produces a type of anemia like the one that also occurs with deficiency of Vitamin B_{12}. Folacin is widely distributed in foods, but is notably found in green leafy vegetables and meats.

Vitamin B₁₂. Known also as cobalamin, Vitamin B_{12} contains cobalt as a part of the molecule. Along wth folacin, it has a role in nucleic acid metabolism. It functions as a co-enzyme and is important in red blood cell formation and the functioning of the nervous system. Vitamin B_{12} deficiency is accompanied by pernicious or megalablastic anemia, changes in gastro-intestinal functions, and neuritis. Absorption of the vitamin is dependent upon presence within the intestinal tract of a specific material, known as the *intrinsic factor*. Vitamin B_{12} derives from foods of animal origin, particularly meats, milk, fish and shellfish.

Vitamin C or ascorbic acid has a role in the deposition in the tissues of a material called collagen, which is important for the framework of bones and teeth and for healing wounds. It aids in the absorption of iron and functions of the adrenal gland. A deficiency of Vitamin C causes scurvy, which is accompanied by swollen, bleeding gums and hemorrhage into the skin and other tissues. Items in the diet providing Vitamin C include citrus fruits and juices, strawberries, melons, broccoli, tomatoes, potatoes, and green leafy vegetables.

FOOD CHOICES AND HEALTH

The person concerned with good nutrition is left with some fairly simple advice: he or she must find ways of ensuring a daily supply of these essential nutrients by maintaining a varied and well-balanced diet.

The facts are that in the United States people do generally eat well and health has improved markedly in the last half century as the science of nutrition has evolved and technologies have developed to make foods of great variety available throughout the year. The United States, however, has moved from nutrient deficiency diseases which were common at the beginning of this era to chronic diseases (primarily cardiovascular disease, the number one cause of death in the United States) associated with nutrient excesses, especially fat, cholesterol, salt, and total calories. The advice that follows will concentrate on what is known concerning nutrition as related to prevention of cardiovascular disease.

In 1961, the American Heart Association began providing information to physicians and the public on the link between high levels of cholesterol in the blood and the development of atherosclerosis, the disease in which fatty deposits or plaques accumulate in the walls of the arteries. Simultaneously there was encouragement of the public to decrease its intake of fat and cholesterol. Such advice has its origin in the research around 1913 by a Russian scientist, Nikolai Avitschev, showing a connection between a high-cholesterol diet and fatty deposits in the arteries (atherosclerosis) of rabbits. This discovery has led to extensive medical research on how blood fats and cholesterol contribute to diseases of the human circulatory system.

Atherosclerosis generally develops gradually, with no symptoms, for anywhere from twenty to forty years or even longer. Then serious clinical complications may suddenly manifest themselves—angina (chest pain), heart attack, stroke, or sudden death. Because of the devastating and insidious nature of atherosclerosis, an understanding of what can be done to prevent it becomes imperative.

It is possible that dietary substances and blood constituents other than cholesterol are also involved in the development of atherosclerosis. From what is known of fat metabolism, however, it is clear that the amount of cholesterol and the fatty substances known collectively as lipoproteins in the bloodstream can be modified by diet, and thus help to prevent heart attacks and other circulatory disease.

Studies of the incidence of coronary disease (see chapter 1 for a detailed account of this research) suggest that certain lipoprotein molecules of low density (LDL) and very low density (VLDL)—the major transport of cholesterol and of triglycerides, respectively—may be a contributing cause of heart attacks. On the other hand, there is some evidence that lipoprotein molecules of high density (HDL) tend to transport cholesterol away from body cells and thus to prevent its accumulation in the arteries.

As of 1970, about 35 percent of all deaths in the United States were the result of coronary heart disease, in which deposits of fat, cholesterol, and calcium occur in the walls of the arteries surrounding the heart. Such arteries can eventually be blocked totally by small clots. This is the event that causes a myocardial infarction, the medical term for a heart attack. Careful and repeated studies of comparative death rates from a number of countries have shown a correlation between differences in nutrition—including total calories, fats, and cholesterol—and the rate of mortality. In one study of seven countries, the highest death rates for middle-aged men as a result of coronary heart disease were recorded for eastern Finland and the United States (where the amount of saturated fat and cholesterol in the diet is highest)—120 and 80 deaths per 1,000 respectively, as compared with about 20 per 1,000, or less, for the Greek islands of Corfu and Crete, for the province of Dalmatia in Yugoslavia, and for Japan—all regions where the amount of fat in the diet is notably lower. Recent reductions in the death rate for heart disease in the United States may possibly be related to changes in the diet.

Since the beginning of this century, the total average daily consumption of fat per capita in the United States has increased by about one-fourth, from 125 to 159 grams. The share of the total calories derived from fat has also increased, from 32 percent in the period from 1909 to 1913 to the current figure of 42 percent. The cholesterol content of the current average diet is about 500 milligrams. The American Heart Association recommends that the daily intake of cholesterol be kept below 300 milligrams, and the proportion of fat to the total caloric intake to within a range from 30 to 35 percent. In addition, the amount of animal fat should be reduced, and vegetable (polyunsaturated) fat be substituted in its stead, as an important way of lessening the risk of atherosclerosis and coronary disease.

REDUCING CHOLESTEROL   A basic principle to keep in mind is that food products from animal sources contain cholesterol. Egg yolks are the most concentrated source, and must consequently be limited. Organ meats—liver, kidney, heart, and sweetbreads—are very high in cholesterol (although liver, because it is so rich in vitamins and iron, should not be eliminated entirely from a fat-modified diet). Unlike most seafood, shrimp is moderately high in cholesterol, and should be eaten sparingly. In general, food products from land animals contain saturated fat, whereas those from aquatic animals contain polyunsaturated oil. Since saturated fats tend to raise the level of cholesterol in the blood, foods containing them should all be limited, and some should be avoided. Whole-milk dairy products, such as cheese and ice cream, and the marbling in red meat are notable examples of food containing saturated fats. The chemical process of hydrogenation changes liquid vegetable oils to a saturated fat, as in solid shortenings and some margarines. Hydrogenated fat is often described as "hardened" or "specially processed." Completely hydrogenated fats are saturated and should be used sparingly, if not avoided altogether.

A few saturated fats are of vegetable origin—coconut, coconut oil, and palm kernel oil. These oils are found in many commercial products—non-dairy coffee creamers, non-dairy whipped toppings, non-dairy sour creams, cake mixes, and commercial cookies. The best way to avoid these oils is to assume that any unidentified vegetable oil in any of these products is a saturated fat of vegetable origin.

In place of animal shortening such as butter and lard, oils of vegetable origin, such as corn, cottonseed, safflower, sesame, soybean, or sunflower seed, are recommended because they tend to lower the level of cholesterol in the blood. As distinct from such polyunsaturated fats, there are certain monosaturated fats, which do not raise or lower the level of cholesterol, and are thus called "neutral fats." The content of olive oil and peanut oil is primarily monosaturated. These two may be used in small quantities for seasoning, but it should be remembered that they do not have the cholesterol-lowering properties of polyunsaturates.

In place of butter, the preferred margarines are those listing *liquid* oils as the first ingredient, followed by one or more partially hydrogenated vegetable oils. Margarines that contain twice as much polyunsaturated as saturated fat are to be preferred. Diet margarines contain water and provide half the amount of fat found in the recommended polyunsaturated margarines; as a consequence, they are labled "imitation." Although usable as seasoning or as a spread, they are not desirable for cooking because of their high water content.

Except for walnuts—which contain a polyunsaturated oil—nuts are primarily "neutral" in their fat content. Peanut butter thus falls in the same category, as do avocados. Commercial salad dressings and mayonnaise are generally acceptable since they are made largely with unsaturated oils.

LABELING OF FAT CONTENT   Assistance in determining the fat and cholesterol content can be found in the labeling of commercially packaged foods. For example, the label of a commercial mayonnaise lists the ingredients used.

Vegetable salad oil, which is listed first, is thus understood to be the main ingredient. It can be also learned from the label that a one-tablespoon serving affords 10 milligrams of cholesterol—a rather small quantity, which comes from the egg yolks listed among the contents. The yolk of a single large egg contains about 250 milligrams. Thus, it can be determined with a little calculation that one would have to consume 25 servings of the mayonnaise in question to obtain the same amount of cholesterol as from eating a single egg.

It is important to read the labels on all premixed, packaged, frozen, dehydrated, and crystallized food products. Unfortunately, manufacturers of commercial cakes, cookies, quick-bread mixes, and similar ready-to-use products often use saturated fats, whole milk, and eggs. (On the other hand, most grains, flours, pastas, ordinary loaf bread and rolls are practically free of fat.) Some packaged and prepared foods now on the market—e.g., vegetarian baked beans and angel food cake mix—contain no fat at all. Cereal products, both cooked and dry, are acceptable with the exception of those that contain coconut.

Convenience foods should be approached with caution. Those prepared with fat are acceptable only if the fat belongs to the polyunsaturated category; for example, sardines packed in cottonseed or soybean oil. Items such as packaged popcorn, potato chips, and French-fried potatoes should be avoided. Frozen dinners and other ready-to-eat, canned, or frozen food mixtures usually contain saturated fat. Dehydrated foods such as potatoes, pancake mixes, and those to which fat is to be added, are usually acceptable—although, for true convenience, no commercial product can equal the potato that bakes in its own jacket, or the apple that needs only washing.

CONTROLLING FATS IN FOOD PREPARATION   With a little study and imagination, it is possible to turn out excellent meals with a minimum of fat. Well-trimmed, lean meat can be prepared by baking, roasting, broiling, or simmering as the cut requires. It can be browned or sauteed with a few drops of oil in a frying pan or a Teflon-coated skillet. The skillful use of herbs, lemon juice, and wines to accent the natural flavors of food will more than compensate for the familiar flavor of butter and other animal fats in food preparation (as is true for salt, which is discussed below). Properly used—but not overused—they can transform a simple dish into an elegant one. Foreign cookery offers wonderful guidance in the use of herbs.

The rich meat essence that drips into the roasting pan or broiler along with the fat from roasts, steaks or other meats may be salvaged for future use by pouring the contents of the pan, fat and all, into a refrigerator dish and chilling it. The dark, protein-rich juice that separates out beneath the fat will add zest to meat pies, brown sauces, hashes, or meat loaf. The hardened fat should be discarded. Gravies can be made by blending clear, defatted broth with a thickening agent. Homemade broth is heartier and more flavorful than the canned variety. It should be made the day before so that it can be defatted after refrigeration. Canned broths, as well as canned soups and stews, are usually relatively free of fat, but the can should be refrigerated before opening so that the visible fat can be removed before using.

Favorite recipes can be used by making appropriate substitutions.

WHEN A RECIPE CALLS FOR	USE
Sour Cream	Low-fat cottage cheese blended until smooth, or cottage cheese plus low-fat yogurt for flavor, or ricotta cheese made from partially skimmed milk (thinned with yogurt or buttermilk, if desired). One can of chilled, evaporated skim milk whipped with 1 teaspoon of lemon juice. Low-fat buttermilk or low-fat yogurt.
Chocolate	Cocoa blended with polyunsaturated oil or margarine (one 1-oz. square of chocolate = 3 tablespoons of cocoa + 1 tablespoon polyunsaturated oil or margarine).
Butter	Polyunsaturated margarine or oil. One tablespoon butter = 1 tablespoon margarine or ¾ tablespoon oil. To substitute margarine for oil, use 1¼ cups of margarine for 1 cup of oil. Use 1¼ tablespoons of margarine for 1 tablespoon of oil.
Eggs	Use commercially produced cholesterol-free egg substitutes according to package directions. Or use 1 egg white plus 3 teaspoons of polyunsaturated oil.
Milk	Use 1 cup of skim or nonfat dry milk plus 2 tablespoons of polyunsaturated oil as a substitute for 1 cup of whole milk.
Buttermilk	One cup lukewarm nonfat milk plus 1 tablespoon of lemon juice = 1 cup buttermilk. Let the mixture stand for five minutes and beat briskly.
Cornstarch	Use 1 tablespoon flour for 1½ teaspoons cornstarch, or 2 tablespoons flour or 1 tablespoon arrowroot for 1 tablespoon cornstarch.
Cream Cheese	Blend 4 tablespoons of margarine with 1 cup dry low-fat cottage cheese. Add salt to taste and a small amount of skim milk if needed in blending mixture. Vegetables such as chopped chives or pimiento, and herbs and seasonings, may be added for variety.

Additional help and ideas can be obtained from the American Heart Association Cookbook.

Changing from a usual diet to a fat-modified one is a matter of re-education of tastes and cannot be accomplished in a day. Habits are reformed slowly. Success is more likely if as few changes as possible are made in the beginning. As one becomes acquainted with necessary substitutes, seasonings can also be altered.

A fat-controlled meal plan that includes restaurant fare can be easily mastered. A few pointers will help. Instead of bacon and eggs for breakfast, fish, chicken, or lean Canadian bacon can provide a welcome change. The variety of hot and cold cereals is almost endless. English, corn or bran muffins, whole wheat, rye or raisin bread are all appropriate substitutes for butter-laden Danish pastries. For lunch, chicken, turkey, fish, lean meat, and large fruit or vegetable salads are good choices.

The dinner menu is replete with possibilities. Thin broths and consommés are the best bets in the soup category. For the entree, broiled, baked, or roasted meat, fish, or poultry should take precedence over fried, grilled, or sauteed versions of the same. On request, chefs are usually willing to serve entrees without fatty sauces or gravies. Meat should be ordered broiled without butter. As a general rule, dishes prepared in wine are acceptable as opposed to those prepared in thick sauces and gravies such as stews. Oriental cuisine offers a great variety of low-fat dishes. Vegetables pose little problem unless they are swimming in butter. One can enjoy the natural goodness of a baked potato while avoiding the sour cream. Salad dressing may be mixed at the table with oil and vinegar. A hard roll is preferable to a rich, buttery dinner or sweet roll. The best choices for dessert are fruits, fruit ice, sherbet, gelatin, and angel food cake without icing. Whipped cream, whipped topping, and custard sauces are to be avoided.

Cooking and eating in a fat-controlled style is an adventure in healthy living.

A GENERAL GUIDE TO FOOD CHOICES

Translating these recommendations into food requires some information about food selection and preparation. It will become apparent that a wide variety of foods is possible and that they can be prepared either simply or with elegance. The fat-controlled diet is a balanced one, and the approach to individualizing it to suit a person's life style can be accomplished by utilizing the following daily food guidelines. They include quantities and kinds of foods necessary for good nutrition. For those for whom these guidelines will not provide sufficient calories to meet daily energy needs, calories may be increased by choosing additional servings from all but the meat group and egg yolks.

General Guidelines for a Fat-Modified Diet to Reduce the Risk of Heart Attack

Every day, select foods from each of the basic food groups in lists 1–5.*

FOOD GROUP	NUTRIENT SUPPLIES	RECOMMENDED	AVOID OR USE SPARINGLY
1. Meat Poultry Fish Dried beans and peas Nuts Eggs	Protein Irons B complex vitamins Fats Cholesterol (from animal sources)	*Chicken, turkey, veal, fish in most of your meat meals for the week.* *Shellfish: clams, crab, lobster, oysters scallops.* Use a 4-ounce serving as a substitute for meat. *Beef, lamb, pork, ham less frequently.* Choose lean ground meat and lean cuts of meat. Trim all visible fat before cooking. Bake, broil, roast or stew so that you can discard the fat which cooks out of the meat.	Duck, goose Shrimp is moderately high in cholesterol. Use a 4-ounce serving in a meat meal no more than once a week. Heavily marbled and fatty meats, spare ribs, mutton, frankfurters, sausages, fatty hamburgers, bacon, luncheon meats. Organ meats (liver, kidney, heart, sweetbreads) are very high in cholesterol. Since liver is very rich in vitamins and

* *This refers to fat equivalents, not protein.*

FOOD GROUP	NUTRIENT SUPPLIES	RECOMMENDED	AVOID OR USE SPARINGLY
		Nuts and dried beans and peas: Kidney beans, lima beans, baked beans, lentils, chick peas (garbanzos), split peas are high in vegetable protein and may be used in place of meat occasionally. *Egg whites* as desired.	iron, it should not be eliminated from the diet completely. Use a 4-ounce serving in a meat meal no more than once a week. Egg yolks: limit to 3 per week, including eggs used in cooking. Cakes, batters, sauces, and other foods containing egg yolks.
2. Vegetables and Fruits (Fresh, frozen, or canned)	Vitamins A & C Minerals Fiber Carbohydrates	*One serving should be a source of Vitamin C:* Broccoli, cabbage (raw), tomatoes. Berries, cantaloupe, grapefruit (or juice), mango, melon, orange (or juice), papaya, strawberries, tangerines. *One serving should be a source of Vitamin A—dark green leafy or yellow vegetables, or yellow fruits:* Broccoli, carrots, chard, chicory, escarole, greens (beet, collard, dandelion, mustard, turnip), kale, peas, rutabagas, spinach, string beans, sweet potatoes and yams, watercress, winter squash, yellow corn. Apricots, cantaloupe, mango, papaya. Other vegetables and fruits are also very nutritious; they should be eaten in salads, main dishes, snacks, and desserts, in addition to the recommended daily	If you must limit your calories, use vegetables such as potatoes, corn, and lima beans sparingly. To add variety to your diet, one serving (½ cup) of any one of these may be substituted for one serving of bread or cereals.

FOOD GROUP	NUTRIENT SUPPLIES	RECOMMENDED	AVOID OR USE SPARINGLY
		allowances of high vitamin A and C vegetables and fruits.	
3. Bread and cereals (whole grain, enriched, or restored)	Iron Niacin Carbohydrates Protein Fiber	*Breads made with a minimum of saturated fat:* White enriched (including raisin bread), whole wheat, English muffins, French bread, Italian bread, oatmeal bread, pumpernickel, rye bread. Biscuits, muffins, and griddle cakes made at home, using an allowed liquid oil as shortening. Cereal (hot and cold), rice, melba toast, matzo, pretzels. Pasta: macaroni, noodles (except egg noodles), spaghetti.	Butter rolls, commercial biscuits, muffins, donuts, sweet rolls, cakes, crackers, egg bread, cheese bread, commercial mixes containing dried eggs and whole milk.
4. Milk products	Vitamins A & D Protein B vitamins Calcium Phosphorus Carbohydrates	*Milk products that are low in dairy fats:* Fortified skimmed (non-fat) milk and fortified skimmed milk powder, low-fat milk. The label on the container should show that the milk is fortified with Vitamins A and D. The word "fortified" alone is not enough. Buttermilk made from skimmed milk, yogurt made from skimmed milk, canned evaporated skimmed milk, cocoa made with low-fat milk.	*Whole milk and whole milk products:* Chocolate milk, canned whole milk, ice cream, all creams including sour, half-and-half, and whipped; whole milk yogurt. Non-dairy cream substitutes (usually these contain coconut oil, which is very high in saturated fat). Cheese made from cream or whole milk. Butter.

FOOD GROUP	NUTRIENT SUPPLIES	RECOMMENDED	AVOID OR USE SPARINGLY
		Cheeses made from skimmed or partially skimmed milk, such as cottage cheese, creamed or uncreamed (uncreamed is preferable), farmer's, baker's, or hoop cheese, mozzarella and sapsago cheeses. Processed modified fat cheeses (skimmed milk and polyunsaturated fat).	
5. Fats and oils (Polyunsaturated)	Essential fatty acids Vitamins A & D	*Margarines, liquid oil shortenings, salad dressings and mayonnaise containing any of these polyunsaturated vegetable oils:* Corn oil, cottonseed oil, safflower oil, sesame seed oil, soybean oil, sunflower seed oil. Margarines and other products high in polyunsaturates can usually be identified by the label, which lists a recommended liquid vegetable oil as the first ingredient, and one or more partially hydrogenated vegetable oils as additional ingredients. Diet margarines are low in calories because they are low in fat. Therefore it takes twice as much diet margarine to supply the polyunsaturates contained in a recommended margarine.	*Solid fats and shortenings:* Butter, lard, salt pork fat, meat fat, completely hydrogenated margarines and vegetable shortenings, products containing coconut oil. Peanut oil and olive oil may be used occasionally for flavor, but they are low in polyunsaturates and do not take the place of the recommended oils.

FOOD GROUP	NUTRIENT SUPPLIES	RECOMMENDED	AVOID OR USE SPARINGLY
6. Other foods to meet energy needs		*Low in calories or no calories:* Fresh fruit or fruit canned without sugar, tea, coffee (no cream), cocoa powder, water ices, gelatin, fruit whip, puddings made with non-fat milk, low-calorie drinks, vinegar, mustard, ketchup, herbs, spices. *High in calories:* Frozen or canned fruit with sugar added, jelly, jam, marmalade, honey, pure sugar candy such as gum drops, hard candy, mint patties (not chocolate); imitation ice cream made with safflower oil; cakes, pies, cookies, and puddings made with polyunsaturated fat in place of solid shortening; angel food cake; nuts, especially walnuts; peanut butter; bottled drinks, fruit drinks, ice milk, sherbet, wine, beer, whiskey.	Coconut and coconut oil, commercial cakes, pies, cookies, and mixes, frozen cream pies, commercially fried foods such as potato chips and other deep-fried snacks, whole milk puddings, chocolate pudding (high in cocoa butter and therefore high in saturated fat), ice cream.

Quantitative Guidelines for Following a Fat-Modified Diet

FOOD GROUP	PRE-SCHOOL	PRE-ADOLESCENTS	ADOLESCENTS	ADULTS
1. Meat Poultry Fish Dried beans and peas Nuts Eggs	No more than 2 servings daily. *One serving is:* 1 tablespoon (½ oz.) for each year of the child's age	No more than 2 servings daily *One serving is:* 2–3 oz. lean meat, fish or poultry 1 cup cooked	No more than 2 servings daily *One serving is:* 2–3 oz. meat, fish or poultry 4 tablespoons peanut butter	No more than 2 servings daily *One serving is:* 2–3 oz. meat, fish or poultry 4 tablespoons peanut butter

FOOD GROUP	PRE-SCHOOL	PRE-ADOLESCENTS	ADOLESCENTS	ADULTS
	for lean meats, chicken, fish, turkey ¼ cup cooked legumes 1 tablespoon peanut butter 1 oz. meat = 1 chicken leg 1½" diameter meatball Fish—1"x3"x½" 1 egg daily	legumes 4 tablespoons peanut butter Hamburger— 3"x½" Chicken leg & thigh Fish—3"x3"x½" 1 egg daily	1 cup cooked legumes 3–4 eggs per week	1 cup cooked legumes 3 eggs per week
2. Vegetables and fruits	4 or more servings *One serving is:* 1 tablespoon or ½ oz. cooked vegetable per year of age ½ cup fruit juice ½ piece medium fruit *Note:* Use small amounts of a variety of fruits and vegetables.	4 or more servings *One serving is:* ½ cup fruit or vegetable juice 1 med. (3") fruit or vegetable ½ cup cooked fruit or vegetable	4 or more servings *One serving is:* ½ cup fruit or vegetable juice 1 med. (3") fruit or vegetable ½ cup cooked fruit or vegetable	4 or more servings *One serving is:* ½ cup fruit or vegetable juice 1 med. (3") fruit or vegetable ½ cup cooked fruit or vegetable
3. Bread and cereals	4 servings *One serving is:* ½ slice bread ½ cup dry cereal ¼ cup pasta, rice, noodles ¼ cup cooked cereal ½ tortilla 1 graham cracker	4 or more servings *One serving is:* 1 slice bread 1 cup dry cereal ½ cup pasta, rice, noodles ½ cup cooked cereal 1 tortilla 2 graham crackers	4 or more servings *One serving is:* 1 slice bread 1 cup dry cereal ½ cup cooked cereal ½ cup pasta, rice, noodles 1 tortilla 2 graham crackers	4 or more servings *One serving is:* 1 slice bread 1 cup dry cereal ½ cup cooked cereal ½ cup pasta, rice, noodles 1 tortilla 2 graham crackers

FOOD GROUP	PRE-SCHOOL	PRE-ADOLESCENTS	ADOLESCENTS	ADULTS
	½ cup popcorn	1 cup popcorn	1 cup popcorn	1 cup popcorn
4. Milk products	(Age 1–3) 2 servings (Age 4–6) 3 servings *One serving (to meet calcium requirements) is:* One 8 oz. glass milk, buttermilk 1 oz. low-fat cheese 1 oz. low-fat yogurt One ⅓ oz. cup low-fat cottage cheese 1 oz. cheese = 3 oz. meat *Note:* Serve small portions more frequently, ¼–½ cup at a time.	Minimum of 3 servings per day (to meet calcium requirements) *One serving is:* One 8 oz. glass milk or buttermilk 1 oz. low-fat cheese One ⅓ cup low-fat cottage cheese One 8 oz. carton low-fat yogurt 1 oz. cheese = 3 oz. meat *	4 or more servings (to meet calcium requirements *One serving is:* One 8 oz. glass milk or buttermilk 1 oz. low-fat cheese One ⅓ cup low-fat cottage cheese One 8 oz. carton low-fat yogurt 1 oz. cheese = 3 oz. meat *	2 or more servings *One serving is:* One 8 oz. glass milk or buttermilk 1 oz. low-fat cheese One ⅓ cup low-fat cottage cheese One 8 oz. carton low-fat yogurt 1 oz. cheese = 3 oz. meat *
5. Fats	2–3 teaspoons	4–6 teaspoons	2–4 tablespoons	2–4 tablespoons
6. Other foods to meet energy needs	1–3-year-olds: The total quantities from food groups meet estimated energy intake of 1300 K cals/day. 4–6-year-olds: Other low-fat, low-cholesterol foods to	Other low-fat, low-cholesterol foods to meet energy needs or increase portions of above foods except meat.	Other low-fat, low-cholesterol foods to meet energy needs; or increase portions of above foods except meat.	Other low-fat, low-cholesterol foods to meet energy needs; or increase portions of above foods except meat.

* *This refers to fat equivalents, not protein.*

FOOD GROUP	PRE-SCHOOL	PRE-ADOLESCENTS	ADOLESCENTS	ADULTS
	meet energy needs or increase portions of above foods except meat.			

THE PROBLEM OF EXCESS CALORIES AND OVERWEIGHT

The heart functions most efficiently in persons who are not obese and who remain physically active. Among the ailments to which overweight persons have been found to be more subject than others are diabetes, arthritis, kidney disease, and cirrhosis of the liver, as well as hypertension and heart disease. The death rate from the latter two diseases among obese persons is estimated to be three times higher than among those who are not overweight. The reason for this alarming discrepancy is not difficult to understand. Since obesity entails an increase in the amount of body tissue and in the blood supply that maintains it, obviously the heart must work harder. The result of this demand is an increase in the size of the heart muscle (the myocardium) and a correspondingly greater expenditure of energy. This increased output is associated with high blood pressure and the danger of heart attacks. Thus the importance of preventing obesity, through diet and regular exercise, can hardly be exaggerated.

Much of modern technology seems to be involved in a conspiracy against every effort that is made in the direction of keeping one's weight down. No one needs to be reminded that the favorite foods of many Americans—notably teenagers, but they are not alone in this—consist primarily of fatty foods, sugars, and sodium-laden snacks and soft drinks. The past decades have brought a multitude of labor-saving devices, which become increasingly important to the individual just at the time in life when added physical exertion is needed to keep weight down. And never before in history has food been so readily at hand as it now is in the United States. In the refrigerator at home, there are foods prepared for immediate consumption; in schools and offices, vending machines dispense all manner of food and drink at the drop of a coin; and fast-food chains have set up shop in every town and along every highway.

For anyone desiring to lose weight, some restriction in caloric intake may be necessary in addition to a program of daily exercise. The simplest procedure is to reduce the intake of calories by about 500 below the standard allowance for a given age, body weight, and height. Over a period of time, cutting down by this amount makes it possible to shed about a pound a week.

It is never too early to begin good nutrition. The earlier the habit of eating sensibly is established, the more likely that it will last a lifetime. We don't have to go far to see proof of this. The extra pounds usually associated with poor nutrition tend to linger and increase with age, so that the overweight child often is overweight as an adult—thus increasing the risk of cardiovascular disease. Equally important is the role of example. A child whose parents are overweight tends to become overweight as well. Although inherited traits may have something to do with this tendency, the fact remains that most cases of overweight are caused by one thing, and one thing only—taking in more food energy than the body is able to use.

THE PROBLEM OF EXCESS SODIUM For a patient with heart failure or any other cardiac malfunction, it is important to cut down on sodium to avoid overworking the kidneys and thus adding to the burden on the heart. In such patients, the accumulation of fluid in the body tissues, causing edema or swelling—usually in the feet or ankles—may signal an excess of sodium. Given the generally recognized connection between hypertension and coronary heart disease, there is enough evidence of a relation between hypertension and excessive amounts of sodium that it becomes prudent to avoid such an excess in the diet. It has been observed that patients with high blood pressure frequently show an improvement when the quantity of salt they consume is restricted. This happens because a decrease in the amount of salt in the blood has the effect of shrinking the volume of fluid in the blood vessels. The decrease in fluid reduces pressure on the interior walls of the blood vessels and lessens the effort which the heart must put into pumping the blood.

CONTROLLING SODIUM IN THE DIET Determining just how much salt we consume is difficult, not only because sodium is a natural constituent of so many foods, but also because the amounts of sodium chloride and other sodium compounds added by food processors tend to vary and are often unknown. Since recent surveys indicate that nearly 15 percent of all adults have hypertension and would benefit from some reduction in sodium intake, a great many people would be assisted by more explicit information concerning the sodium content in commercially processed foods. U. S. Food and Drug Administration regulations permit the inclusion of sodium content in labeling. For example, among the natural constituents of a cup of whole milk are 120 milligrams of sodium.

Anyone concerned with limiting the intake of sodium should be alert to the fact that most seasonings—e.g., soy sauce, catsup, relishes, seasoning salts, and bouillon cubes—are rich in salt or other sodium compounds, as are many common foods: cheeses (except dry cottage cheese), luncheon meats, frankfurters, corned beef, bacon, ham, canned soups, bakery goods, and many canned or frozen vegetables. These foods are to be avoided or, at most, consumed in strictly limited quantities. Attention is to be paid to the list of ingredients given on the label to determine whether salt is among them. The use of flavoring agents such as spices, herbs, and lemon can help reduce the use of salt while imparting zest to meals.

FOODS FOR ALL AGES By adopting good nutritional practices in early life, it is likely that the onset of a number of diseases common to later life can be avoided or delayed. The following guidelines take into account the requirements for the various stages of life.

INFANCY Breast feeding for at least six months is without doubt to be preferred. The breast-fed infant should be provided with supplements of iron and Vitamins A, D, and C beginning at about six weeks. Supplemental feedings of infant formula and other simple foods need not be started until the fourth or fifth month. For mothers not wishing to breast-feed the physician can provide a prescription that includes the necessary nutrients, to be supplemented in the same way as for a breast-fed infant.

	Average Calorie Allowances	
Infant	Per Kilogram Body Weight	Per Pound Body Weight
0- 6 months	117 calories	53
6-12 months	108	49
Child		
1- 3 years	100	46
4- 6 years	90	41
7-10 years	80	36

CHILDHOOD   At the age of one year, a child is ready to eat most of the foods prepared for other members of the family. It is best to keep servings small, so that the younger child is not under pressure to overeat. Equally important is to encourage the child to be active physically, so as to avoid becoming overweight and to aid in developing strong muscles. The calorie needs of childhood are importantly determined by the rates of growth and levels of physical activity. *See chart.*

To avoid dental caries, which begins in childhood, drinking water should be fluoridated; otherwise children should be given daily supplements of fluoride. Foods that contain much sugar are best avoided entirely or given infrequently and in small amounts.

ADOLESCENCE   This is the period when the rate of growth and the manufacture of new skeletal and muscle mass are greatest. It can also be a time of aberrant behavior, which may be expressed in food habits. The adolescent who is withdrawn and inactive may find satisfaction in snacking, frequent visits to the refrigerator, and a full stomach, with obesity as the result. On the other hand, especially in girls and young women, there may be a tendency to reject food, impeding growth and leading to anorexia nervosa, a disorder that can be life-threatening. Adolescent youngsters with a major interest in sports, or in developing a trim figure, can be encouraged to take an interest in nutrition, in avoiding fats, and in following the diet recommended in this chapter.

ADULTHOOD   The major requirement after the body has reached maturity is for energy to meet its metabolic needs. The basal metabolic rate for the body at rest is directly related to body size, is greater in men than in women, and decreases with age. For a young adult male of average size, the basal metabolic rate is of the order of 1,800 calories per day. For a young woman, it is about 1,600 calories per day. As a general guide, about 25 calories per kilogram, or 12 calories per pound of body weight, are utilized daily by both males and females for the metabolic process. In addition to these amounts the diet must provide further calories to meet the cost of physical activity. Recommended allowances provide an additional 800 or 900 calories for this purpose in relatively inactive young men and about 350 or 400 calories for women. The costs of physical activity relate to body weight, the amount of work done, and the length of time it is engaged in.

A woman who is pregnant or who is breast-feeding an infant has a notable need for extra calories and nutrients. The energy cost of a normal and uncomplicated pregnancy is about 45,000 calories. When a woman is eating appropriately during pregnancy, she can expect to gain from 22 to 30 pounds. The infant at term should weight in the range of 3.0 to 3.5 kilograms, or between 6½ and 7½ pounds. To accomplish this, an expectant mother should add to her usual daily diet an additional 300 calories, 30 grams of protein, and iron in a pill or capsule. During periods of breast-feeding, she will need 500

PRINCIPLES

1. *Habitual excesses in eating habits— especially of fats, salt, and possibly sugar—are high on the list of controllable factors that have been linked to cardiovascular disease. Obesity is directly related to such excesses and is another leading risk factor, controllable by attention to the diet.*

2. *The heart functions most efficiently in persons who are not obese and who remain physically active. Since among obese persons the death rate from heart disease and hypertension is estimated to be three times as high as among those who are not overweight, prevention of obesity through exercise and attention to diet can hardly be exaggerated as a means of alleviating the risk of heart attacks.*

3. *More than one-third of all deaths in the United States are the result of coronary heart disease, in which deposits of fat, cholesterol, and calcium occur in the walls of the arteries surrounding the heart.*

4. *The connection between fatty deposits in the arteries (atherosclerosis) and a*

diet high in cholesterol has been well established through medical research. Atherosclerosis develops gradually, with no symptoms, over a period of many years. Because of the devastating and insidious nature of the disease, controlling the intake of cholesterol is emphasized as a major concern in the prevention of heart attacks.

5. *It is recommended that the daily intake of cholesterol be kept under 300 milligrams. In addition, it is recommended that the proportion of fat to the total caloric intake be kept to somewhere between 30 and 35 percent, and that vegetable (polyunsaturated) fat be substituted for that from animal sources as an important means of lessening the risk of atherosclerosis and coronary disease.*

6. *The excessive consumption of sodium, mainly in the form of table salt (sodium chloride), has been linked with hypertension, a leading contributor to the risk of heart attacks. For this reason it becomes prudent to limit the amount of salt in the diet. Patients with high blood pressure frequently show an improvement when the quantity of salt they consume is restricted.*

7. *Most people in the United States consume more protein than they need, in the form of meat, fish, eggs, and dairy products. To lessen the risk of cardiovascular disease, the balance should be shifted in favor of more complex carbohydrates, such as are found in fresh fruits and vegetables. On the other hand, overindulgence in the chemically simpler sugars, in the form of desserts, soft drinks, and snack foods, is to be avoided as contributing to obestity.*

8. *Currently about 4 percent of the average caloric intake by adult Americans is in the form of alcohol. Most alcoholic drinks contain few nutrients other than calories, and should be recognized as potent contributors to obesity. For anyone with symptoms of coronary disease or hypertension, a strict embargo on alcohol is recommended.*

calories, 20 grams of protein, 2,000 International Units of Vitamin A, and 400 I.U. of Vitamin D in addition to what her usual diet provides.

OLD AGE   By the age of 55 or 60, life and patterns of living have changed for most persons. Even though body weight may not have changed, the proportion of fat will have increased in relation to lean body mass or metabolizing tissue. With this there is a reduction in the basal metabolic rate. Accordingly, the total energy needs are reduced by from 10 to 20 percent of what they have been in middle life. In elderly people the pleasure in the taste and smell of food is blunted, and appetites may begin to fail. Although energy requirements are less, the need for other nutrients is unchanged, and special care should be taken to encourage consumption of small and nutritious meals. Attention should be given to foods providing bulk or fiber, as an aid to avoiding the constipation that often plagues older persons.

For whatever age, a wisely chosen diet will avoid foods that may contribute to the causes of disease, especially cardio-vascular disease. This means, above all, learning to eat in moderation so that overweight is avoided.

4

EXERCISE

Michael M. Dehn, M.S.
Jere H. Mitchell, M.D.

Theories about exercise and physical fitness, especially in relation to a healthy heart, have abounded in the decades following the first studies of the origins of cardiovascular diseases among the general population in the United States. At one extreme, exercise in the form of jogging or bicycling is extolled as an almost inpregnable defense against coronary artery disease and a cure for hypertension. At the other extreme is the less fashionable but still popular notion that any extensive physical exertion after the age of forty is dangerous. Those looking for guidance from pseudoscientific publications come away starry-eyed from miracle claims of fitness without effort, while others are frightened away from the whole idea of exercise by reports of sudden death on the tennis court or joggers' dropping permanently by the wayside. Perhaps a more rational approach can be achieved by examining the meaning of the concept of "physical fitness," the differences between the basic types of exercise, and the effects of physical activity on the whole body and the cardiovascular system in particular. Such information can provide the guidelines necessary for working out a program of exercise or sports best suited to a person's age, physical condition, and daily activity.

FITNESS Although "fitness" is difficult to define in the abstract, broadly speaking it is the capacity to perform a specific task. Fitness therefore varies, depending on the nature of the task to be done. For the weight lifter, fitness is the capacity to lift ("pump" or "press" are more accurate terms) specific heavy objects. In general, strength alone is necessary to qualify as a weight lifter. For the gymnast, an additional element, flexibility, is needed for a physically taxing but also graceful performance on parallel bars. For the marathon runner, fitness must include endurance as the essential element. For the average, noncompeting adult, fitness is the ability to carry out daily activities without undue fatigue and to respond to sudden physical and emotional stress without an excessive increase in heart rate and blood pressure. This capacity to adapt is most closely related to the endurance and stamina that come with cardiovascular fitness—the ability of the heart and blood vessels to supply the oxygen needs of body tissues. The fit person is able to work or exercise longer and harder and with less effort than the person who is not physically fit. To understand the relationship between cardiovascular fitness and exercise it is important to know how the body responds to different kinds of exercise and how a well-designed exercise program results in beneficial adaptations.

KINDS OF EXERCISE There are two basic types of muscular activity—static and dynamic. Static or isometric exercise involves the development of tension within muscle fibers and results in little or no movement of joints and bones. Dynamic or isotonic exercise shortens the muscle fibers and moves the joints and bones, even at low levels of muscle activity. Most forms of exercise are actually a mixture of both static and dynamic, with one type more dominant than the other. Walking, running, and swimming, for example, are predominantly dynamic, while weight lifting and water skiing are primarily static. The difference in the effect on the body can be seen by comparing predominantly static water skiing with predominantly dynamic rowing. Both activities involve the muscles of the arms, shoulders, back, and legs, and both clearly develop tension and contraction in these muscle groups. During rowing, however, the

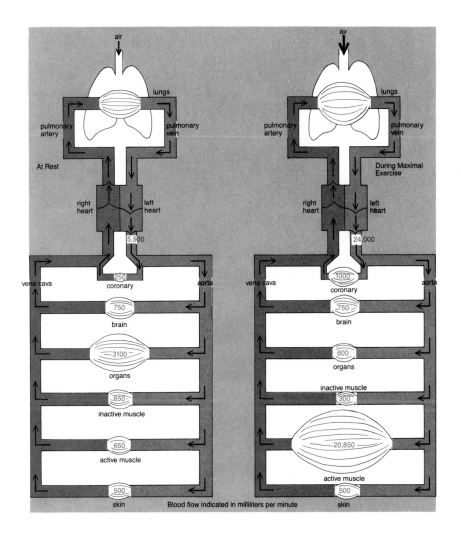

muscle action produces considerable body movement; during water skiing the body remains in a relatively fixed position. This distinction between static and dynamic is important, because the body's physiological response to the two kinds of exercise varies substantially. Moreover, the results of physical conditioning are considerably different when one kind of exercise is more dominant than the other. Only certain kinds of exercise, when performed regularly, can promote cardiovascular fitness; it is crucial, therefore, to engage in the right kind of exercise.

During static exercise there is less oxygen used in the body than in dynamic **Static Exercise** exercise. Although static exercise causes a marked increase in blood pressure, the increase in the amount of blood pumped by the heart is relatively small in comparison to that pumped during dynamic exercise. In static exercise, the pressure of tensed muscles squeezes blood vessels, so that less blood can pass through. The rise in blood pressure happens abruptly and at low levels of tension, even at the level of tension equivalent to carrying an average suitcase. The added pressure means, however, that the heart must work harder to overcome the resistance. The heart muscle itself is thus subjected to a large increase in demand for oxygen because it must accommodate the "pressure load" of static exercise. For the average person with no underlying heart condition, this extra demand does not present any physiological hazard. For the patient with coronary artery disease, however, static exercise presents a significant risk of developing irregular heart rhythms or temporary impairment of the heart's pumping capacity, or perhaps both. Also for the patient with high blood pressure, the added rise during static exercise may be excessive.

While weight lifting and other forms of static exercise increase the strength, size, and tone of the muscles being used, little if any cardiovascular fitness results from this kind of conditioning. This kind of exercise is nevertheless of value, especially for anyone whose occupation requires heavy manual labor. Static exercise can also prevent and even treat orthopedic injuries, and when used in conjunction with dynamic conditioning it can be of benefit in developing physical fitness. It is important to stress that patients with known heart disease should not participate in static exercise without a doctor's approval. Anyone who may be considered at high coronary risk or is suspected of having coronary heart disease should approach this kind of exercise with caution and preferably only after consultation with a doctor. (For a discussion of risk factors, see chapter 24.)

Dynamic Exercise   Dynamic exercises, such as walking, running, swimming, rowing, and bicycling, involve large numbers of muscles and therefore generate a great demand for oxygen in the cells of these muscles to provide the energy for the physical activity. The oxygen is supplied to the working muscles by the coordinated effort of the heart and the circulatory system. Basically, three physiological changes take place in order to accomplish this task:

(1) The heart pumps more blood per minute. In a young normal se-

The volume of blood pumped by the heart to meet the demands of various activities. At rest, the heart pumps approximately 5 to 6 quarts (5 to 6 liters) of blood each minute. That amount can increase twentyfold to meet the requirements of strenuous exercise.

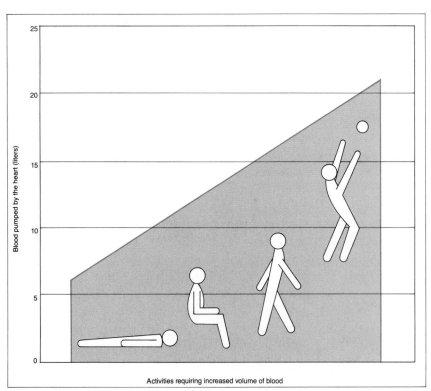

Blood pumped by the heart (liters)

Activities requiring increased volume of blood

dentary man (weighing approximately 154 lbs) the amount of blood pumped each minute (cardiac output) is increased from the average resting value of around 5.9 liters (6 quarts) to about 24 liters (25 quarts) during maximal exercise, thus increasing by 4 times the amount of available oxygen to the body. The increase in cardiac output is achieved by an increase in the number of heartbeats in a minute and an increase in the volume of blood ejected by the heart with each beat (stroke volume), which rises from around 66 milliliters (2 ounces) to 126 milliliters (4 ounces) per beat. In a well trained enduranced athlete, cardiac output and stroke volume will be much higher.

(2) A greater portion of blood is directed to the working muscles. The increased cardiac output is redistributed to guarantee more efficient circulation and oxygen supply to the areas of greatest demand. This is accomplished by constriction of the blood vessels in the visceral organs (kidneys, liver, spleen, and gastrointestinal tract), as well as those in the muscles that are not being used in the activity. At the same time, the blood vessels in the working muscles dilate. Through these adaptations, the blood supply to the working muscles increases from 20 percent of 5.9 liters (6 quarts) a minute pumped by the heart at rest to nearly 90 percent of 24 liters (25 quarts) a minute at maximal exercise. The blood supply to the working muscle is much higher in the endurance trained athlete.

(3) Working muscles extract a greater percentage of oxygen from the blood. There are about 20 milliliters of oxygen in each 100-milliliter unit of blood leaving the heart. During resting conditions as much as 14.4 milliliters of oxygen still remain in the blood when it is returned via the venous system to the heart. That means that at rest only 5.6 milliliters of oxygen per 100 milliliters of blood are extracted—less than 30 percent of the amount delivered to the body tissues. The difference is called arteriovenous oxygen difference.

During maximal exercise, physiological changes in the body result in a widening of the arteriovenous oxygen difference. The blood carries nutrients and oxygen to every cell in the body to fuel the output of energy. In the working muscle, the exchange of oxygen for waste materials—the metabolic process —is accelerated, and more oxygen is extracted from the blood. The ability of muscle cells to extract oxygen is further enhanced by chemical changes such as increased acidity and elevated body temperature. The net result is that the arteriovenous oxygen difference is widened to 15.8 milliliters of oxygen per 100 milliliters of blood. Instead of using less than 30 percent of the oxygen delivered, as at rest, the tissues consume more than 75 percent during heavy exercise. This almost threefold increase in oxygen extraction provides a convenient "oxygen transport reserve" which spares the heart considerable work, even during mild physical effort. The maximal arteriovenous oxygen difference is not much higher in the endurance trained athlete than in a sendentary man.

The entire oxygen transport operation is dependent on the body's ability to increase the oxygen supply to meet the demands imposed by dynamic exercise. The maximum amount of oxygen that can be transported from the lungs to the muscles and other tissues is called the maximal oxygen uptake. Except in patients with severe lung disease or in persons exercising at high altitudes, the capacity of the lungs to replenish the blood with oxygen does not limit maximal oxygen uptake. Maximal oxygen uptake, which physiologi-

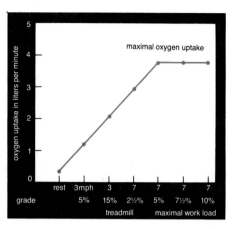

Progressive increase in oxygen uptake as determined by increased work tests on a motor-driven treadmill. Work load can be increased beyond the point of maximal oxygen uptake, but this oxygen debt must be repaid during rest.

cally sets the upper limit of endurance, is a standard measure of cardiovascular fitness and functional capacity of circulation, not of lung capacity. A decrease in maximal oxygen uptake occurs in persons who lead a sedentary life and is a natural part of the aging process. It is not clear whether or not this deterioration is noticeably slowed by physical conditioning.

Maximal oxygen uptake is measured by performing a series of work tests on a motor-driven treadmill or a stationary bicycle (bicycle ergometer), during which the heartbeat, electrocardiogram, blood pressure, and sometimes the amount of oxygen consumed are monitored. The exercise is made progressively harder, and the uptake of oxygen per minute rises steadily until the maximal uptake s attained. After this point, most people can still exercise harder, but the oxygen uptake cannot rise higher. The increase in work load is accomplished through a process known as an oxygen debt.

Oxygen debt is a mechanism which allows the person performing the exercise to live temporarily beyond his capacity to transport oxygen to active muscles. During rest after exercise, however, the individual must compensate for being "overdrawn." The phenomenon of oxygen debt is what causes oxygen uptake to take some time after vigorous exercise before it can return to normal resting levels.

The amount of oxygen debt that can be contracted is limited by the ability of the muscle fibers and blood to absorb acidic waste products of metabolism without an unduly large change in its acidity. Some degree of oxygen debt always builds up during a short, hard burst of exercise. Sprinters breathe hard for several minutes after they cross the finish line, a period during which they pay back the debt. Endurance and marathon runners, however, can complete a long race with a relatively small oxygen debt as a result of achieving what is called "steady state." This term is used by exercise physiologists to define a rate of work that can be performed for considerable periods of time without an oxygen debt. During a continuous period of activity, such as walking steadily at 3 miles an hour for several hours, the oxygen debt builds up rapidly at first and then levels off; it may then remain virtually unchanged for some hours. During violent activity, however, the oxygen debt builds up rapidly and continuously until the activity ceases.

The contraction of an oxygen debt has natural limitations, however, for a person cannot work or exercise hard for long periods of time without experiencing the exhaustion that comes from an inadequate oxygen supply. Ideally, the process of adaptation to exercise is adjusted to the work load so elegantly that the oxygen debt incurred is kept at a minimum. Contracting a small oxygen debt is a normal part of the adaptation. A large oxygen debt is an emergency mechanism that is invoked only in the case of dire need. In most sedentary persons, the mechanism is far from fully used.

Conditioning Effects of Dynamic Exercise

An increase in the maximal oxygen uptake is the most important physiological adaptation that takes place with a well-designed program of dynamic exercise. This increase is experienced as increased stamina and diminished fatigue during prolonged work or exercise at submaximal levels. The heart muscle fibers, like those of any muscle that is exercised, become stronger with conditioning. This stronger heart muscle is able to pump more blood with each beat, thereby requiring fewer beats to deliver the same amount of blood and oxygen as before conditioning. Many athletes, especially those for whom endurance is critically important, have a resting heart rate of approximately 45 beats a minute, compared to the average person's rate of from 72 to 80. The heart of such an athlete may actually have the capacity to pump twice the volume of blood per beat as that of the average person.

Physical conditioning thus results in a lower heart rate, not only at rest but all the time, regardless of activity, except at maximal levels. If physical conditioning lowered the heart rate only 10 beats a minute, the heart would beat 15,000 fewer times a day and 5 million fewer a year. Although medical science has not determined whether a slower heart rate actually extends the life span, it is certain that the fewer heart beats per minute, the less work for the heart. In addition, the period of rest between beats is longer, and prolongation of that interval provides more time for blood to flow through the coronary arteries which supply the heart muscle with oxygen. The vigorous contraction of the heart during each beat interrupts the flow of blood in the coronary arteries, and if interruptions are fewer more oxygen can be brought to the heart muscle itself.

The degree of cardiovascular fitness does not, however, necessarily describe the state of cardiovascular health. Cardiovascular fitness can compensate for the effects of coronary artery disease without having a direct influence on its cause. Some people with known heart disease have been able to compete in marathon races, while highly conditioned individuals can and occasionally do show manifestations of coronary artery disease and have heart attacks. Studies show, however, that conditioned individuals experience heart disease less frequently than do the sedentary.

Ideally, physical conditioning should be accompanied by a program of modifying coronary risk factors, so that the chances of developing a heart problem are reduced to a minimum. It is, moreover, fairly certain that many of the known risk factors are affected by habitual physical exercise and activity. There is still a good deal of controversy about the exact relationship between exercise and risk factors, but tentative findings indicate that some risk factors are diminished by physical conditioning.

BLOOD FATS   Since high levels of cholesterol in the blood—and possibly also of triglycerides, the main fatty substance in the body—seem to be important in the development of heart attacks, it is prudent to lower these levels, but the effect of exercise in this respect is controversial. A few studies have shown that either cholesterol or triglycerides, or both, have been reduced by a physical conditioning program. Other investigations have found little change unless weight loss (which in itself can reduce blood fats) also takes place. The increased expenditure of 400 calories a day during exercise, repeated four times a week, can result in a weight loss of 2 pounds a month, assuming caloric intake is held constant. If the goal of a weight-loss program is 2 to 3 pounds a week, exercise alone is not the solution; nor is exercise alone likely to solve the problem of increased cholesterol and triglycerides. But in conjunction with dietary restrictions on saturated fats, cholesterol, and caloric intake, exercise is unquestionably of great benefit.

BLOOD PRESSURE   Some studies have shown modest reductions in blood pressure after physical conditioning. As with blood fats, weight loss and dietary changes can be contributing factors. Although a physical conditioning program alone does not normalize high blood pressure, hypertensive patients who undertake such programs are often able to reduce the dosages of medicines required to control their blood pressure.

PSYCHOLOGICAL FACTORS As is well known, stress can have physiological effects on the body and may be a contributing factor in many health problems, including heart disease. Exercise provides a good outlet for reducing tension and promoting a sense of well-being and a good self-image. Conditioned individuals seem to tolerate stressful situations with small increases in heart rate and blood pressure better than do those who have not undergone a conditioning program.

LONGEVITY Although physical conditioning clearly makes a person feel better and thereby improves the quality of life, there is insufficent evidence that it significantly affects the life span. Studies do show lower rates of heart attack and higher rates of survival afterward in physically active as opposed to sedentary individuals. Claims have been made that exercise induces the formaton of new blood vessels (collaterals) to the heart muscle and also helps expand existing vessels, but no scientific evidence has unequivocally shown that such phenomena occur in humans. This area is still being investigated, and technical advances may produce significant information in the near future.

GUIDELINES FOR DYNAMIC PHYSICAL CONDITIONING

Regular participation in an exercise program is more than justified by the well-documented physiological adaptations that come from some forms of conditioning. However, such benefits are neither immediate nor easily achieved. Certain cautions are also necessary: although more heart attacks actually occur during rest than during exercise, even the rare coronary emergency during exercise might be prevented if exercise were approached with the caution usually reserved for prescribed medications. The basic principles and guidelines described here will increase the potential benefit of the effort put into exercise and also minimize the risk of orthopedic or cardiovascular complication.

Every physical conditioning program should involve three phases: warm-up, work-out, cool-down. Warm-up usually should be for a minimum of 3 to 5 minutes of walking and limbering-up exercises, gradually increasing in intensity. Cardiac patients and individuals over forty-five years of age should increase the warm-up period to 5 or 10 minutes. Warm-up allows for gradual circulatory adjustment and increases in muscle temperature, reducing the chances of orthopedic injury and enhancing muscle efficiency and oxygen exchange between blood and tissues. The net effect is a greater work capacity, less fatigue, and a lower risk of injury or irregular heart rhythms, particularly in the cardiac patient. The length of warm-up should be extended after a lengthy layoff and particularly during cold weather. Clothing should be adequate to guard against chill.

Following the work-out, described in the following paragraphs, the cool-down phase prevents a rapid fall in blood pressure which might precipitate fainting, irregular heart rhythms, or more serious complications.

Dilated blood vessels in exercising muscles may cause a fall in blood pressure, pooling of blood in the veins, and a diminished return of blood to the heart if exercise is terminated abruptly, especially if the individual stands motionless after exercise. When the person walks or engages in other activity involving rhythmic contraction of the leg muscles during the cool-down phase, blood is "milked" out of these vessels and the circulation is aided. Continuous movement until sweating ceases, pulse and respiration approach pre-exercise levels, and fatigue dissipates (usually after 5 to 10 minutes of walking or other mild exercise) insures readjustment of circulation, dissipation of the heat developed normally by exercise, and removal of metabolic waste products.

INTENSITY OF EXERCISE Research has shown that the work-out phase need not be exhausting in order to achieve the desired physiological adaptations. The intensity of exercise—usually related to the speed of walking, jogging, bicycling, and swimming—should be in the range of from 60 to 80 percent of maximal oxygen uptake if a cardiovascular training effect is desired. This effect, also known as an aerobic effect, means an improvement in the capacity of the cardiovascular system to deliver oxygen to the working muscle.

Because of the relationship between heart rate and the relative intensity of exercise, checking the immediate post-exercise heart rate is a good means of monitoring intensity. A heart rate of 70 to 85 percent of the maximal heart rate achieved on a maximal exercise test correlates well with the desired level of intensity. Thus an individual with a maximal heart rate of 180 would have a training range of from 126 to 153. It should be emphasized that one does not need a heart rate of 150, as some have claimed, or even the target heart rate before conditioning is initiated. Some benefit, even if minimal, is probably achieved from prolonged activities that require as little as 25 percent of maximal oxygen uptake.

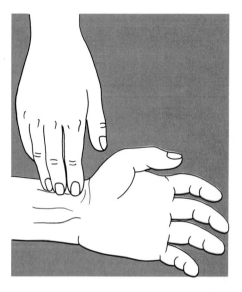

Heart rate is found by counting the pulse at the wrist. Press lightly with the first three fingers on the inside of the wrist near the bone that protrudes below the thumb. Count for 10 seconds and multiply by 6 to obtain the heart rate for one minute.

DURATION OF EXERCISE The time required to produce a desirable cardiovascular conditioning effect is to a great extent dependent on the intensity of the exercise: the lower the intensity, the longer the necessary duration. It might, for example, take an hour of walking at 50 percent of maximal oxygen uptake to equal jogging for 20 minutes at 75 percent of the maximal. If cardiovascular fitness and endurance are the goals, the duration should probably be at least long enough to produce sweating, mild fatigue, and breathlessness (usually from 8 to 12 minutes). Obviously, the longer the work-out, the better the conditioning effect.

FREQUENCY OF EXERCISE Frequency is also an important factor in an exercise program. A work-out three or four times a week stimulates a significant rise in maximal oxygen uptake, although five or six days a week may produce a more rapid initial increase. Once a desired level of fitness is achieved, three work-outs a week are probably sufficient to maintain this level. Reaching a level of fitness is one thing; staying there is another. The only way to do that is by keeping to a regular schedule. Cutting back on the number of work-outs each week will have a direct result on the level of fitness. Exercise physiologists estimate that cutting back from three periods a week to one a week will result in a loss of half of the fitness level within ten weeks. If the work-outs are eliminated completely, all the gains will be wiped out in about three or four months. When illness or other unavoidable circumstances make it necessary to cut back or eliminate exercise, the work-outs must be re-established gradually to give the body time to adjust.

PROGRESSION IN EXERCISE   The body will adapt to a given overload by increasing maximal oxygen uptake gradually over a period of several weeks or months. As maximal uptake increases, the same work load becomes a lower percentage of it; that is, the relative intensity of the work load diminishes. Thus, in order to maintain an optimal conditioning level, the work load must become heavier. Fortunately, this is not an open-ended progression, since every individual has naturally imposed limits to strength and endurance. The goal of every fitness program is to let the individual reach the level of fitness that is ideal for him.

VARIETIES OF EXERCISE   A weekly program of three to four exercise sessions of from 20 to 30 minutes' duration (not counting the 5- to 10-minute warm-up and the 10-minute cooldown periods), at an intensity of 60 to 80 percent of maximal oxygen uptake, will probably provide the greatest benefit for the least amount of time and effort. In a lower-intensity program, the person must compensate by increasing the duration and the frequency of the activity.

Many different kinds of exercise and recreational activity can be used in a physical conditioning program. Walking and jogging provide the most direct benefits for cardiovascular fitness, but other kinds of exercise can also be beneficial. Some forms of dynamic exercise and the important factors that should be considered in selecting among them are discussed in the following paragraphs.

WALKING   Practically everyone can enjoy walking, perhaps the best all-purpose form of dynamic exercise available. It requires no special skill, equipment, or facility and can be undertaken on a moment's notice in almost any environment. Walking is a particularly good exercise for some cardiovascular patients, because the finite limit on walking speed prevents overdoing. However, younger or more fit persons will often derive more benefit from an exercise program of greater intensity. Walking for an aerobic effect should be brisk and at a good stride, averaging from 3 to 4 miles an hour for a young person but less fast for an older person.

JOGGING   This has probably become the most popular means of achieving a dynamic exercise work-out in the least amount of time. Since the speed of jogging will greatly affect the heart rate and blood pressure response, particular attention should be given to the precautions and recommendations discussed later. Joggers have been known to become slaves to the stop watch, trying to shave seconds off their time. They would no doubt benefit more if they relaxed and let the exercise release tension rather than create it.

CYCLING   Both as a form of transportation and as a dynamic exercise program, cycling is increasing in popularity. Since one can cover a greater distance in a shorter time, some people get a greater sense of accomplishment from it. Because of the great variations in gearing mechanisms, bicycle weights, and terrain, it is difficult to prescribe the amount of cycling neces-

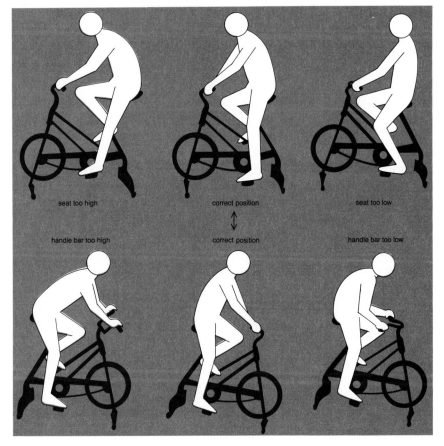

seat too high

correct position

seat too low

handle bar too high

correct position

handle bar too low

Arrows indicate correct seat height and handlebar position. The knee should be slightly bent when the toes are on the lower pedal. The body should be relaxed and leaning slightly forward.

sary to produce the desirable intensity. Monitoring the heart rate is an effective way of determining this. Stationary bicycles eliminate some of the variables and permit exercise indoors during inclement weather or when city traffic and pollution threaten to cancel out the benefit of the exercise. Ergometers should have calibrated controls for setting the resistance at a reproducible level.

SWIMMING This exercise is excellent for training muscles of the arms, back, and shoulders, which many people must use in their occupations. Dynamic exercise of these muscles also promotes cardiovascular fitness. The great variation in swimming ability from individual to individual makes it difficult to give exact prescriptions for duration and intensity, however. Here again, checking the heart rate response provides the individual with an accurate gauge of his performance. Any exercise that must be continued for long periods of time is likely to become a bore; to overcome this, and to involve as many muscle groups as possible, the swimmer should use a variety of strokes.

Swimming also provides an excellent form of dynamic exercise for persons with bad knees, bad backs, or other orthopedic problems that prevent them from jogging, cycling, or engaging in other similar sports. Walking or jogging in chest-deep water is a good way for those with orthopedic problems to exercise the lower part of the body, since buoyancy lessens the strain normally imposed on the joints.

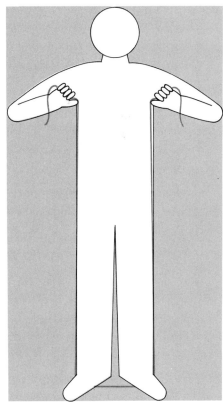

Rope should reach to the armpits when held down by the feet.

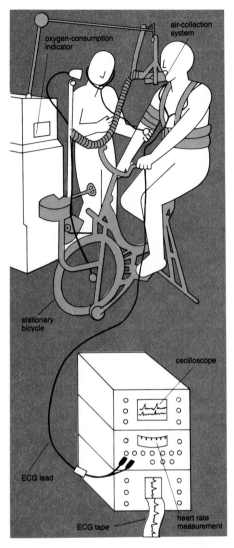

oxygen-consumption indicator

air-collection system

stationary bicycle

oscilloscope

ECG lead

ECG tape

heart rate measurement

Oxygen intake and heart rate are monitored as the subject pedals until stopped by fatigue, breathlessness, or chest pain.

RACQUET SPORTS Tennis, racquets, badminton, and squash can provide a conditioning effect, while the challenge of competition provides a stimulus to stick with a long-term exercise program. The conditioning element of such sports depends on the intensity of play, which in turn depends on the skill of the players. With opponents of equal or slightly greater skill and by minimizing rest between points, racquet games can provide good cardiovascular conditioning. But while competition encourages lifetime participation in such sports, it may lead to frustration and stress.

ROPE JUMPING Once relegated to schoolchildren and prize fighters in training, this exercise has regained popularity. Its value as conditioner is based on several considerations: a minimum of equipment is necessary, the rope can be packed and used when traveling, and except for running in place, few other exercises provide as much aerobic effect in such limited quarters. While rope jumping actually requires more skill than is usually thought, almost everyone can become proficient at it in a relatively short time. Contrary to popular belief, 10 minutes of rope jumping is not equal to 30 minutes of jogging. Assuming the intensity of each produced the same heart rate and oxygen uptake, each activity would be equally beneficial. Above 80 percent of maximal oxygen uptake, increasing the intensity of exercise—jumping harder, running faster, for example—will not increase conditioning significantly. Within the realm of rhythmic, continuous dynamic activities, the response of the body is more important than the nature of the activity. Rope jumping has one final plus value however: you do not even need a rope! Many people actually begin by simulating rope jumping, a technique that is very much like shadow boxing.

CALISTHENICS These exercises can be performed in structured programs that are designed to develop strength, muscular endurance, and flexibility. However, beneficial as these results are, significant improvement in cardiovascular fitness rarely results. Calisthenics serve as excellent adjuncts to a cardiovascular conditioning program, particularly as warm-up exercises before jogging or swimming, but they are not an adequate substitute. Certain calisthenics involve a high degree of static exercise. These should be approached cautiously by those suspected or known to have a heart condition.

PRECAUTIONS AND RECOMMENDATIONS Always consult a physician before embarking on a vigorous exercise program. This is particularly important for anyone who has been sedentary for several years, is overweight, has a heart problem, or has a known risk factor such as high blood pressure, diabetes, high cholesterol or triglycerides, a family history of heart disease, or cigarette smoking. A careful history taken by a physician is extremely important in uncovering latent heart disease.

An exercise test should be taken in a further attempt to exclude the possibility of underlying heart disease, which might rule out certain forms of exercise without medical supervision. Such an exercise test will assist the physician in prescribing a safe and effective exercise program adjusted to the person's fitness level and health. An exercise test is conducted on a treadmill or stationary bicycle; the subject is monitored on the electrocardiogram while exercising to the limits of fatigue, breathlessness, or chest pain. An electrocardiogram taken at rest is usually not sufficient to determine

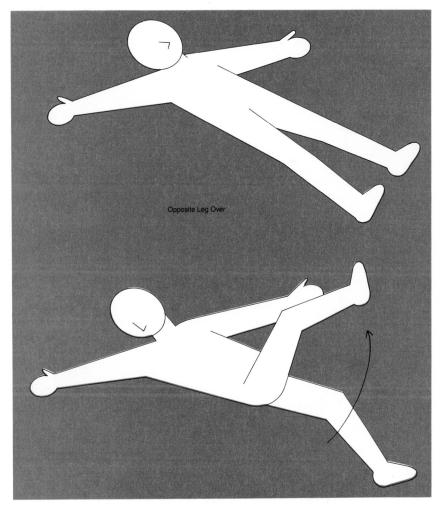

Opposite Leg Over

Lie on back with arms outstretched at shoulder level and palms up. Kick right foot to left hand; exhale. Return to starting position. Kick left foot to right hand; exhale. Return to starting position.
Level 1, 3-5 times; level 2, 6-8; level 3, 9-12.

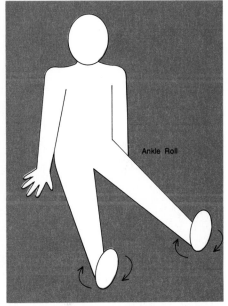

Ankle Roll

Sit on floor with hands on floor alongside hips. Rotate ankles clockwise in complete circle. Repeat 360-degree rotation of ankles in counterclockwise direction.
Level 1, 3-5 times; level 2, 6-8; level 3, 9-12.

Plan to spend 4 weeks at each level of activity, progressing from the lowest number of repetitions to the highest within each level before proceeding to the next level. After reaching the greatest number of repetitions in level 3, include this standard in a maintenance program.

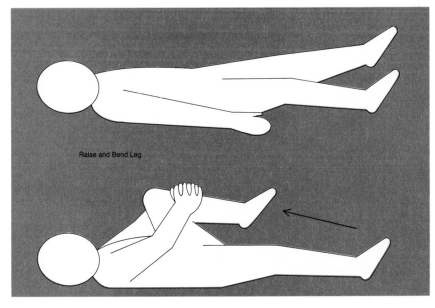

Raise and Bend Leg

Lie on back with legs straight, feet together, and arms at sides. Raise left leg about 10 inches, keeping it straight. Bend knee and bring knee as close to chest as possible, using abdominal, hip, and leg muscles; clasp both hands below knee and pull slowly closer to chest. Straighten leg, keeping it 10 inches off the floor. Return to starting position. Repeat with right leg.
Level 1, 1-4 times; level 2, 5-8; level 3, 9-12.

Sit erect with legs straight, feet shoulder-width apart and hands on waist. Keeping legs straight, bend trunk forward and down with arms extended. Try to touch lower legs or toes with fingertips. Return to starting position. Perform exercise slowly, stretching and relaxing at intervals.
Level 1, *2-4 times;* level 2, *5-8;* level 3, *9-10.*

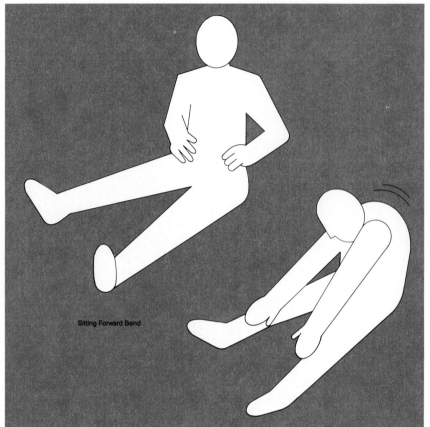

Sitting Forward Bend

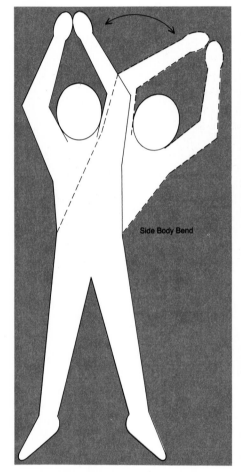

Side Body Bend

Stand with feet shoulder-width apart, arms extended over head, and fingertips touching. Bend trunk slowly to left as far as possible, keeping arms straight and fingertips together. Return to starting position. Repeat, bending to right.
Level 1, *2-5 times;* level 2, *6-9;* level 3, *10-12.*

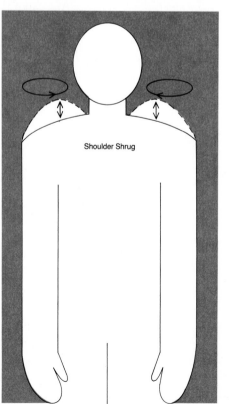

Shoulder Shrug

Stand in relaxed position, arms hanging at sides. Shrug shoulders high into neck; relax and stretch shoulders down. Rotate shoulders front to back, making a complete circle; repeat, rotating shoulders back to front.
Level 1, *5-10 times;* level 2, *5-10;* level 3, *5-10.*

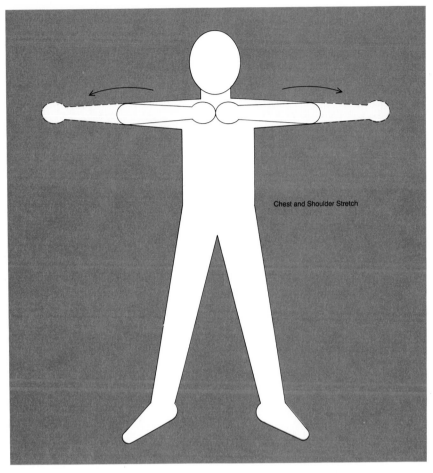

Chest and Shoulder Stretch

Stand erect with bent arms in front of chest at shoulder height, fingertips touching. Pull elbows back as far as possible, keeping arms at shoulder height. Return to starting position. Do chest stretch 3 times, then swing arms outward at shoulder height with palms up. Return to starting position. Do these 4 steps to a rhythmic count of 1-and-2-and-3-and-4.
Level 1, 3-6 times; level 2, 7-10; level 3, 11-15.

the existence of any limit on an individual's ability to engage in a program of vigorous exercise.

When a physician has approved an individual for exercise, the program devised should follow some basic, commonsense principles of training. Following these simple procedures will avoid many of the most frequently encountered mishaps.

START OFF SLOWLY   Avoid the tendency to undo many years of inactivity in a few days or weeks. The body is certain to rebel against such an experience, and sore muscles and stiff joints may be the least of the complications. No one should attempt to run a mile, play three sets of tennis, or swim forty laps on the first time out. A pre-training period of one or two-weeks at sub-training intensity is recommended to acclimate the body. This gradual introduction is particularly important for persons who are forty years of age or older.

WARM UP AND COOL DOWN ADEQUATELY   These steps are critically important in avoiding not just muscle and joint injuries, but more serious complications, such as cardiac arrest. Violation of this rule, one of the oldest in athletics, is probably the single largest cause of exercise complications. Low-intensity exercise for 5 to 8 minutes at the start of the program and 10 minutes at the end should be the minimum allowed. If lack of time forces shortening the

PRINCIPLES

1. Physical fitness is the ability to carry out daily activities without undue fatigue and to respond to physical or emotional stress without an excessive increase in heart rate and blood pressure. Cardiovascular fitness is the ability of the heart and blood vessels to supply the oxygen needs of body tissues. The degree of cardiovascular

Stand erect with feet shoulder-width apart and hands on hips. Rotate head from left to right, then right to left, using slow, smooth motion. Close eyes to avoid dizziness and loss of balance.
Level 1, 2-4 times; level 2, 5-8; level 3, 9-10.

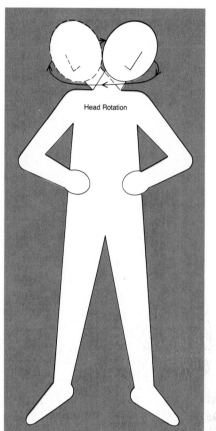

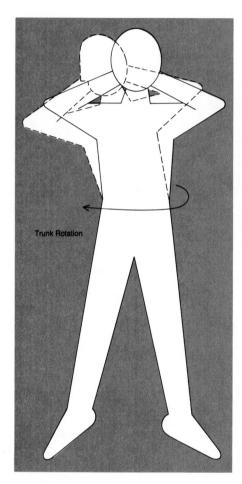

Stand erect with feet shoulder-width apart and fingers locked behind head. Rotate trunk to right, keeping feet flat on floor. Return to starting position. Rotate trunk to left, keeping feet flat on floor. Return to starting position.
Level 1, 2-4 times; level 2, 5-8; level 3, 9-10.

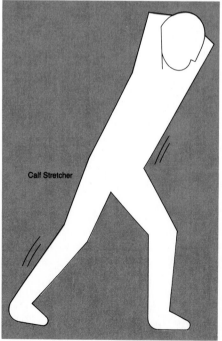

Place one foot about 24 inches ahead of the other in stride position with forward leg bent at knee, rear leg straight. Clasp hands behind neck, elbows close to head. Carefully lean trunk forward, continually stretching rear calf; hold 8 to 10 seconds. Change leg positions and repeat. Breathe freely while stretching.
Level 1, 2-4 times for each leg; level 2, 4-6 for each; level 3, 4-6 for each.

program, it's probably better to shave minutes from the exercise itself rather than at either end.

DRESS APPROPRIATELY   In jogging, wear running shoes with slightly elevated heels, well-supported arch, lightweight body, and solid rubber soles. Such shoes will minimize or avoid altogether the muscle and joint problems many get from jogging. To reduce the risk of knee or back injury, jog on a prepared track or on grass or earth rather than on asphalt or concrete. In cold weather, wearing sweat shirts and pants may be necessary to avoid chills. Substitute lightweight clothing in warmer weather, but always avoid plastic or rubber suits, which cause excessive sweating and provide no means for the accumulated heat to escape into the atmosphere.

CHOOSE THE BEST TIME   Avoid exercise for at least an hour and perhaps two hours after eating, and avoid the heat of the day, particularly during periods of high humidity. Food in the stomach and high external temperatures require significant redistribution of blood flow to the stomach for digestion and to the skin for heat dissipation. Both add substantially to the stress on the heart.

RETURN GRADUALLY TO THE PROGRAM AFTER A LAYOFF   A substantial loss in maximal oxygen uptake is suffered in as little as one week to three weeks of inactivity, particularly after bed rest for illness or injury. Trying to resume the same exercise program after a layoff might result in a hazardous strain on the body and a greater risk of cardiovascular and musculo-skeletal complications. It is reasonable to reduce the intensity of exercise and gradually work back to the previous level in equal increments over a period of time equal to the duration of the layoff.

AVOID ALL-OUT EFFORT   Many exercisers have the misconception that they must become totally exhausted in order to obtain a training effect. The truth of the matter is that all-out effort greatly increases heart rate, blood pressure, the amount of stress on the heart, and the risk of complications.

AVOID HOT SHOWERS, STEAM BATHS, OR SAUNAS IMMEDIATELY AFTER EXERCISE The external heat these supply can put too much burden on the circulatory system. It is important to wait until the internal heat generated by exercise can be dissipated and the circulation restored to normal. Otherwise, the demand on the body may result in a rapid fall in blood pressure and an inadequate return of blood to the brain and heart. Such severe circulatory stress should be avoided, particularly by the person with heart disease. The cooling-off period, with low-intensity exercise or brisk walking rather than sitting or standing still, is essential before showering. The shower should be neither very hot nor very cold. If light-headedness or nausea develops after exercise, it helps to contract the leg muscles rhythmically by walking or wriggling the toes, or to lie supine with the legs elevated.

AVOID EXERCISE DURING ILLNESS   Certain illnesses decrease blood volume, increase heart rhythm disturbances, and decrease lung efficiency. Other illnesses are aggravated by exercising. If you feel unusually tired or weak, it is best to omit exercise until you recover. On the other hand, it is not a good idea

fitness does not necessarily describe the state of cardiovascular health, although a very high correlation could be expected.

2. *There are two types of muscular activity—dynamic and static. Static or isometric exercise involves the development of tension within muscle fibers, with little change in muscle length or movement of joints and bones. The abrupt rise in blood pressure during static exercise subjects the heart to a large increase in demand for oxygen to accommodate this "pressure load." For the person with coronary artery disease, static exercise presents a risk of irregular heart rhythms or temporary impairment of the heart's pumping activity.*

3. *Dynamic exercise, or isotonic exercise, shortens muscle fibers and moves joints and bones. Walking, running, and swimming generate a great demand for oxygen in the cells of the muscles to provide energy for physical activity: the heart pumps more blood per minute, a greater portion of blood is directed to the working muscles, and the working muscles extract a greater percent of oxygen from the blood.*

4. *During heavy exercise, the body tissues consume more than 75 percent of the oxygen delivered. This almost threefold increase in oxygen extraction spares the heart considerable work. The body can increase the oxygen supply to meet the demands of dynamic exercise. The maximum amount of oxygen that can be transported from the lungs is called the maximal oxygen uptake. Maximal oxygen uptake is a standard measure of cardiovascular fitness and functional capacity of circulation. A person exercising beyond his capacity for transporting oxygen to active muscles is able to do so by a process called "oxygen debt." Steady state is a term used to define a rate of exercise that can be performed for considerable periods of time without building up an oxygen debt.*

5. *An increase in the maximal oxygen uptake is the most important physiological adaptation that takes*

place with a well-designed program of dynamic exercise. This increase is experienced as increased stamina and diminished fatigue during prolonged work or exercise. The heart muscle becomes stronger, requiring fewer beats to deliver the same amount of blood and oxygen as before conditioning.

6. *Physical conditioning should be accompanied by a sound program of coronary risk factor modification. Tentative findings indicate that some risk factors are diminished by physical conditioning. Exercise alone is not likely to solve the problem of blood fats or high blood pressure, but in conjunction with diet changes it is unquestionably of great benefit.*

7. *Regular participation in an exercise program is more than justified by the well-documented physiological adaptations that come from some forms of conditioning. Every physical conditioning program should involve three phases: warm-up, workout, and cooling down. The warm-up phase is especially important for cardiac patients and those over 45 years of age. Cooling down prevents a rapid fall in blood pressure.*

8. *Among the most effective dynamic exercises are walking, jogging, cycling, swimming, racquet sports, rope jumping. Each involves techniques that should be learned to derive the maximum benefit and enjoyment from the exercise.*

9. *A physician should be consulted before any vigorous exercise program is begun. Basic, commonsense principles of training include: starting off gradually, warming up and cooling down adequately, dressing appropriately, choosing the best time for the exercise, returning gradually after a layoff, avoiding all-out, exhaustive effort, and exercising during illness.*

to discontinue working-out every time you have a sore muscle or feel a little under the weather, since resuming an exercise routine is twice as hard once the habit is broken.

If chest pains develop, they should be reported to the doctor at once; delay in treatment is the major cause of death in heart attacks. In most healthy persons, chest pains are usually muscular and are related to the stress of the exercise itself rather than to any underlying cardiovascular disease. However, if chest pain does occur, the only sensible procedure is to stop the exercise and get help at once, for even a normal exercise stress test cannot totally exclude the possibility of heart disease.

5

LIVING WITH
CARDIOVASCULAR DISEASE

Nanette K. Wenger, M.D.

Twenty-eight million Americans have some type of heart disease, and yet a great many of them are able to lead normal or near-normal lives. Heart disease, like most other illness, is best controlled when the patient participates in the management of the problem and in the program for recovery. As Dr. Lawrence Weed of the University of Vermont has said, "The most powerful of all medical and paramedical personnel is the patient—highly motivated, not costing anything, even willing to pay—and there is one for every member of the population." Thus the patient with heart disease is often a most important member of his or her own health-care team.

Training for the position begins with learning a few basic facts. The patient should know, for instance, that heart problems can best be cared for when they are diagnosed early. That means early recognition of symptoms and early consultation with a doctor. Today, most heart conditions respond to proper treatment, which may include diet, medication, surgery, and rehabilitation. Even after severe cardiovascular incidents, many patients can resume work and normal daily activities. Naturally, the length of time this takes, and the limitations imposed on former activity, vary from patient to patient, but with the great advances in medical and surgical therapy, a heart patient does not have to be a heart "victim" or a lifelong invalid.

GUIDELINES FOR TAKING MEDICATION Since taking medications is often part of long-term recovery routines, certain ground rules should be learned at the beginning.

1. Learn the name of each medicine prescribed and its purpose. No doctor is too busy to explain, and no patient should be too shy to ask, how a drug works and why it is prescribed.

2. Follow the doctor's prescription exactly by taking the ordered amount of medication at the times specified. Taking more or less than the prescribed amount and taking drugs at random intervals can interfere with their effectiveness and may actually be harmful. Greater than prescribed dosage of some medicines can be dangerous because of toxic effects. Do not discontinue medication simply because you feel better. Stop medication only when your doctor tells you to do so; some medications must be taken for long periods of time.

3. Renew prescriptions in time to avoid interruptions in dosage schedule. But don't stock medicines for excessively long periods—some drugs lose their strength and even become dangerous after several months. Check with your doctor if your medication is several months old.

4. Never use another person's prescription, even if it is for treatment of the same illness or symptoms. Medications are prescribed on a highly individual basis and should not be exchanged.

5. Some drugs interfere with the actions of others. Do not take nonprescription, over-the-counter medications without checking with your doctor.

6. If you are taking several drugs, keep each in a separate container, with the name of the drug and the directions for taking it clearly marked on the label.

7. Store medications in a place that is not accessible to children.

There are many kinds of heart disease and many kinds of drugs and therapies for dealing with them. The major cardiovascular diseases are discussed in detail in individual chapters of this book and can be easily located in the contents. This chapter is concerned with some of the problems confronting the person with heart disease and the best ways to live with them.

One out of six adults in the United States has high blood pressure (hypertension) with a greater incidence reported among black males than among white, and a greater likelihood of its developing among those with a family history of the disease. Therefore, members of the family of anyone who has high blood pressure should also have periodic blood pressure measurements. The cause of hypertension is, in most cases, unknown, and there is as yet no cure, although the condition can be controlled effectively through proper treatment. Emotional stress or tension in itself does not cause hypertension, but it can raise the blood pressure of those who already have the condition. It is advisable, therefore, to avoid as much as possible all situations that create excessive tension. Being relaxed, however, is no guarantee against hypertension.

One of the most significant facts about hypertension is that usually there are no symptoms. Some patients do experience headache, dizziness, and nosebleeds, but these symptoms do not indicate the level of blood pressure. The only way to detect the disease is by actual measurement of blood pressure with an instrument designed for that purpose. The instrument, called a sphygmomanometer, is the familiar inflatable rubber cuff connected to a gauge that registers blood pressure. The same device is used to check on how well the treatment program is able to control hypertension. Control does not mean cure, however. If treatment is halted, blood pressure will often rise again and with it the risk of the complications of the disease: stroke, heart attack, eye problems, and kidney failure. Appropriate medical treatment can maintain pressure at normal or near-normal levels, but it is a lifelong procedure requiring constant treatment and medical surveillance.

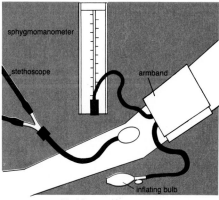

Blood Pressure Measurement

Physical examination, in addition to blood pressure measurement with the sphygmomanometer, includes a careful check of the eyes, kidneys, and heart to determine if these organs have been affected by hypertension. The frequency of visits to a physician's office for blood-pressure measurement is generally greater in the initial period, until control is achieved. The doctor will prescribe one or several drugs; some work to rid the body of excess fluid and salt (diuretics); some act by relaxing the narrowed blood vessels which cause hypertension; some by preventing narrowing of the blood vessels. Some of the drugs must be used in combination with other medications; for example, many diuretics eliminate potassium as well as fluid, and supplementary potassium medication or dietary potassium may also have to be taken.

The best medication, or combination of medications, for any patient must be worked out in a trial period. The patient must have a chance to adjust to the medication that is most effective in controlling blood pressure with the fewest side effects. The possible side effects include nasal stuffiness, heartburn and other gastrointestinal upset, and occasional dizziness. If these symptoms are present, they should be reported to the doctor. However, some time and considerable patience may be required before the right combination of medications in the right dosage is achieved, but the effort is worthwhile because the treatment, once tailored to the patient, becomes a long-term program of proved efficacy.

Diet can be as important as routine medication in controlling hypertension. Statistics show that the disease is more likely to be present in obese or overweight persons than in those of normal weight, and weight reduction often results in lowered blood pressure. A well-planned diet to reduce weight and keep it off can therefore be a significant part of the program. Reducing the amount of salt (sodium) in the diet may also help to lower blood pressure, so patients are cautioned to avoid foods with a high salt content and to refrain from adding salt to food either during preparation or at the table. The patients family members can salt their food at the table. Another commonly recommended change in diet is to reduce or eliminate certain fats (saturated, animal fats). These fats are associated with an increased risk of heart attack, and many patients with hypertension are already prone to coronary atherosclerosis (fatty deposits in the wall of blood vessels that supply the heart) and heart attack. Other changes in daily life that a doctor recommends are of great value in maintaining general health, as well as being important in controlling hypertension itself. Adequate sleep is important, since blood pressure levels are lowest during sleep. Relaxation is of value; seek out pleasurable and relaxing activities. Exercise is of value in weight reduction and in reducing stress and tension. However, the doctor should be consulted before any program of physical exercise is begun, because an exercise test may be needed to determine the patient's physical condition and the type and extent of exercise that would be most beneficial. The doctor will also advise about drinking alcoholic beverages, which may be acceptable in moderation, and cigarette smoking, which usually is not. Although cigarette smoking is not specifically linked with hypertension, it is a risk factor for cardiovascular diseases and for diseases of the lung and should be avoided.

Many doctors recommend that patients with high blood pressure learn to take their own blood pressure and keep a daily record. Blood pressure cuffs are now readily available, and the technique is learned quickly. Remember, a record of blood pressure measurement is the only way to determine if hypertension is present and whether medication and diet are keeping it under control. It is encouraging to know that, although the cause of hypertension is unknown, treatment can keep the disease under control and decrease the likelihood of life-threatening complications.

THE CORONARY – PRONE INDIVIDUAL

Certain apparently healthy individuals have an increased risk of developing coronary artery disease (coronary atherosclerosis), the narrowing and eventual obstruction of the coronary arteries which can lead to interruption of the blood supply to the heart muscle and eventual heart attack (myocardial infarction). The typical high-risk person has high blood pressure and a high blood-cholesterol level, smokes cigarettes, and has a family history of premature coronary

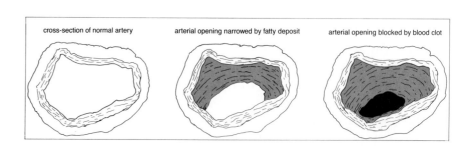

cross-section of normal artery   arterial opening narrowed by fatty deposit   arterial opening blocked by blood clot

disease or early death from heart attack. A number of precautionary or re-medial measures are recommended for these "coronary-prone" individuals, in-cluding blood pressure control, restricted consumption of saturated fats and high-cholesterol foods, and elimination of cigarette smoking. Regular medical checkups are advised, with attention to weight control and a program of reg-ular exercise.

The importance of diet has become increasingly evident, particularly for those who have an increased risk of developing atherosclerosis. There are some simple, general principles to follow in planning a prudent diet; reduce the amount of red meat and saturated animal fat and increase the use of fish, poultry, and veal in the weekly menu; trim all fat from meats. Eggs and other cholesterol-rich foods should be restricted, and vegetable (polyun-saturated) oils should replace animal (saturated) fats. Use skim milk instead of whole milk and whole-milk products. (The guidelines for such a diet, whether eating at home or dining out, are given in greater detail in Diet and Nutrition, chapter 3.)

Another important aspect of prevention is to recognize the warnings—the symptoms of an impending heart attack. Early recognition of the warn-ings and being prepared to take appropriate action can often make the difference between disability or death and life itself. In most cases the early warning is clear and dramatic—prolonged, oppressive pain or unusual dis-comfort in the center of the chest. The pain is sometimes mistakenly labeled indigestion, but it is persistent and cannot be relieved by change of position or antacid medication. The pain may radiate to the arm, shoulder, neck, or jaw; it may be accompanied by sweating, shortness of breath, nausea, or vomiting. When such symptoms occur, it is always best to err on the side of caution. Call a doctor at once; if none is available, call for emergency police or ambulance assistance. Many hospitals and many communities are now equipped with mobile rescue units that are prepared to deal with the immedi-ate emergency of a heart attack and the critical period that follows. Keep emergency numbers handy. Everyone who is of age and physically capable should be trained in emergency cardiac care—cardiopulmonary resuscitation (see Cardiac Emergencies, chapter 6.) This immediate aid to the victims of heart attack is credited with saving the lives of thousands of people. If im-properly used, however, the techniques can damage an unconscious victim; therefore, no one who has not received instruction from qualified teachers should attempt to give such first aid. Courses in basic life support are given in most communities. Ask your local Heart Association, Red Cross, YMCA or similar organization for more information on such courses.

The pain or discomfort of angina pectoris is felt under the breastbone and is usually transient. It signals a temporary imbalance between the demands of the heart and the supply of oxygen-carrying blood that it is receiving. Angina is usually brought on by exertion or emotional stress and is relieved by rest and certain drugs, particularly nitroglycerin. In most cases, angina is not dis-abling, and many patients can lead active and productive lives by following appropriate medical recommendations. Control of body weight and blood pressure is essential; when these are achieved angina may be significantly de-creased or eliminated completely. For some, a prescribed exercise program helps decrease the frequency and severity of anginal attacks. Patients are

Angina Pectoris

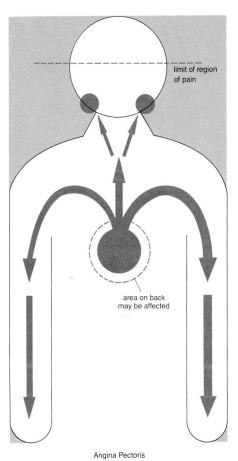

limit of region of pain

area on back may be affected

Angina Pectoris

urged to avoid situations which can precipitate angina—cold, excessive exertion, heavy meals, emotional flareups.

Nitroglycerin, the medication most frequently used to relieve anginal pain, differs from most "pain killers" in that it is not habit forming and the body does not develop a tolerance to it. The same amount of nitroglycerin should be as effective months and years from now as it is currently. Therefore, if the anginal pain is not relieved by nitroglycerin or if pain relief is considerably slower or less complete than usual, notify the physician immediately. Nitroglycerin does, however, deteriorate if kept too long, and small amounts should be purchased every several months to make sure the drug will be effective. It should be stored in an airtight, moisture-proof dark-glass container. Nitroglycerin works best if taken at the onset of angina; it can also be taken preventively before any activity that is likely to provoke an attack or that has been associated with attacks in the past. Patients are instructed to place a tablet under the tongue before any such activity, whether it is walking up a steep flight of steps, watching an exciting ball game, or sexual intercourse. Most patients with angina soon learn that pacing their activities, working more slowly, and avoiding long periods of high-intensity work or play are the most effective means of coping with the problem. Extremes of temperature and humidity are other factors requiring adjustments of activities, because of the added burden they place on the heart. When attacks of angina are severe or frequent, other medications may be prescribed, among them long-acting nitroglycerin-like preparations such as tablets or ointments and/or a potent drug called propranolol or metoprolol. None of these drugs should be discontinued and the dosage should not be changed without directions from a doctor, because interruption in treatment may produce serious chest pain and other complications.

The doctor must rely on the patient's own description of anginal symptoms and precipitating factors to guide the recommendations for treatment. Angina is seldom associated with an abnormal electrocardiogram or abnormal findings on the physical examination; therefore it is important to report all changes in pain pattern or intensity to the doctor. Changing or worsening angina, or angina that fails to respond or responds poorly to medication, may indicate the need for further diagnostic study. A doctor often recommends a test called coronary angiography if he suspects the existence of serious obstruction to blood flow in the arteries supplying the heart. Very often, the severity of pain does not parallel the severity of the disease, and physicians are increasingly doing coronary angiography to determine which patients with angina will benefit from coronary bypass surgery. Angiography is an X-ray procedure that outlines the arteries of the heart and makes pictures of them, revealing any obstruction to blood flow. On the basis of this and possibly other tests, and the symptoms, a patient may become a candidate for coronary by-pass surgery, a procedure which relieves angina by, in effect, creating new and clear passages for the needed blood supply to the heart.

Myocardial Infarction Heart attack, the layman's terms for myocardial infarction, is often a major crisis. Yet recent studies indicate that most patients who have recovered from an uncomplicated heart attack can and do return to a normal life, including resumption of their previous work. Naturally, in more severe cases, patients have had to modify their activities and adjust their work and living habits to the new limits imposed by their disease. Guidance in making such adjustments, particularly for changes in jobs and careers, can be obtained from a number of federal, state, and local government and nongovernmental agencies, including vocational rehabilitation agencies.

For the patient who has had a myocardial infarction, the doctor usually recommends certain alterations in life style. Weight should be kept at normal levels, elevated blood pressure should be controlled, and diet may have to be changed, particularly as far as the fat content, and often the sodium content, are concerned. Because the digestive process itself imposes a work load on the heart, patients are advised to avoid excessively heavy and large meals and to avoid exercise immediately after eating. Emotional upset and excessively stressful situations should also be avoided. As far as coffee and alcohol are concerned, recommendations vary widely, and the patient's own doctor is the best qualified person for suggestions about how much, if any, should be consumed. Cigarette smoking, on the other hand, must be discontinued. Recent evidence indicates that patients recovering from myocardial infarction who continue to smoke cigarettes are more likely than their nonsmoking counterparts to die suddenly. Regular exercise is essential in regaining physical fitness following a heart attack. Physicians often recommend exercise stress testing both to determine safe levels of work and to prescribe a specific exercise program. But exercise should be approached in the same way as medication: taking the amount prescribed is good; taking more can be as dangerous as taking none at all. No substantial changes in the exercise program should be made unless the doctor is consulted.

Suggestions for patients with heart failure or heart rhythm disturbances (arrhythmias) and those who are taking anticoagulant drugs as treatment are given in chapter 2.

Many of the recommendations for the post-myocardial-infarction patient serve just as well for the patient recovering from coronary by-pass surgery. Cornerstones of the recovery program are control of weight and blood pressure, a fat-controlled diet, cessation of cigarette smoking, and a regular physical fitness routine.

In general, women are less likely than men to develop coronary atherosclerotic heart disease, but even young women may have angina and myocardial infarction. Moreover, there is a significant increase in the risk for heart attack among women who use oral contraceptives. This is particularly the case among women who have a family history of coronary disease, who smoke cigarettes, or have hypertension or high blood-fat levels. Such women should consult a doctor about the advisability of using oral contraceptives. Estrogen compounds, particularly those administered for post-menopausal symptoms, should not be taken without consulting a doctor, because of the increased risk of coronary disease.

One important question in the minds of many patients after myocardial infarction is how the attack and the course of recovery can be expected to affect sexual activity. Contrary to myth, sexual intercourse places only a modest work load on the heart; research has shown an increase in heart rate at orgasm to about 120 beats a minute (the normal average heart rate is 65 to 85 beats a minute). Most people who have recovered from myocardial infarction or who have cardiovascular diseases can engage in sexual intercourse without difficulty or impairment of heart function. Any patient who does experience chest pain, shortness of breath, or abnormal palpitations during sexual activity should consult a doctor. Because of the intimate nature of this subject and because of the concern of many patients after heart attack, doctors generally try to allay any unnecessary anxiety or feeling that a normally active sexual life is no longer possible by discussing the subject with the patient and his or her spouse.

ARTIFICIAL PACEMAKERS Several kinds of heart disease cause an abnormally slow heart rate. When the heart no longer functions adequately to keep a steady, normal rate, an artificial pacemaker may be implanted to take over the task. The pacemaker, a small battery-powered unit, is usually implanted under the skin and wired to the heart to control its rate and rhythm of contraction. Significant advances have been made in these devices, making them much longer lasting than before. The batteries still require replacement, however, with the length of time between replacements varying according to the type of pacemaker and battery.

A pacemaker imposes very few restrictions on normal daily life. The battery packs are fully protected against contact with water, so baths, showers, and swimming present no problem. The ordinary electrical household appliances and television sets do not interfere with a pacemaker, but some caution is necessary. The doctor should be informed if the patient is in contact with heavy-duty electrical motors, generators, and poorly shielded microwave ovens. The person who has had a pacemaker inserted can resume sexual activity without problems. Although the limitations on physical activity are few, patients should consult the doctor about the kinds and extent of physical exercise and recreation permitted. Pacemakers do not interfere with travel by air, train, or bus, but there are occasional restrictions on driving a car.

Living with a pacemaker may require counting and recording the heart

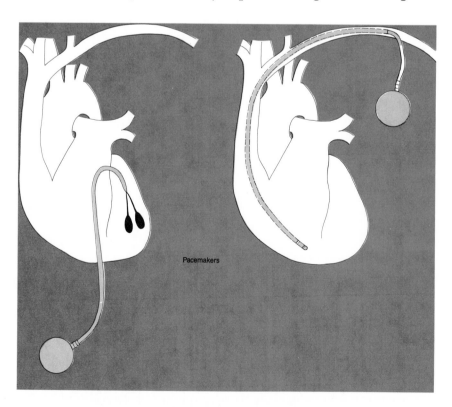

Pacemakers

rate daily or at less frequent intervals. The patient should, therefore, know the heart rate for which the pacemaker is set, learn how to count the pulse accurately, and report any variation in rate to the physician. Some patients with pacemakers attend clinics or transmit pacemaker recordings by telephone to a central service as a method of pacemaker surveillance. When dental work or other medical care is to be performed, or when a different physician is consulted, the patient should be sure to tell these doctors about the pacemaker. Colleagues at work, school personnel, and all persons in daily contact with the patient should also know that the person has a pacemaker. The American Heart Association supplies a pacemaker identification card which should be carried at all times. The card lists information that is essential in an emergency —in addition to data on the patient, it lists the doctor's name and the name, type, date of implant, and rate of the pacemaker.

Acute rheumatic fever occurs most commonly in children and young adults, but it also occurs in adult life. Moreover, anyone who has ever had the disease is at an increased risk of subsequent recurrence. The most common result of rheumatic fever is damage to the heart valves; in some cases the heart muscle itself may be weakened. Increased damage occurs with recurrent attacks of rheumatic fever. Rheumatic fever is almost always the result of a streptococcal infection of the throat and its recurrence can be prevented by long-term treatment with penicillin or other antibiotics. Treatment, either by monthly injection or daily oral dosage of antibiotics, is often a lifelong precautionary measure, particularly for patients who may be exposed to streptococcal infections. The parents of school-age children, teachers, and health-care personnel are especially likely to be exposed. Any sore throat should be promptly reported to a doctor, so that appropriate tests and treatment can be instituted. A "strep throat" cannot be diagnosed simply by looking a it; swabbing the throat with a sterile applicator is needed to determine if "strep" are present. If a streptococcal sore throat is diagnosed, antibiotics are necessary.

RHEUMATIC FEVER AND RHEUMATIC HEART DISEASE

Bacterial endocarditis, an infection of the heart lining, is a potential danger in anyone who has rheumatic fever or rheumatic heart disease. As an essential precaution against this infection, antibiotics must be taken before and after all dental work and many surgical procedures, including childbirth. An identification card stating that "endocarditis prophylaxis" is required should be carried at all times. The information alerts health personnel and all dentists and physicians treating the patient to order appropriate medication.

Heart damage is not an inevitable result of rheumatic fever. Some patients show no evidence of permanent damage, and other than long-term medication to guard against a recurrence, they need no special management and have no restrictions of activity or daily life. The medication is taken as a safeguard and is not evidence of chronic illness. The state Crippled Children's Service, Vocational Rehabilitation Agency, and other government agencies can provide referral to proper medical facilities for additional diagnostic or medical services when needed, and many furnish financial assistance for this care.

No "miracle drug" is available which can cure rheumatic heart disease. Some patients with moderately severe illness may require only medication and restriction of occupational or recreational activities, as recommended by a physician. At times an exercise test is performed as a basis for advising levels of work and activity. State vocational rehabilitation agencies may be able to help with job counseling and retraining when necessary.

The outlook for patients with severe rheumatic heart disease has been vastly improved in recent decades by advances in cardiac surgery. The decision for surgery is based on symptoms, such as shortness of breath, decreased exercise tolerance, chest pain, *and* fatigue, and diagnostic tests, especially heart catheterization (examination of the heart and valves by means of a thin tube inserted into the heart chambers). After damaged heart valves are repaired, or replaced with artificial valves, most patients have fewer restrictions on activity than before surgery; many can lead completely normal lives and women can complete pregnancies successfully. Some patients with artificial heart valves may have to take anticoagulant medication for varying periods of time; all require endocarditis prophylaxis.

CONGENITAL HEART DISEASE

Every year approximately 25,000 babies born in the United States have heart defects (congenital heart disease), but very little is understood about the causes of abnormal heart development before the baby is born. Some defects are associated with drugs taken during pregnancy and with cases of German measles (rubella) in the mother during the first three months of pregnancy. On the basis of these statistics, all young women who have not had rubella are advised to be vaccinated against the disease prior to pregnancy, and no medications should be taken during pregnancy without the advice of a doctor. Moreover, even though most congenital heart defects do not seem to be hereditary, any woman who has given birth to a baby with a defect should consult a doctor about the advisability of future pregnancies.

Many children with mild congenital heart defects require only minimal medical supervision and can lead completely normal lives. In other cases, corrective surgery may be required even though the child appears completely well, because many defects become more serious in adult life, with a greater risk of heart failure or heart infections. Parents can get help from various government agencies that provide referral services for diagnosis and surgery and sources of financial aid. The standard immunizations and the usual treatment of illness for all children also apply to the child with a heart defect. Certain symptoms, however, should be brought to the doctor's attention; these include failure to thrive or gain weight, difficulty in feeding, shortness of breath, chest pain, dizziness, fainting, and limited capacity for physical activity. Children with certain heart defects may have a bluish tint to the skin (cyanosis) as a result of decreased amounts of oxygen in the blood. Cyanosis in itself is not life-threatening and often disappears after corrective surgery. Fortunately, most children tolerate heart surgery well and many are completely cured of the defect, and within several months there are few or no restrictions on activity. During convalescence, however, activity may be restricted and home teaching may be recommended until the child is able to return to school.

Protection against bacterial endocarditis is essential for patients with congenital heart defects during surgery or dental work. All such patients should carry an identification card to alert health-care personnel to the needs of the patient for endocarditis prophylaxis.

Some congenital heart defects still cannot be cured, and some people are severely limited in activity as children and in career opportunity as adults.

PRINCIPLES

1. Cardiovascular disease does not have to be incapacitating, nor does the person with a heart condition have to become a heart "victim" or a lifelong invalid. Leading a normal or near-normal life is possible if certain

Information on special educational and career training can be obtained from various federal, state, and local organizations. In consultation with the child's physician, personnel from these agencies evaluate the child's activity tolerance, conduct tests to determine skills and aptitudes, and offer career counseling and vocational planning and training.

In spite of its ominous sound, heart failure does not mean that the heart has ceased to beat. A failing heart continues to beat, but at a below-normal pumping level. Because the heart cannot pump as well as it should, fluid collects in the lungs, legs, and body tissues. Heart failure is thus not a specific disease but the result of a variety of heart problems, among them hypertension, heart valve disease, and coronary artery disease. Control and treatment of the underlying disease, by medical management or surgical intervention, can improve heart function and decrease heart failure.

A number of measures are taken to strengthen a failing heart. Digitalis is usually prescribed to improve the heart's pumping function. Diuretic drugs (water pills) increase the kidneys' ability to eliminate excess water and salt, thus ridding the body of excess fluid. Because many diuretic drugs also cause the body to lose potassium, the patient may be given potassium-supplement medication or may be advised to increase consumption of such potassium-rich foods as bananas, raisins, and orange juice. A salt-restricted diet is very important; patients should also avoid medications such as laxatives, headache preparations, and cough medicines, which may contain sodium. Check with a physician before using any medication not specifically prescribed.

Adequate rest is essential, and the patient may require specific rest periods during the day, as well as pacing of work. Excessive weight places an added burden on the heart, so weight reduction to ideal body weight is a vital part of treatment. The doctor should be alerted to the appearance, which is often very gradual, of such symptoms of heart failure as increased fatigue, shortness of breath, limited capacity for activity, and swelling of the legs and ankles.

Arrhythmias (disturbances of heart rhythm) may occur with or without evidence of heart disease. Some arrhythmias produce no symptoms and are detected only by physical examination or electrocardiograms. Others may cause palpitations, dizziness, fainting, or chest discomfort. The patient who becomes aware of an abnormal heartbeat should try to note whether the heartbeat is fast or slow, regular or irregular, gradual or abrupt in onset and temination, of short or long duration, and whether it is caused or increased by some activities. This information, along with any associated symptoms, helps the doctor determine the type of rhythm disturbance. The patient may have to wear a device similar to a tape recorder to monitor heart rhythm over long periods of time in order to document rhythm abnormalities during usual daily activities or to detect intermittent arrhythmias.

Some arrhythmias require no treatment; others may have to be treated with a variety of medications used to regularize heart rhythm, among them digitalis, quinidine, procainamide, and propranolol. The drugs are sometimes taken in combination, and it may take several weeks before the type of drugs and the dosage are adjusted to the individual requirement of the patient. These drugs must be taken precisely as prescribed and often for long periods

basic facts are learned and practiced as soon as a condition is diagnosed.

2. *Taking medication, a common part of long-term recovery routines, requires following some simple and*

CONGESTIVE HEART FAILURE

commonsense procedures. These include learning the name and purpose of prescribed medicines, following the prescribed dosage exactly, renewing prescriptions in time to avoid interruption in dosage schedule, avoiding use of other drugs that may interact with prescribed medicines, and learning proper storage methods.

3. *Hypertension, which afflicts one out of six adults, requires special attention to daily regimen, since often there are no overt symptoms. Control of hypertension is achieved by regular visits to the doctor's office for pressure measurements, use of antihypertensive drugs, and careful attention to diet. Excessive weight must be avoided, and the use of salt and certain fats regulated.*

4. *Coronary artery disease afflicts certain high-risk individuals—those with high blood pressure, high blood-cholesterol levels, a family*

ARRHYTHMIAS

history of premature coronary disease or death from heart attack, and a smoking habit. Eliminating avoidable risks by changes in habits and diet and recognizing early warning signals can minimize the danger of coronary artery disease.

5. *Angina pectoris, a sign of imbalance between the heart's demand for oxygen and its supply, can be relieved by rest and, in some cases, medication. Control of weight and blood pressure, together with avoidance of situations that precipitate attacks, permit many patients to function well.*

6. *Heart attack is usually a major crisis, yet many victims can and do return*

to normal life and work. Alterations in life style are often necessary, particularly in eating habits.

HEART DISEASE AND PREGNANCY

Cigarette smoking must be discontinued and a regular program of exercise undertaken—but only under the control and direction of the physician.

7. *The patient with an artificial pacemaker experiences few restrictions in daily life, but a doctor should be consulted before engaging in strenuous exercise. The patient must learn to count and record the heart rate, and family members and associates should be advised that a pacemaker has been inserted. The wearer should carry a pacemaker identification card.*

8. *Rheumatic fever does not inevitably result in heart damage, but anyone who has had the illness is at increased risk of subsequent attacks. Prevention of recurrences of streptococcal infections is achieved by long-term treatment with antibiotics. Special precautions are required during dental work and surgical procedures, as well as childbirth, to avoid bacterial infection of the heart lining. Advances in cardiac surgery have improved the outlook of patients with severe rheumatic heart disease.*

9. *Congenital heart defects may require only minimal medical supervision or may require corrective surgery to avoid serious complications in later life. Parents should learn to recognize childhood symptoms of heart defects, such as failure to thrive, chest pain, dizziness, fainting, and limited physical stamina.*

10. *Congestive heart failure is not a specific disease; it is the result of a variety of heart problems, including hypertension, valve disease, and coronary heart disease. Control of the underlying condition can improve heart function and decrease*

ANTICOAGULANT THERAPY

of time. Some arrhythmias are best controlled by the insertion of an artificial pacemaker.

During pregnancy, as the baby grows, the demand on the mother's heart to pump blood increases. Because of this extra work required of the pregnant woman's heart, all women who know they have heart disease, who have had rheumatic fever, who have high blood pressure, or who have been told they have a heart murmur should discuss with their physician the advisability of becoming pregnant, any special care requirements during a pregnancy, and the choice of contraceptive methods if these are desired.

Many people are concerned about inheritance of heart disease. Rheumatic heart disease is not inherited; women with rheumatic heart disease have babies with perfectly normal hearts. Congenital heart disease is not generally considered to be inherited; having congenital heart disease is not a reason for concern that a pregnancy will result in a child with congenital heart disease. However, a woman who has already had a child born with heart disease should discuss with her doctor the likelihood that a future pregnancy will result in a child with congenital heart disease. Remember, though, that rubella (German measles) in the mother during pregnancy is likely to cause congenital heart disease in her baby; if a woman has not had German measles as a child, the doctor will recommend vaccination against German measles before becoming pregnant.

Recommendations for rest and limitations of activity during pregnancy vary according to the severity of the heart condition. The same can be said for changes in diet and in salt consumption. Some women who have not previously taken medications for a heart condition may require digitalis or diuretics to offset the increased work load imposed on the heart by pregnancy. Most women are advised to take supplementary iron and vitamins during pregnancy whether or not heart disease exists. No pregnant woman should smoke, because women who smoke tend to have smaller babies and more premature babies. Although medical recommendations concerning alcohol consumption in pregnancy vary, excessive alcohol consumption is clearly undesirable. Pregnant women should never take any medication without the explicit approval of a doctor. For women with rheumatic heart disease, rheumatic fever prophylaxis will be continued during pregnancy.

Women with heart disease who have tolerated one pregnancy without complications rarely have difficulty during normal labor and delivery. In patients with rheumatic heart disease, the doctor prescribes an antibiotic before and a few days after delivery to guard against endocarditis. Heart disease does not prevent a mother from breast feeding, but women who are taking oral anticoagulant drugs cannot breast-feed because the drugs are secreted into the milk and may cause bleeding problems in the infant.

The choice of contraceptive agents should be made in consultation with a doctor, because oral contraceptives predispose to blood clotting, particularly in some patients with heart disease; an alternate method of contraception may be recommended. Oral contraceptives are also not recommended for women with hypertension. Studies show that these agents may be associated with an increased risk of heart attack, particularly in women over the age of forty.

Anticoagulant, or blood-thinning, drugs may be prescribed to prevent recurrence of a blood clot, especially in the legs or lungs, or to prevent clots from developing as a result of heart failure, arrhythmias, or when an artificial valve has been implanted in the heart. Anticoagulant drugs do not really "thin" the blood; they prolong the time needed for blood to clot and thereby prevent blood-clotting problems. Cooperation by the patient is essential in oral anticoagulant therapy. Periodic blood tests (prothrombin time determinations) are necessary to determine the appropriate dosage. The patient must be sure to take the medication exactly as prescribed, at the time prescribed. Certain other medications can interfere with the action of an anticoagulant, increasing or decreasing its potency. The result can either be excessive delay of clotting, with bleeding complications, or inadequate anticoagulant activity, with clotting problems. Among the medications that should not be taken simultaneously with anticoagulant drugs are many cold remedies, sedatives, patent medicines of any kind, and headache preparations, particularly aspirin. If necessary, the doctor can prescribe an aspirin substitute.

A person who is taking anticoagulants is apt to bleed or bruise easily. Any injury and any excessive or unusual bruising should be reported to the doctor. Blood in the urine or stool may also be a danger sign which should be reported at once. Women sometimes have some increase in menstrual flow; any excessively heavy flow should be called to the doctor's attention. Anticoagulants do not pose any problem for sexual intercourse.

The length of time that anticoagulant therapy is needed varies from several months to several years and in some cases may be required for indefinite periods. During pregnancy anticoagulant therapy poses special problems but usually does not interfere with successful completion of pregnancy and delivery. All patients who take anticoagulants should carry an identification card and should inform a dentist or any other doctor that they are taking these drugs, which may have to be temporarily discontinued for some surgical and dental procedures.

Although varicose veins are not directly related to heart disease, the condition may cause a predisposition to the formation of blood clots in the legs. In most cases, there is some leg discomfort or swelling, and although the problem is primarily a cosmetic one, periodic medical checkups are recommended and day-to-day care is essential. Elastic stockings or support hose should be worn during the day to maintain good circulation. Tight clothing, such as girdles, garters, or rolled stockings, should be avoided. Exercise generally helps to improve circulation, and long periods of sitting or standing should be avoided. It is helpful to interrupt long periods of sitting, as in a car or on an airplane trip, every half hour to stand or walk about to restore circulation. Sleeping with the foot of the bed elevated is also sometimes recommended to help circulation. These measures usually suffice to control ordinary cases of varicose veins; corrective surgery may be advisable for more serious cases.

Stroke may result in weakness, in partial or complete paralysis, and in difficulty with speech, memory, understanding, or vision. The extent of disability and the speed of recovery vary considerably from patient to patient. Early rehabilitative care is crucial, and restoration of impaired functions, when this is possible, usually involves the cooperation of the patient, the family, trained rehabilitation personnel, and the doctor. In the first days of illness, massage

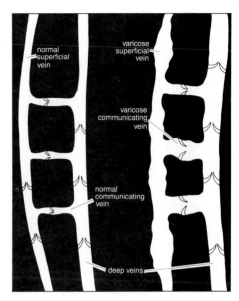

Swellings in the superficial veins of the legs, varicose veins, are not directly related to heart disease. The condition, however, requires periodic medical checkups and day-to-day care to maintain and improve circulation.

heart failure. Digitalis, diuretic drugs, salt-restriction, weight control, and adequate rest are essential aspects of control of congestive heart failure.

VARICOSE VEINS

11. Arrhythmias, disturbances in heart rhythm, are not in themselves evidence of heart disease. Some arrhythmias are treated with medications, while other more severe arrhythmias require insertion of an artificial pacemaker.

12. Pregnancy places special stress on women with heart disease, rheumatic fever, high blood pressure, or heart murmurs. Limitations on

STROKE

activity vary according to the severity of the condition. Certain oral contraceptives have been linked with increased risk of heart attack, especially in women over forty, and

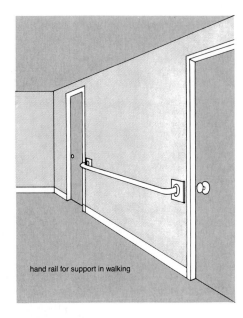

hand rail for support in walking

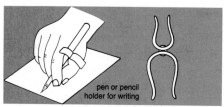

pen or pencil
holder for writing

Rehabilitation aids for the Stroke Victim

should not be taken without consultation with a doctor.

13. *Anticoagulant therapy involves taking drugs to prevent recurrence of blood clots or the formation of blood clots resulting from heart failure, arrhythmias, or following implantation of an artificial pacemaker. Many common drugs such as cold remedies, sedatives,*

SUMMARY

aspirin, and other over-the-counter medications interfere with anticoagulants and should not be taken with them.

14. *Strokes resulting in partial or complete paralysis and impairment of speech, memory, understanding, or vision require early rehabilitative care. The cooperation of family, doctor, patient, and trained rehabilitation personnel is essential if the patient is to learn to care for daily needs.*

and exercise are important in preventing weakness and shortening or distortion of muscles from extended bed rest and inactivity.

Training stroke patients to care for their daily needs begins in the hospital and is continued at home. Many community agencies are available to help stroke patients learn to care for themselves and to resume independent activity in spite of some loss of function. Nurses, physical and occupational therapists, speech therapists, vocational counselors, and career advisors are all part of the rehabilitation team. Many communities have stroke clubs where stroke patients and their families get mutual aid and support. Advice is available from the physician or hospital and from such agencies as the public health nurse and visiting nurse associations and state departments of vocational rehabilitation regarding physical aids to help a stroke patient regain independence—wheelchairs, walkers, canes; walking rails and support bars in the house; special bath, shower, bed, and other household arrangements. Participation on the part of the patient's family is vital to recovery; this includes learning how to communicate with the patient whose speech or understanding has been affected and encouraging the redevelopment of speech. By understanding the recovery process, the family can give support during the long and often frustrating period of convalescence. With such help many stroke patients recover a great portion of their mental and physical capacities and are able to return to normal or nearly normal living. Even when faculties have been considerably impaired, many can be retrained to care for themselves and even to manage a household, drive a car, and do certain kinds of work.

During convalescence, the doctor tries to keep blood pressure under close control to prevent a recurrence of stroke. Weight control will be advised when appropriate. Gradually increasing physical activity is beneficial. The patient must report to the doctor any signs of transient weakness, paralysis, numbness, or disturbance in speech or vision.

Both the doctor and the family should be aware of the emotional effects of stroke. The patient may develop a sense of guilt over inability to care for his or her needs. Depression often develops as a result of the long period needed for recovery and the inadequate restoration of some faculties. Aid is available from many sources, both public and private. Stroke patients and their families should understand that such problems are not unusual or a cause for guilt.

A great many persons with various kinds of heart disease are leading full and active lives today. Patients who once would have been incapacitated have been restored to normal life by the advances in medical and surgical treatment in the last few decades. Although many patients with severe heart problems require intensive long-term care, restrictions of activity, or restructuring of life style, increased knowledge about the heart and heart disease has opened up new approaches to treatment and rehabilitation. For best results patients and their families must work in partnership with the health personnel in the treatment of the disease and to prevent recurrence or complications.

6

CARDIAC EMERGENCIES

Malcolm R. Parker, M.D.

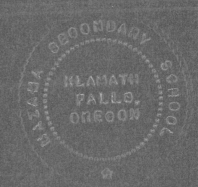

Most people have no difficulty in recognizing an obvious medical emergency: loss of consciousness, broken bones, extensive bleeding. But some emergencies, including those occasioned by cardiovascular diseases, are accompanied by more subtle symptoms that can be overlooked or even ignored. The result can be tragic: one out of two victims of heart attack dies before receiving any emergency treatment. Although death from heart attack is immediate in some situations, there are many more in which death could be prevented if early warning signals were recognized. These warnings come from the heart itself, from blood pressure levels, or, in the case of stroke, from impairment in such body functions as sensation, vision, speech, or movement. The warning signals of stroke are discussed in chapter 19; this chapter is concerned with heart rhythm irregularity and heart attack and with emergency treatment, particularly the techniques of cardiovascular resuscitation (CPR).

Except when under some unusual physical or emotional strain, the average healthy person is unaware of the heart's activity. Quietly and efficiently, the heart goes about the task of pumping oxygen-rich blood through the entire arterial system, bringing the nutrients that sustain the body's organs. The circulating blood then carries the waste products of this process to the kidneys and lungs for elimination. The heart's labor is truly prodigious; it beats some 60 to 100 times a minute, 3,600 times an hour, 31,536,000 times a year, pumping out about 1.5 gallons of blood each minute under normal conditions and more than quadrupling that volume when necessary. And while the healthy heart functions quietly and with a steady rhythm, a threatened heart signals danger by a disturbance in rhythm, by pain, or by other symptoms of heart attack.

KINDS OF HEARTBEATS
Normal Heartbeat

The techniques for checking the rhythmic beat of the heart include feeling the pulse, listening to the heart with a stethoscope (auscultation), or taking an electrocardiogram, a graphic record of the heart's electric impulses which cause contraction of the heart muscle. Using these techniques, a physician is able to detect any disorders of rhythm, including shifts to faster or slower rates or a change in the regularity of the beat, which may involve occasional alteration in rhythm or complete absence of a regular pattern. The normal rate varies from 60 to 100 beats a minute at rest. (In infants, the resting heart rate is faster—from 90 to 130 a minute.) Physical condition and general health influence the rate, and very often well-trained athletes will have resting rates as low as 45 to 50 beats a minute. With physical activity or emotional stress, the rate of the beat can increase dramatically, giving the heart and the body a great reserve of energy to draw upon in emergency situations. Occasionally, however, the heart rate increases when there is no apparent need for it to do so.

Rapid Heartbeat

The most common occurrence of suddenly increased heart rate in apparently normal hearts is called paroxysmal atrial tachycardia (PAT). In this regular, rapid rhythm, the heartbeat may go as high as 150 to 180 pulses a minute. Although periods of rapid heart rate may sometimes be due to coronary artery disease or chronic rheumatic disease, and call for special attention, in the average healthy adult the major effect of an episode of PAT is weakness and sometimes a feeling of breathlessness. The "spell" usually is of brief duration and ends as abruptly as it begins, but in some cases it lasts for hours or days. Fortunately, the normal heart can easily tolerate the increased rate for periods of up to several days without damage.

PAT is treated either by digitalis or beta-blocking drugs (see Cardiovascular Drugs, Chapter 21) or by a physical movement called the Valsalva Maneuver (named after the Italian anatomist Antonio Maria Valsalva, 1666-1723, who devised it). In the Valsalva Maneuver, the patient inhales deeply, holds his breath, then attempts to blow the breath out forcefully. The essential part of the maneuver is the length of time during which pressure is exerted on lungs and chest; it should last 15 to 20 seconds and never less than 10 seconds. If the maneuver does not work at first, it should be tried again, with the full straining effort kept up for the full period.

Slow Heartbeat

In contrast to rapid heart rates are the abnormally slow rates referred to as bradycardia, which are under 60 beats a minute. A slow heart rate is not uncommon among well-trained athletes and is a sign of a very efficiently operating cardiovascular system. In elderly persons, however, a slow rate may be due to arteriosclerosis, which can cause weakness and fainting. A very slow pulse accompanied by symptoms of weakness and fainting is then an emergency signal, and a physician should be notified. In such cases, an artificial pacemaker may be needed.

Irregular Heartbeat

In addition to being fast or slow, heart rhythm can also become irregular. Such episodes can involve either single irregular beats of varying frequency or a totally irregular rhythm of fast or slow beats. The single irregular beat, usually felt as a skip or momentary stop of the heartbeat, is actually an early or extra (ectopic) beat. When the electric impulse that triggers the contraction of the heart chambers is fired prematurely, the chamber, not yet adequately filled with blood, contracts and pumps that inadequate volume of blood out into the circulatory system. A pulse taken at this moment will be either weak or seemingly nonexistent. The premature beat is, however, usually followed by a slight pause while the basic rhythm is re-established. The next normal beat will then be a full one, felt as a kind of thump. With a longer time to fill, the heart has more blood to pump than usual, which is why the thump is felt. This kind of irregularity of rhythm, which may occur every third or fourth beat, or once every hour, or with varying degrees of frequency, does not of itself signal danger to the heart, but if the episodes are frequent or increase with physical exertion, a physician should be consulted. For those with cardiovascular disease, however, frequent irregularities in heartbeat require immediate medical attention. If the irregularities are accompanied by other symptoms of heart attack, emergency medical assistance must be obtained at once.

A totally irregular heartbeat (atrial fibrillation) can result in an increase of pulse rate to 110 to 140 beats a minute, with the pulse alternating between strong and weak beats in random fashion. The degree of emergency, as with other disturbances of heart rhythm, depends on the health of the individual and the other associated symptoms. Ordinarily, in persons who have no underlying heart disease, no cardiac symptoms are evident. If, on the other hand, some form of cardiovascular disease exists, fibrillation can be a distinct medical emergency, requiring the prompt attention of a physician and emergency medical units. The extent of the emergency is often judged on the basis of associated symptoms: a feeling of lightheadedness or breathlessness, especially when standing upright, or a loss of consciousness. Much more serious is ventricular fibrillation, which may be due to blockage of a coronary artery. Unless immediately reversed, ventricular fibrillation results in sudden death (see Arrhythmias, chapter 12).

Disturbances in heart rhythm are not necessarily warning signals of a coronary emergency. The following guidelines are helpful in making a preliminary evaluation of such symptoms. The pulse should be taken for a full minute, but if this is impractical, taken for 30 seconds and multiplied by two. An approximate, rather than an exact, figure is what is needed. The regularity of the pulse should also be determined. Other symptoms to be observed include lightheadedness when standing upright; heaviness or squeezing sensation in the chest; difficulty in breathing, especially when lying flat; shortness of breath with activity; pallor; and nausea. While it is important to distinguish between severe and minimal symptoms, it is usually wiser to err on the side of caution in determining whether a physician should be called. If all the danger signals are present, or if there is a previous history of heart disease, a physician should be informed at once and an emergency rescue unit alerted.

HEART ATTACK The major medical emergency of the cardiovascular system is a heart attack, or myocardial infarction. There are about 650,000 deaths from heart attack each year in the United States alone. More than 350,000 of these deaths occur before the person reaches the hospital; most of them within the first hour after the attack. However, survival rates for those who are immediately placed under advanced cardiac life-support care are very encouraging (from 85 to 90 percent). This kind of care, given by specially trained teams or paramedics, working in mobile units, should be a part of every hospital's emergency service system.

In order to respond to the medical emergency of a heart attack, one must be able to recognize the early warning signals. As described in How the Heart Functions, chapter 8, the heart muscle requires an adequate blood supply to bring oxygen and food and to remove its waste products. The coronary arteries supply the heart muscle with blood. These arteries are the heart muscle's sole source of oxygen and nutrients: the heart does not receive these essentials directly from the blood it pumps through its chambers. Under normal conditions, coronary arteries are capable of supplying all the blood the heart needs, even when its work rate increases to two or three times the normal resting rate. This ability is often compromised by the development of coronary atherosclerosis, a disease process that results in thickening and narrowing of the inner walls of the arteries through an accumulation of fatty tissue (see Coronary Artery Disease, chapter 11). The supply of blood to the heart muscle is reduced by the narrowing of the arteries, resulting in injury to the muscle cells if there is prolonged angina or an infarct occurs. If the lack of blood supply is severe and prolonged, the muscle cells suffer irreversible injury and die. This is a myocardial infarction.

The injury and death of the heart muscle cells can also result in disruption in the rhythm of the heartbeat, particularly in the first few hours after the cells are affected. Such radical changes in heart rhythm, commonest in the first hours after an attack, are the most frequent cause of death from myocardial infarction and are almost always the cause of sudden death. If death does not occur, the heart's natural resistance to changes in rhythm gradually asserts itself, and stability is regained within the first 48 to 72 hours after the attack. Fortunately, rhythmic changes can be detected and stabilized. The work of the advanced cardiac life support units responsible for monitoring patients in this condition is discussed at the end of this chapter. All who are confronted by a heart attack emergency should be aware of the vital importance of such aids.

Early Warnings

The most common signal of heart attack is an uncomfortable pressure, squeezing, fullness, or pain in the center of the chest behind the breastbone which may radiate to the shoulder, neck, or arms.

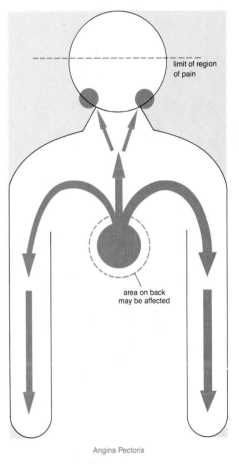

limit of region of pain

area on back may be affected

Angina Pectoris

It may last 2 minutes or longer and may come and go. It need not be severe. There may be such signs as sweating, nausea, shortness of breath, or a feeling of weakness. The person does not necessarily have to "look" ill or to have all the symptoms before action is taken. Sharp, stabbing twinges of pain are usually not signals of a heart attack. The common signals can occur in either sex, even in young adults, at any time and in any place. Contrary to popular belief, physical or emotional stress is not necessarily a precipitating factor of a heart attack.

If the typical chest discomfort lasts 2 minutes or more, the action plan outlined below should be initiated. An exception would be a person who has heart disease and has instructions from his physician to take nitroglycerin first. Even in patients with heart disease, if typical symptoms persist for 10 minutes despite rest and administration of 3 nitroglycerin tablets, the action plan should follow.

ACTION PLAN

NO HISTORY OF CORONARY HEART DISEASE	HISTORY OF CORONARY HEART DISEASE (NITROGLYCERIN PRESCRIBED)
1. Recognize the signals.	1. Recognize the signals.
2. Stop activity and sit or lie down.	2. Stop activity and sit or lie down.
3. If pain persists for 2 minutes or more, activate the emergency system for survival.	3. Take 3 nitroglycerin tablets within 10 minutes.
4. Call the emergency rescue service or go at once to the nearest hospital emergency room which offers 24-hour emergency cardiac care.	4. If signals persist, activate the emergency system for survival.
	5. Call the emergency rescue service or go at once to the nearest hospital emergency room which offers 24-hour emergency cardiac care.

Denial Response

The first tendency of a victim of heart attack is to deny the possibility of its occurrence. The most common reactions are to asume the symptoms are due to indigestion or that the person is too healthy to be having a heart attack. Very often the victim is reluctant to call a doctor because he does not wish to disturb him if a heart attack is not taking place. In other cases, fear of alarming family members deters the victim from taking action. The search for reasons to deny that a heart attack is in progress is a signal for positive action. Because the patient (in spite of his best intentions) is unlikely to act in his own interest, it is essential that those nearest to him at the time activate the system for survival and be prepared to render basic life support if necessary.

If you are with someone who is having the warnings, and if they last 2 minutes or longer, act at once. Expect a denial, but insist on taking prompt action:

1. Call the emergency rescue service, or

2. Take the patient to the nearest hospital emergency room which offers 24-hour emergency cardiac care.

3. Be prepared to give cardiopulmonary basic life support (mouth-to-mouth breathing and chest compression) if necessary. You will need to be trained to do this properly.

Most communities have some type of emergency medical response system provided by private or municipal ambulances, police or fire department, or a combination of these. It is important to know in advance how to reach such aid in an emergency and also to know the location of the nearest medical facility with a special coronary care unit. The monitoring facilities available at such an institution are of critical importance in the first hours and days after a heart attack, when the patient is most in danger from the risk of heart failure, fatal rhythm disturbances, and shock.

CARDIOPULMONARY RESUSCITATION

If the victim has collapsed, has no detectable pulse, and is not breathing, cardiopulmonary resuscitation (CPR) may be necessary to maintain life until emergency medical aid can be summoned. *Only those who have received instruction in CPR from qualified personnel should attempt to revive an unconscious person suspected of having a heart attack.* Since CPR can make the difference between life and death, all who can do so are urged to receive instruction in the techniques. Information on training programs can be obtained through local chapters of the American Heart Association.

Cardiopulmonary resuscitation is an emergency technique that combines artificial respiration and manual artificial circulation to maintain life in cases of cardiac arrest until advanced cardiac life support care is available. There are many causes of sudden death: poisoning, drowning, suffocation, choking, electrocution, and smoke inhalation. Basic CPR deals with three principal concerns: airway, breathing, and circulation.

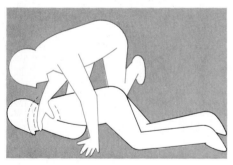

Establishing Unresponsiveness

When a collapsed person is discovered, the rescuer must determine whether he is conscious. *Gently* shake the victim's shoulder and ask, "Are you all right?" Violent shaking may compound injuries, particularly those of the neck. If the victim does not respond, he is unconscious and may be in need of immediate CPR.

The first thing the rescuer should do is to call out for help, even though no one may be in sight. Someone who can assist may be within earshot.

If the victim is crumpled up and lying face down, he is not in position for the start of resuscitation efforts. While the call for help is being made, the rescuer should roll the victim on his back. This should be done with great care, since broken bones or other injuries could be complicated by improper handling.

The victim should be rolled over as a unit, the head, shoulders, and torso moving simultaneously with no twisting. To accomplish this, the rescuer must kneel beside the victim a few inches from his side. Then, raising the arm nearest to him, the rescuer straightens it out above the victim's head. The legs should be adjusted so that they are nearly straight.

One hand is then placed on the back of the victim's head and neck to prevent it from twisting. Using the other hand, the rescuer grasps the victim under the arm to brace the shoulder and torso. This is the major point on the body where pull is exerted to roll the victim over. If the pull is carefully and evenly exerted, the torso and hips will follow the shoulders with minimal twisting, thus avoiding any possible complications involving the neck, head, and spine. The victim should end up flat on his back in a position to begin CPR.

The tongue is the most common cause of airway obstruction in the uncon- scious victim. Since the tongue is attached to the lower jaw, moving the lower jaw forward lifts the tongue away from the back of the throat and opens the airway. As long as there is enough tone in the jaw muscles, tilting the head back will cause the lower jaw to move forward and open the airway.

HEAD TILT–NECK LIFT This maneuver is accomplished by kneeling at the victim's side and placing one hand beneath his neck and the other hand on his forehead. The rescuer then lifts the neck with one hand while tilting the head by backward pressure on the forehead. The rescuer must be very careful in performing this maneuver, because too much force may cause injury to the upper (cervical) spine. Since the specific movement used is extension of the head at the junction of the head and neck, rather than the furthest extension of the cervical vertebrae, the hand lifting the neck should be placed close to the back of the head. When the hand is positioned properly, extension of the cervical spine is minimized.

Sometimes the victim's airway becomes obstructed by loosened dentures. In that case, the dentures may be removed or the rescuer may solve the problem by performing the head tilt-chin lift maneuver.

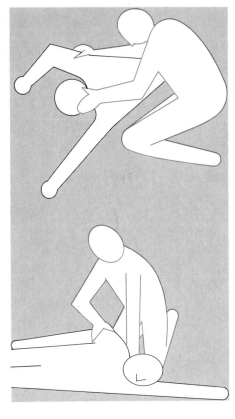

HEAD TILT–CHIN LIFT When an unconscious person attempts to breathe in, pressure in the airway may result in the tongue's acting as a valve and closing the passageway. Even when the head is tilted back and the neck extended, the lower jaw may have to be supported to lift the tongue and open the airway. To accomplish this, the rescuer places the fingers of one hand under the lower jaw on the bony part near the victim's chin, lifting the chin to bring it forward while supporting the jaw and helping to tilt the head back. The soft tissue under the chin must not be compressed, however, since this might obstruct the airway. The other hand presses the victim's forehead to tilt the head back. The thumb is never used to lift the chin; it is only used to depress the lower lip lightly.

The chin should be lifted so that the teeth are nearly brought together,

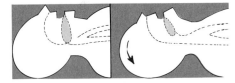

but *the mouth should not be completely closed.* If the victim has loose dentures, holding them in position will decrease the possibility of the lips' obstructing the airway. The mouth-to-mouth seal in rescue breathing, discussed later, is easier when dentures are in place. If they cannot be held in place, remove them.

Establishing Breathlessness

While maintaining the open airway position, the rescuer can determine whether the victim is breathing by placing his ear over the victim's mouth and nose and looking toward the victim's chest and stomach. He then looks for the chest to rise and fall, listens for air escaping during exhalation, and feels for the flow of air on his cheek. If none of these signs is present, the victim is not breathing. If opening the airway has not caused the victim to begin to breathe spontaneously, the rescuer must provide rescue breathing.

Rescue Breathing

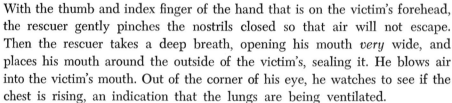

With the thumb and index finger of the hand that is on the victim's forehead, the rescuer gently pinches the nostrils closed so that air will not escape. Then the rescuer takes a deep breath, opening his mouth *very* wide, and places his mouth around the outside of the victim's, sealing it. He blows air into the victim's mouth. Out of the corner of his eye, he watches to see if the chest is rising, an indication that the lungs are being ventilated.

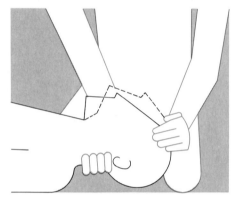

Ventilation should be limited to the extent required to cause the chest to rise. In most adults, this is usually a minimum volume of 800 centimeters; adequate ventilation does not need to exceed 1200 centimeters. To provide this volume of air, the rescuer gives *four quick, full breaths* without allowing time for full lung deflation between breaths, quickly taking in air after each ventilation by turning his head toward the victim's chest. Throughout the time required to give the four breaths, air pressure to open the airway should not exceed 2 liters, since pressure above that level may force air into the stomach by way of the esophagus, the tube leading from the back of the throat into it. If breathing has stopped, even for a short time, some of the small air sacs of the lung will collapse, and these are filled and ventilated more effectively by maintaining positive pressure (2 liters) in the lungs during the four initial full breaths.

One of the most common problems in learning mouth-to-mouth breathing is inadequate sealing of the victim's mouth, which results in air leaks. Applying a great deal of pressure is unnecessary; the seal can be made by the very lightest touch of the rescuer's mouth against the victim's.

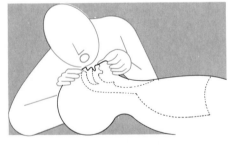

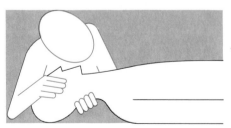

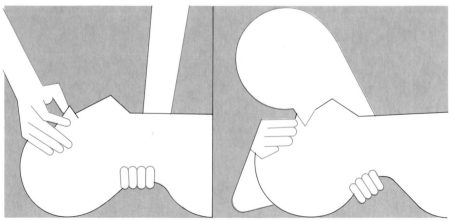

Dentures in the rescuer's mouth may also create a problem by loosening under the pressure. This can be overcome by a very light mouth-to-mouth contact. Occasionally, air is forced between the rescuer's upper denture and palate. If light contact with the victim's mouth does not solve this problem, the rescuer may have to hold his denture in place by pressing against it with his tongue. Removal of the rescuer's dentures is the last resort; mouth-to-mouth contact is more difficult under these circumstances, and some leakage of air is unavoidable. However, the rescuer can provide adequate ventilation after removing his dentures by exerting minimum pressure in closing the victim's nostrils. They should be lightly pinched together between the thumb and forefinger at the nasal openings.

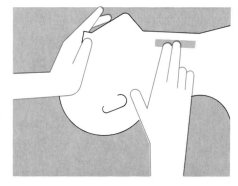

Establishing Presence of Pulse

The pulse in the carotid artery in the neck is the most accessible place to determine whether the heart is beating. It lies in a groove between the wind-pipe and the large neck muscles.

Kneeling at the victim's side, the rescuer keeps his hand on the forehead to maintain the correct head position and uses the other hand to feel the carotid pulse. The pulse is felt on the side of the victim's neck nearest to the rescuer. The rescuer locates the pulse by placing the tips of his fingers gently on the windpipe and then sliding the fingertips to the *side nearest him*, gently pressing the soft part of the neck next to the windpipe. Pressure on the windpipe must be avoided, because it will impede the passage of air. The rescuer should not check the pulses on both sides of the neck at the same time, because doing so would decrease blood flow to the head and brain.

The absence of a pulse indicates that the heart has stopped beating (cardiac arrest).

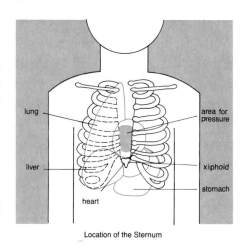

Location of the Sternum

Emergency Medical Service

When no pulse can be felt, artificial circulation must be provided. If the rescuer is not alone, one person should be sent to call the local emergency telephone number to set the emergency medical services system in action.

If the rescuer is alone, he should begin CPR and continue for at least 4 or 5 minutes. After that, if a telephone is immediately available, he should call to activate the emergency system, returning to resume CPR after the briefest possible interruption (less than 2 minutes). If no telephone is nearby, the only option is to continue CPR.

Artificial circulation is provided by external cardiac compression. In effect, **Cardiac Compression** when the rescuer applies rhythmic pressure on the lower half of the victim's breastbone the heart is squeezed against the spine, forcing it to pump out blood. To perform cardiac compression properly, the rescuer kneels at the victim's side nearest the chest and locates the notch at the lowest part of the sternum.

The heel of one hand is placed on the sternum 1½ to 2 inches above the notch, and the other hand is placed on top of the hand in position. The fingers must be kept off the chest wall; this is made easier by interlocking the fingers.

Keeping his arms straight and his shoulders directly over the sternum, the rescuer compresses downward, about 1½ to 2 inches for an adult victim.

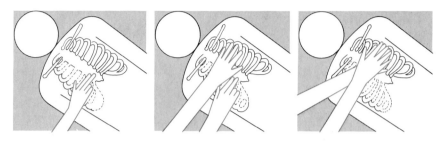

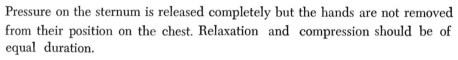

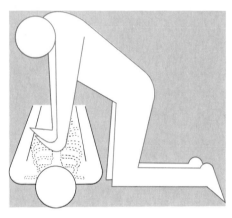

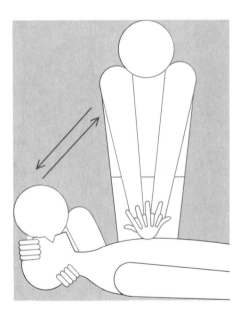

Pressure on the sternum is released completely but the hands are not removed from their position on the chest. Relaxation and compression should be of equal duration.

ONE-RESCUER CPR   If there is only one rescuer, he must provide both ventilation and cardiac compression, at a ratio of 15 chest compressions to 2 quick breaths working alone, compressions are made at a rate of 80 times a minute.

TWO-RESCUER CPR   When a second rescuer arrives, he should take over the ventilation, positioning himself on the opposite side of the first rescuer near the victim's head. He immediately interposes a breath during the upstroke of any chest compression. The first rescuer then changes the rate of compressions from 80 to 60 compressions a minute. A simple method for maintaining this rate accurately is to count as follows: one-one thousand, two-one thousand, three-one thousand, four-one thousand, five-one thousand, one-one thousand, two-one thousand, and so on.

The rescue breathing is then interposed during the upstroke of each fifth compression. In the two-rescuer procedure, mouth-to-mouth positioning should occur at the end of the fourth compression. In effect, this means that the airway should be "pressurized" during the fifth downstroke, so that a breath may be quickly interposed during the upstroke of the fifth compression. The second rescuer may find it easier to establish this pattern of ventilation if he thinks of the rescue breathing as lifting the compressor's hands during the fifth upstroke.

The rescuer who is providing ventilation should feel for the carotid pulse frequently during chest compressions to assess their effectiveness. Every 4 to 5 minutes, ventilation and compression should be interrupted to check for return of spontaneous breathing and pulse.

After a time the rescuers may begin to tire and need to change the procedures they are performing. The rescuer performing chest compressions signals the rescue breather that he wishes to change by saying, "One-one thousand, two-one thousand, three-one thousand, four-one thousand, five-one thousand, *change—after—the—next—breath.*"

Using the middle and index fingers of one hand, the rescue breather quickly locates the lower margin of the victim's rib cage and runs his fingers up the rib cage to the notch where the ribs meet the sternum in the center of the lower chest. Holding one finger on the notch, he places the other finger next to it on the lower end of the sternum. After the third chest compression, he slides his other hand into the proper position on the sternum, sweeping the compressor's hands off the chest. He should pick up the fourth and fifth compressions. The chest compressor must not leave the chest until his hands are pushed off. He then moves directly to rescue breathing, interposing a a breath during the upstroke of the fifth chest compression. If he is not in time for the fifth compression, he should give the ventilation on the upstroke of the first or the second compression and then again on the next fifth upstroke to get back into the rhythm.

Artificial ventilation frequently causes gastric distension or air in the stomach. Although it is more common in children, distension also occurs in adults and is usually caused by excessive pressure exerted in rescue breathing and obstruction in the victim's airway. The distension can be minimized by limiting the volume of air interposed into the victim's lungs to the point at which the chest rises.

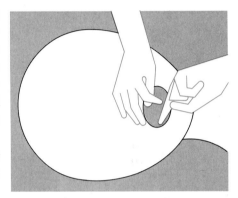

Marked distension of the stomach may be dangerous because it promotes regurgitation of substances in the stomach and reduces lung volume by elevating the diaphragm. When the stomach becomes distended during rescue breathing, the rescuer should recheck and reposition the airway, observe the rise and fall of the chest, and avoid excessive airway pressure. Rescue breathing should be continued, and no attempt to expel the stomach contents should be made. Manual pressure over the upper abdomen almost invariably causes regurgitation, and the stomach contents may enter the lungs.

In the event that regurgitation does occur, the rescuer should turn the victim's entire body on the side, open the mouth, and scoop out the debris with his fingers before continuing CPR.

If the victim's mouth does not open readily, the rescuer may have to pry it open with his fingers. The even pressure that is necessary to open an unconscious person's mouth is accomplished by the crossed-finger technique. The rescuer crosses his thumb under his index finger, braces his fingers against the upper and lower teeth, and pushes his fingers apart to separate the jaws.

The basic life support technique in CPR must be adapted to the special needs of infants and young children, persons with suspected neck injuries, and victims of severe obstruction of the airway by a foreign object.

There are a few important differences in administering CPR to infants and small children:

AIRWAY Since an infant's neck is extremely flexible, the rescuer must be careful to avoid exaggerating the backward position of the head tilt. Forceful backward tilting may block breathing passages rather than open them.

BREATHING If the infant or small child is not breathing, the rescuer should not pinch the nose shut. He should cover the victim's nose and mouth with his mouth and give one small breath every 3 seconds. The volume of air to inflate the lungs should be less than for an adult.

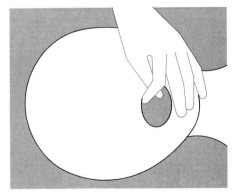

PULSE The absence of a pulse may be more easily determined by feeling over the left nipple.

CARDIAC COMPRESSION Although the technique for cardiac compression is different for infants and for small children, only one hand is used in both cases. The other hand may be slipped under the child to provide firm support for the back.

For infants, the rescuer uses only the *tips* of the index and middle fingers to compress the chest at mid-sternum. The sternum should be depressed ½ to ¾ inch at a fast rate—100 to 120 times a minute.

For small children, the rescuer uses only the *heel* of one hand to compress the chest. Depending on the size of the child, the sternum is depressed between ¾ inch and 1½ inches. The rate should be 100 to 120 times a minute.

For both infants and small children, breaths should be administered during the relaxation following every fifth chest compression.

Neck Injury The possibility of neck injury should be considered for victims of automobile and diving accidents. If neck injury is suspected, the techniques described in the section on opening the airway should be modified to prevent further damage. The rescuer should keep the victim's head in a fixed, neutral position and open the airway by using the jaw thrust maneuver. This is accomplished by grasping the angles of the victim's lower jaw and lifting with both hands, one on each side, to bring the jaw forward while tilting the head backward. The rescuer's elbows should rest on the surface on which the victim is lying.

When mouth-to-mouth breathing is necessary, the victim's nostrils are closed by the rescuer's cheek pressed tightly against them. If the victim's mouth is closed, the thumb of one hand is used to retract the lower lip.

Choking Emergency relief for the victim whose airway is completely obstructed by a foreign object varies according to whether the victim is conscious or unconscious and the amount of training the rescuer has had.

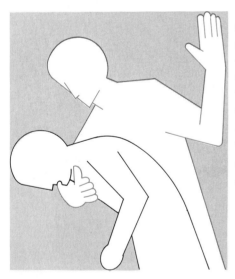

CONSCIOUS VICTIM A choking person who is unable to speak clearly and is attempting to dislodge and expel a foreign object should not be interfered with. The rescuer should be prepared to take immediate action, however, when any of the following signs are present: weak, ineffective coughing; bluish color of the skin or lips; clutching the throat; and inability to speak. The first step, then, is to deliver 4 back blows rapidly and forcefully to try to dislodge the object. The back blows are delivered while the rescuer stands beside and slightly behind the victim. One hand is on the chest for support while the other is used to deliver 4 sharp blows between the shoulder blades with the heel of the hand.

If the back blows do not dislodge the object, the rescuer should then try manual abdominal thrusts. In this procedure, the rescuer stands behind the choking victim, wraps his arms around the waist, and locates the navel with the fingers of one hand. Making a fist of the other hand, the rescuer presses the thumb against the victim's abdomen about 1 inch above the navel. The other hand is then placed on top of the fist, and 4 quick thrusts are exerted upward and inward.

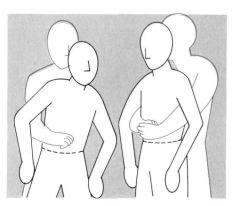

The 4 back blows and the 4 manual thrusts should be continued until the object has been expelled. This procedure may also be followed when the victim is sitting in a chair. If the victim becomes unconscious, the following sequence of procedures should be attempted.

UNCONSCIOUS VICTIM Sudden collapse and loss of consciousness is a grave emergency, since a lack of air for 4 to 6 minutes may result in irreversible brain damage. When this emergency occurs while a person is eating, the collapse may be due to other causes besides obstruction of the airway by a foreign object. The victim may have fainted or suffered a heart attack or

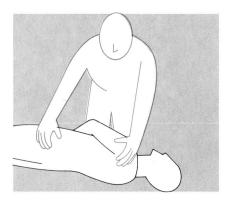 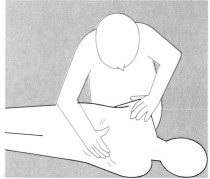

stroke. However, the first priority for an unconscious victim, regardless of the cause of the collapse, is to insure an open airway and to call for help.

If the victim is not breathing and can be ventilated, the rescuer should proceed with mouth-to-mouth rescue breathing. If there is no pulse, he should proceed with cardiopulmonary resuscitation.

If the rescuer has found an unconscious victim, called for help, opened the airway, and attempted to ventilate but cannot, the following procedures should be performed immediately: Reposition the victim's head and try again to ventilate. If this attempt fails, the rescuer should roll the unconscious person on his side and administer 4 back blows. Rolling the victim is accomplished by placing one hand on his shoulder and the other on his hip. The unconscious victim is rolled toward the rescuer so that his weight is supported by the rescuer's thighs; the hand on the victim's shoulder remains in position to keep the body steady. The other hand should be raised about 12 inches from the victim's back and a blow struck with the heel of the right hand between the shoulder blades. Four forceful blows should be administered in rapid succession.

If these measures fail to dislodge the obstruction, 4 manual thrusts should be given. Manual thrusts are of two kinds: chest thrusts and abdominal thrusts. The chest thrust is used for obese or obviously pregnant victims and is the safer technique. The correct position of the hands on the chest is the same as for administering CPR and should be followed explicitly. Once the correct position has been located (see illustration for cardiac compression), the rescuer should administer 4 downward thrusts in rapid succession to compress the chest cavity. This maneuver creates pressure in the victim's windpipe and pushes the obstruction further up so that it can be cleared by the rescuer's fingers.

To administer abdominal thrusts, the rescuer must turn the victim face upward from the side position he was in when the back blows were delivered. The rescuer should take a position facing the victim's head, his body parallel to the unconscious person's and his knees close to his hips. The heel of one hand is placed on the victim's abdomen about 1 inch above the navel, and the other hand is placed over it.

The rescuer should begin the abdominal thrust with elbows bent, then sharply straighten his arms to push his hands into the abdomen. (The hands should never push down on the victim's abdomen.) Four manual abdominal thrusts should be given to accomplish the same purpose as for chest thrusts— to force the obstruction up to where it can be cleared from the victim's

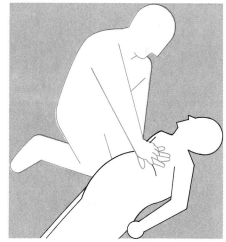

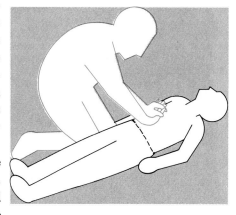

PRINCIPLES

1. Signals of heart attack are sometimes so subtle they are ignored. The alarming ratio of one out of two deaths from heart attack could be changed if symptoms were recognized

and emergency care administered in the first hour of the attack.

2. *Although not necessarily warnings of a cardiac emergency, disturbances in the rhythm and rate of the heartbeat should not be ignored. Pulse rate should be taken for a full minute and the regularity of the pulse determined. Radical changes in rhythm demand immediate emergency care.*

3. *The most common signal of heart attack is pain or pressure under the breastbone that lasts 2 minutes or longer. There may also be sweating, nausea, shortness of breath, or a feeling of weakness, but these symptoms are not always present.*

4. *If danger signals persist for 2 minutes or longer, all physical activity should cease and the victim should sit or lie down, depending on which is more*

ADVANCED CARDIAC LIFE SUPPORT

comfortable. Emergency rescue action must begin promptly.

5. *Emergency rescue units available in most communities or through police and fire departments should be contacted immediately, even though there is doubt that a heart attack is occurring. A nearby hospital offering emergency cardiac care can provide life-saving services if the victim of heart attack is taken there quickly. Advance knowledge of how to reach such emergency rescue units is of critical importance, and telephone numbers should be readily available.*

6. *Cardiopulmonary resuscitation (CPR) may be necessary if the victim of heart attack has collapsed, has no pulse, and is not breathing. However, only those who have received instruction in CPR from qualified personnel should attempt to revive an unconscious person suspected of having a heart attack.*

7. *Training in CPR is available through local chapters of the American Heart Association. All persons are urged to receive instruction in these life-saving techniques, which are reviewed in this chapter.*

mouth. If the obstruction is not dislodged, the cycle should be repeated: 4 back blows, 4 manual thrusts, and a finger probe.

It is important to note that as a victim becomes more deprived of oxygen (anoxic), muscles will relax and previously unsuccessful attempts to remove an obstruction may become effective. When the muscles relax or the obstruction is partially dislodged and the airway partially open, slow, full, and forceful ventilation may keep the person alive while bypassing the obstruction.

If the rescuer is successful in removing the foreign body, he should begin mouth-to-mouth ventilation or cardiopulmonary ventilation if necessary. Any vomit in the victim's mouth should be removed by turning the head to the side and wiping it out quickly with the fingers before proceeding.

The sequence of manual maneuvers is the same for adults, children, and infants whose airway is obstructed by a foreign object. The positioning of an infant or small child and the method of applying back blows are slightly different, however. The rescuer holds the victim face down over his forearm, with the child's head and chest in a dependent position. Back blows are delivered between the shoulder blades. If the back blows are ineffective, 4 manual chest thrusts should be administered while the child is being held. The chest thrusts are the same as those used in cardiac compression.

A heart attack victim's chances of surviving the period immediately after the attack are greatly increased by special care units designed to provide maximum surveillance and therapy. When combined with cardiopulmonary resuscitation, these emergency measures are called advanced cardiac life support. An advanced cardiac life support unit provides equipment and instruments that open and maintain the airway, provide artificial ventilation and circulation, monitor changes in heart rhythm (usually through an oscilloscope, which translates the heart's electric impulses into visual terms), provide intravenous infusion, and defibrillate the heart (stop uncoordinated rhythms and restore a normal beat).

The specially trained and equipped members of such a unit, called paramedics or emergency medical technicians, first attempt to stabilize the victim's condition by assuring regular breathing. In the absence of spontaneous breathing, artificial means are employed. Circulation is maintained by cardiac compression, and a stable heart rhythm is sustained, usually by administration of drugs. Only when the patient's condition is considered stable will he be transported to a hospital for additional care.

Advanced life support systems are in operation throughout the United States; they are mobile units which come to the scene of a heart attack or other medical emergency. In the event that emergency aid is not available, it is usually wise to move the victim of a suspected heart attack to a place where such care is available. The period immediately following a heart attack is so critical, and expert monitoring and treatment so essential, that no time should be lost. It is important to learn the location of a facility providing advanced life support before a cardiac emergency arises. Such information can be obtained from the American Heart Association or a physician. Concerned individuals might well consider working for the creation of an emergency medical system in any community that does not have one. The value of such a system in reducing the tragic death toll from heart attack has been proved time and again.

7

THE ANNUAL CHECKUP

Donald F. Leon, M.D.

Ask any owner of a valuable piece of machinery whether a regular checkup by a competent mechanic is likely to keep his costly investment operating smoothly for a longer period of time, and chances are he'll answer "Yes." Indeed, many manufacturers' guarantees are contingent on regular inspections for possible adjustments. During these routine checkups, the expert may notice mechanical defects that were not obvious to the owner. He may spot wear and tear on a fan belt, for example, which could cause it to break without warning and possibly damage the engine by overheating. The owner may become aware of slight changes in performance—sluggishness in pickup or an occasional unfamiliar noise—not so severe as to warrant calling a repairman but significant enough to report at the routine inspection. And because of his training and experience the expert will be expected to locate the source of trouble and determine whether it indicates an impending serious malfunction, requires repairs, or is normal considering the length of time the equipment has been in use.

Although conscientious attention to the care and maintenance of a manufactured product cannot guarantee that trouble will not occur, the chances of a breakdown are appreciably decreased and in many instances avoided. The same principle applies to the human body and in particular to that vital pumping organ, the heart, and the arteries and veins that together compose the cardiovascular system. Regular checkups are essential to detect conditions that may lead to a breakdown in the cardiovascular system, and they can often signal the need for "repairs" before a problem progresses from a simple annoyance into a serious threat to health. But unlike a piece of machinery, the body cannot be traded in for a new model, and malfunctions must therefore be regularly monitored if they are to be corrected or kept from doing further damage.

The examination is best performed by the doctor who is primarily responsible for your long-term health, although occasionally other experts may be consulted. Your doctor will set the schedule for the checkups, taking into account such individual factors as your age, past illnesses, and present condition. In general, yearly checkups are recommended, but more frequent evaluations are advisable in a large number of cases. There are five major components of a cardiac evaluation: a medical history, a physical examination, a chest X ray, an electrocardiogram, and certain special tests. The first four are basic to a proper examination; the special tests are a matter for professional decision in each case.

MEDICAL HISTORY   A history—a careful review of symptoms, complaints, past illnesses, habits, and family history of illness—is a vital aspect of the initial evaluation. The doctor must make a thorough search to uncover clues to aid the diagnosis as well as to estimate the limitation produced by a heart condition. At subsequent checkups only the intervening history will be added to the medical record. This later information is of the utmost importance because it indicates the succcess of treatment or the possible deterioration of the condition. The initial medical history consists of six parts: the patient's profile, his or her chief complaint, the history of the present illness, the past history, the family history, and a review of symptoms related to the various body systems.

THE PATIENT'S PROFILE The doctor begins his examination by asking questions about age, marital status, and number of children. He will want to know whether you are working or retired. What is the nature of your job? What do you do when you are not working? What stresses in your life might affect a heart condition? All these factors contribute to the effect of a heart condition on the patient and the family. And as patterns of long-term evaluation and care develop between patient and physician, the profile assumes an important role in all decisions about tests and treatments.

CHIEF COMPLAINT The symptomatic patient—that is, the person whose heart condition manifests itself in identifiable symptoms—usually has one symptom which causes more distress than any other. This most troublesome symptom, called the chief complaint, is the one that the patient thinks requires most attention. However, many people with active, significant cardiac conditions have no symptoms sufficiently troublesome to classify as a chief complaint.

PRESENT ILLNESS High on the list of chief complaints are chest pain; shortness of breath; palpitations (rapid or fluttery heartbeats); swelling of the legs, ankles, or feet; fatigue; and fainting. Other chief complaints, reported rarely, are a bluish discoloration of the skin known as cyanosis and coughing up small amounts of blood. While these complaints do not point directly to any specific diagnosis, they do serve as a starting point for detailed inquiries. A patient whose chief complaint is chest pain, for example, might also complain, but to a lesser degree, about palpitations or ankle swelling or some other cardiovascular manifestation. Chest pain can be of several types, and only after learning all the characteristics of the pain is it possible to draw any conclusions regarding its significance.

PAST HISTORY Once a chief complaint has been identified, the doctor will want to know its history. If it is chest pain, he will want to know when the pain first occurred. Where is it located? What does it feel like? Are there any factors that seem to bring it on? How long does it last? What helps it disappear? Has it changed any since it first began? The doctor may also want to know whether temperature, meals, or physical activity seem to influence the pain. A similar series of questions must be explored for each complaint, for a complete history includes information on whether the patient has previously suffered any of these complaints or has ever had a heart attack, a heart murmur, rheumatic fever, or any other indicators of heart disease earlier in life. The doctor will also want a record of surgery and of illnesses, including the common diseases of childhood. To the patient this may seem like ancient history and unrelated to the heart problem, but in fact many clues to the cause of heart conditions are to be found in earlier illnesses.

Personal habits are significant factors, too, and the doctor will try to identify risk factors by asking: Do you smoke? Cigarettes, cigar, a pipe? How much and for how many years? What are your dietary habits? How much salt, fat-containing foods, sugars, starches, and protein do you ordinarily consume? How much alcohol do you drink? What is your total calorie intake for an average day? How much exercise do you get? Is it conditioning exercise, such as walking, cycling, or swimming? Or do you engage in muscle-building exercise, such as push-ups or weight lifting?

FAMILY HISTORY   Additional important clues can be provided by the kinds of illnesses found among the patient's blood relatives, both those living and those who have died, and the causes of their deaths. A family history of heart disease, high blood pressure, high blood cholesterol levels, diabetes, rheumatic fever, or nephritis (a kidney ailment) may influence the way a physician will evaluate and treat a related condition in the patient.

REVIEW OF SYMPTOMS   To complete the initial medical history, the doctor tries to determine whether any other symptoms are present by asking key questions about each of the major body systems. He will inquire about headaches, visual or hearing problems, difficulties in breathing, problems with swallowing and digestion, bowel habits, urinary problems, and bone, joint, or muscle complaints.

After assembling all the historical information, the doctor will have a good idea about what troubles you, what might have caused the problem, how much you are actually suffering at present, and how the illness might influence your family and associates. Compiling a good medical history can consume considerable time, but fortunately it has to be done only once, provided you remain in the care of the same doctor.

PHYSICAL EXAMINATION

Another important aspect of a periodic checkup is a thorough physical examination of the cardiovascular system. When coupled with the medical history, the information gained from physical findings leads to an accurate diagnosis. Moreover, certain physical findings are indicators of the seriousness of a cardiac problem. When these findings do not change from one examination to another, they indicate that your condition has probably not worsened and any therapy appears to be on the right track.

The physical examination includes checking blood pressure, pulse count, and rate of breathing. It also includes feeling (palpating) the key pulses, the chest wall that overlies the heart, and the right side of the upper abdomen. The doctor carefully examines the artery and vein pulses in your neck and, with a stethoscope, listens to your heart, lungs, and perhaps over your abdomen and selected pulses. He also checks your liver and examines your feet and ankles for swelling due to fluid accumulation.

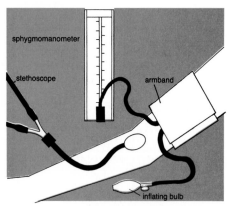

Blood Pressure Measurement

Blood Pressure Measurement
A flat, rubber bag wound around the arm is inflated until circulation in the main artery of the arm is cut off. As air pressure in the armband is gradually released, the sound of blood returning at its maximum pressure (systole) is heard through a stethoscope. As the air pressure slowly diminishes, the sound disappears at the low point of blood pressure (diastole).

BLOOD PRESSURE   Blood pressure is measured with an instrument known as a sphygmomanometer. During the pumping stroke of the heart, when the heart muscle contracts (systole), the pressure in the arteries will rise to peak blood pressure, and the figure registered on the gauge of the sphygmomanometer is called the systolic pressure. During the phase in which the heart muscle relaxes (diastole), blood pressure drops to its low point; this figure is known as the diastolic pressure.

PULSE RATE   Traditionally, the pulse is taken by feeling the pulsations in the artery on the thumb side of the wrist and counting the number of beats in a fifteen-second period. The number is then multiplied by four to get the number of heartbeats per minute. With heart patients, however, the pulse is often counted for a full minute. If there is any irregularity, the pulse at the wrist may not be accurate, especially in a brief time span. Therefore, to get an accurate reading, the doctor listens over the heart with a stethoscope. In that way he can identify minor irregularities in the heart rate which cannot be picked up by feeling the pulse with his fingers. The pulse rate—eighty per minute, for example—is put into the medical record along with a description of any irregularities.

BREATHING   The doctor observes your breathing pattern to see whether it is labored—that is, requires more effort than normal—and whether it is regular or irregular. He also counts how many breaths you take in a minute. He listens for wheezing and watches the motion of the chest cage during several breaths. He studies your fingernails, earlobes, and the tip of your nose for cyanosis, which is caused by less-than-normal amounts of oxygen in the blood. The many causes of cyanosis include lung and heart problems.

KEY PULSES   The next step is to check the major arterial pulses to see if they are present and of normal fullness. The most important pulses lie in the two carotid arteries, the blood vessels which run up each side of the neck, and the femoral arteries, one on each side of the groin. The carotid pulses are important because they are closest to the heart and provide many clues to how the heart is working. The femoral pulses give some important clues about high blood pressure and about hardening of the arteries in and around the abdomen.

HEART   Usually, a heart examination is performed with the patient lying down on an examining table, clothed in an examining gown or covered with a sheet. Before listening to your heart with a stethoscope, your doctor feels with his hand various areas of the chest wall overlying your heart. By palpating, he can tell whether there is any enlargement of the heart or increased pressure in its chambers, and he can also identify "thrills"—that is, murmurs that can be felt—and very prominent heart sounds. A doctor who is skilled in cardiac palpation is able to make very specific and accurate determinations based on his findings.

Listening to the heart through a stethoscope is called auscultation. It is a highly refined technique which provides valuable information that often cannot be found in any other way. Careful auscultation of the heart takes time, several minutes at least, and involves listening over many specific areas of the heart and during various phases of breathing. The doctor may ask you to turn on your side so that he can hear certain sounds better, or he may want you to squat down from a standing position.

The patient's end of the stethoscope has two or three listening pieces, and the doctor uses these to detect high-pitched or low-pitched sounds when these are soft and difficult to hear. Normally, he hears two distinct sounds each time the heart beats—a first sound and a second sound. Actually, there are several components of the first sound, which are almost simultaneous, and two components of the second sound, which are very close to each other but can be distinguished in most patients. The various components of the first and second heart sounds represent closure of each of the valves of the heart. These two sounds as heard through the stethoscope have been described as "lub, dub."

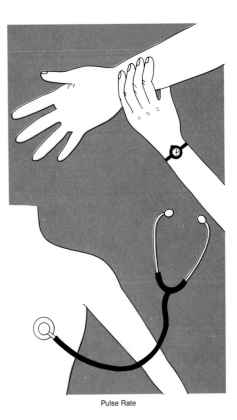

Pulse Rate

Pulse rate is measured by counting the number of pulsations felt in the artery on the thumb side of the wrist or, more accurately, by listening to the heartbeat through a stethoscope.

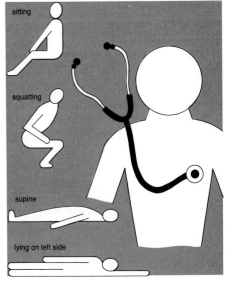

sitting

squatting

supine

lying on left side

Positions for Auscultation

The closing of the heart valves can be heard through a stethoscope as two distinct sounds, described as "lub, dub."

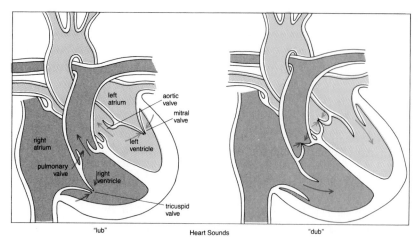

"lub"   Heart Sounds   "dub"

Sometimes a whishing sound, called a murmur, is heard, even in people with normal, healthy hearts, as blood flows through the heart chambers and valves. These sounds are called functional murmurs or innocent murmurs, and they are particularly common among children and teenagers and in young women, especially during pregnancy. But they are found in most other age groups as well. Cardiac murmurs result from turbulence in the bloodstream, which causes vibrations that produce sound waves. The turbulence may be caused by blood being forced through a narrowed, roughened heart valve, or through a deficit in the wall (septum) separating two chambers. It also occurs when the valves do not shut completely, allowing a backflow of blood into the upper heart chambers (atria) or the lower chambers (ventricles).

Abnormal extra heart sounds called gallops, as well as abnormal heart murmurs, are usually readily identifiable by the doctor. The term gallop is used because the cadence of such a sound resembles that of the gallop of a horse. Some abnormal sounds and murmurs are very soft, which is why the modern stethoscope, capable of picking up soft sounds, was developed. The intensity of abnormal sounds and murmurs does not, however, necessarily indicate the seriousness of a heart condition, and there are some types of heart conditions that do not produce any such abnormal sounds.

LUNGS   In ancient times, merchants thumped casks to see how much wine they held. They knew that the sound produced from an empty cask is different from one that is full. Using the same principle your doctor can tell if there is congestion in your lungs by examining the front and back of your chest during various breathing phases. He will thump (percuss) your chest, listening and feeling for areas of dullness representing fluid between the lungs and the chest wall. He also locates your diaphragm in this way and checks to see that it moves properly during respiration. As you breathe in and the lungs expand, both sides of the diaphragm should move down.

In the next step, the doctor places his hands over different parts of your chest while you utter certain high-pitched sounds, such as the word "ninety-nine." Ordinarily these sounds transmit strongly to the outside of your chest and can be easily felt. However, when a portion of the lung is heavily congested or when fluid has accumulated between the lung and the chest wall, the impact of spoken words is decreased and therefore not felt. With the stethoscope, the doctor listens at points that cover the entire area of the lungs as you breathe in and out. If a lung is congested, typical extra breath

The faint sounds of breathing are magnified by the stethoscope and the doctor listens to different areas of the chest.

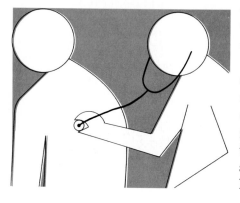

sounds, called rales, will be heard, usually over the lower portion of the chest. Louder, scratchy sounds, called rhonchi, are made if there is excess mucus in the large airway tubes. These sounds, which are quite different from rales, are usually caused by the kind of congestion that results from cardiovascular disease.

LIVER   The next organ to be examined for signs of a heart problem is the liver. This very large organ, sitting in the upper right-hand portion of the abdomen under the rib cage, enlarges under certain circumstances, one of which is congestion caused by heart problems. Therefore, the doctor will ask you to breathe deeply in and out so that he can locate the lower edge of the liver by pressing with his hands on your abdomen. He notes whether or not it is tender and whether it is smooth or lumpy (nodular) and then finds the top margin by thumping. A normal liver is four to five inches (ten to twelve centimeters) long from top to bottom, and is smooth and is not tender. A congested liver will be longer than usual and will probably be tender and yet smooth.

FEET AND ANKLES   The pulses in the feet and those behind the ankles and knees are the final checkpoints. Swelling (edema) which can be dented with the fingertip (pitting edema) around the feet and ankles indicates fluid accumulation and congestion. Your doctor checks your lower legs for normal warmth, which serves as an index of the adequacy of your circulation. While doing that, he also looks for swollen or dilated (varicose) veins.

All these checks constitute the bare essentials of a cardiovascular examination. A careful physician frequently conducts a more encompassing examination, looking carefully, feeling, and auscultating many other areas.

Another major component of a thorough cardiac evaluation is getting a clear picture of the size and shape of the heart and the general condition of the lungs. This is obtained through one or more X-ray techniques, including fluoroscopy. The objective is to obtain a good visual image of the structures inside the chest, using the technique best suited for that purpose. In many cases, ordinary chest X rays, when properly taken in two views, provide sufficient information and a permanent picture which can be kept and compared with subsequent X rays. The ability to compare pictures over the years is a valuable asset for diagnosis. In a routine chest X ray—the back-to-front view—the front of the chest is placed against the film, which is in a container called a cassette. The tube, the source of the X rays, is usually situated six feet behind the subject. At that distance, X rays travel in parallel lines when they pass through the chest and strike the film, thereby reducing the distortion of the shapes on the final picture. The lateral, or side-view, X-ray film is exposed in the same way. This view is frequently important and should be routinely taken.

In a few instances, most notably during pregnancy, it may be desirable to avoid exposure to X rays. If a chest X ray during pregnancy is really necessary, it should be done after the first three months, and a lead shield should be hung across the lower back, between the patient and the X-ray tube, to protect the fetus from exposure. Actually, a single picture can be taken with relative safety during the first three months of pregnancy if it is absolutely

X-RAY TESTS

X rays are emitted from the tube in which they are produced, passing through the chest and onto a film which, when developed, outlines the inner structures of the body.

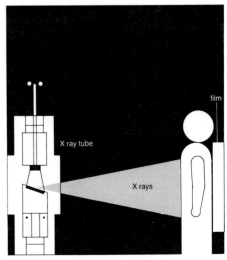

Routine Chest X Ray

necessary and the shielding is carefully done. The X-ray dose for a single view is very small.

The picture obtained from X-ray exposure shows dense or hard structures like bones as white, thick structures like the heart as white, and air-filled structures like the lungs as gray. Areas where no structure lies between the X-ray source and the cassette show up as black. When the doctor reviews the X-ray pictures, he examines every structure reflected on the film: the soft tissues, the ribs and other bones, the lungs, and the heart. When looking at the heart, he can judge its overall size and determine whether any chamber or vessel is enlarged. Abnormal calcification of tissue in the heart can sometimes be seen. When looking at the lungs, he can see whether the lung arteries and veins are normal. Abnormal fluid accumulation between the lung and the chest wall shows up, particularly if the patient takes a proper deep breath. In some cases, lung congestion is visible.

The doctor may order an oblique (angular) chest X ray for a better view of one or another heart chamber. Ordinarily, the accuracy of this technique is enhanced if the esophagus, the channel which leads from the mouth to the stomach and lies directly behind the heart, is filled with barium. Barium, a chalky thick liquid, shows up very white on an X ray and improves the outline of the chamber on the back of the heart (the left atrium). Barium is not pleasant to the palate in spite of various artificial flavorings, but its reputation is worse than its actual taste.

Much additional information about the function of the heart can be gained through the use of fluoroscopy, an X-ray technique which provides moving pictures of the internal structures of the body. The doctor can observe the contraction and expansion of the chambers of the heart and the large vessels by means of shadows cast on a screen as the structures are being X-rayed. In the past, the quality of the fluoroscopic image was not always optimal, because it was viewed on a faint glass screen in a dark room. Higher X-ray currents improved the image, but exposing a patient to more than a few moments of fluoroscopy was undesirable. Recent electronic advances now permit the use of very low currents, with very faint images electronically brightened many times over. Television cameras transmit this brightened picture, and the final image on a large screen can be easily displayed in a lighted room. Image-intensified fluoroscopy allows better identification of abnormal calcification inside the heart, and the various movements can be seen clearly. The disadvantage of modern fluoroscope viewing is that it requires very expensive machinery which is generally available only in a hospital or an X-ray specialist's office.

ELECTROCARDIOGRAM   An electrocardiogram (ECG), the recorded markings made by electric charges in contracting heart muscles, is the fourth major component of a good cardiac checkup. An easy test, the ECG takes about ten minutes and is completely safe. Over the years, as ECG recording and analysis have improved, some people have concluded that a normal ECG necessarily means a normal heart and that an ECG alone may be enough for a checkup. Neither conclusion is correct. Many people with normal electrocardiograms have heart problems. Neither an ECG nor any other single test can take the place of a thorough evaluation.

How exactly does electrocardiography work, and what does it show? Each time the heart beats, it does so because of minute changes in sodium and potassium in the heart muscle cells. There are literally thousands of such cells in a heart, and these cells beat in a specific sequence which takes a little less than three-quarters of a second. Each case contains many particles of sodium and potassium, and each particle has a minute electron charge attached to it. If the number of sodium and potassium particles in each cell are multiplied by the number of cells, it becomes evident that literally millions of particles change their electron charges during the three-quarters of a second that it takes a heart to beat once. The very tiny electrical current caused during each beat can be recorded on the surface of the body, amplified in an instrument called the electrocardiograph, and printed, on a paper chart. The ECG leads, which are small metal contacts connected by wires to the electrocardiograph, do not put any current into the patient's body; they simply pick up the current transmitted to the skin surface as a result of the heartbeat. The electric power used in the ECG is only that needed to run the amplifier and the motor which moves the strip of paper on which the markings are recorded.

Normally, the heart beats in a certain sequence. First the two upper chambers of the heart (the right and left atria) contract. The muscles of these chambers are small, and their contraction causes a small ECG wave

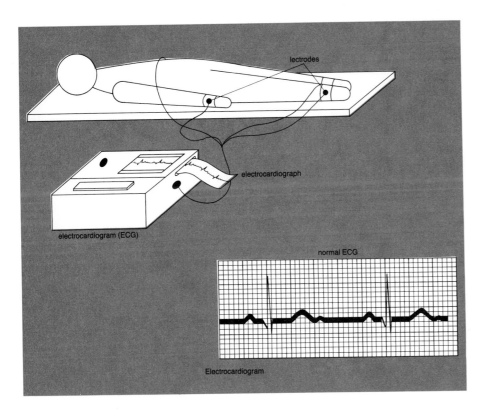

Electrocardiogram
Electric impulses produced by the heart are amplified and printed with a heated stylus on a strip of paper.

which is called a P wave. After a moment, the two major pumping chambers (the right and left ventricles) contract. Their muscle mass is comparatively much greater, and as the contraction spreads through this muscle mass, a large wave form called a QRS appears. As the sodium and potassium in the cells of the ventricles readjust to get ready for another heartbeat, they form a T wave on the graph. The normal ECG complex thus contains a P, a QRS, and a T wave for each heartbeat, and each beat therefore shows the same pattern on the graph. Modern electrocardiography is designed to analyze the P, QRS, and T waves from twelve different directions. Standards for normal appearance on the graph paper have been set for each of the twelve leads, and the specific criteria for identifying abnormalities are well known.

A correctly done ECG reveals several facts about the heart. By reading the graph, the doctor can tell what the heart rate is and whether the rhythm is normal. If it is abnormal, he usually can identify the abnormal rhythm with accuracy. He can detect enlargement of any of the four chambers with a good degree of reliability. He can also locate any significant scars in the heart muscle; such scars often result from heart attacks. He can detect an under-supply of blood to any part of the heart muscle, and he can see evidence of certain drugs and medications which the patient may be taking. The graph will also show whether the sequence of the contraction wave through the heart is normal. With all the information available from the ECG, a comparison of tracings over the years can provide data about the progress of a heart condition which cannot be obtained otherwise. A skillful doctor realizes, however, that an ECG is a laboratory test and subject to some of the vagaries that limit all laboratory tests in medicine and therefore that it must always be considered in the light of other findings.

SPECIAL TESTS The fifth and last major subdivision of the cardiac evaluation consists of special tests. As the word special implies, not everyone requires such tests, since in most periodic checkups all the information the doctor needs is obtained from the medical history, physical examination, X-ray tests, and electrocardiogram. In certain cases, however, special tests are required; among them exercise stress testing, ambulatory electrocardiography, heart-sound recordings, ultrasound tests, cardiac catheterization, and X-ray vascular contrast tests.

EXERCISE STRESS TESTS The purpose of these tests is to determine whether evidence of coronary heart disease is uncovered during exercise and, if such evidence is disclosed, to determine the level of exercise tolerance at which such changes occur. An ECG is taken during and after levels of exercise determined by age and physical condition.

The Master Two-Step Test, devised more than forty years ago by Dr. Arthur M. Master of Mount Sinai Hospital in New York, uses a two-step apparatus over which the subject walks at a specific rate of speed. The subject walks to the top step and then down to the other side; this is counted as one trip. The number of trips is standardized for age, sex, and weight, and the prescribed number of trips should be completed in as close to three minutes as is possible. An ECG is taken before and after this simple test, which can be given in a doctor's office.

More modern exercise stress testing employs a treadmill or sometimes a bicycle exercise unit called an ergometer. Electrocardiographic tracings are recorded before and during exercise. The exercise work load is progressively increased until the subject either demonstrates an abnormal response or reaches the level of exercise considered maximal for his or her age and physical condition. The tracings continue to be recorded during the time of recovery from stress. This system has the advantage of providing tracings at any time during the exercise. In addition, the exercise work load is known at all times during the test and can readily be reduced at a later date. Stress testing, properly performed, has become a valuable tool in the diagnosis of coronary heart disease and in measuring the exercise load necessary to provoke an abnormal response. The latter can be useful in evaluating the success of treatment as time passes.

Very recently a new level of diagnostic accuracy has been achieved by coupling radioactive isotope scannings of the heart with exercise stress testing. When a portion of the heart is insufficiently supplied with oxygen during stress, the picture obtained by radionuclectic imaging may identify the precise area of inadequate blood supply and distinguish it from the surrounding normal heart muscle.

AMBULATORY ELECTROCARDIOGRAPHY In recent years, with improved equipment, it has become possible to record an ECG continuously for a number of hours during which the person being tested goes about normal daily activity at work or while eating or resting. The technique, called ambulatory electrocardiography or dynamic electrocardiography, requires the patient to carry a small ECG tape recorder. Most such devices use high-quality magnetic tape to register the ECG wave complexes. The tape can be played back rapidly, and thus every heartbeat can be analyzed later by a doctor. The magnetic tape reveals exactly what disturbances in cardiac rhythm occurred during the recording period. Usually the subject is asked to keep a diary of activities during the recording period so that various levels of activity can be related to specific rhythm disturbances. The disadvantage of this method, which requires a small computer, is the high cost of the equipment needed to analyze the tape. Because of that expense, many doctors send the tapes to an analyzer rather than purchasing an expensive, infrequently used piece of equipment. Large medical centers are more likely to have their own analyzers because of the large number of tapes recorded in the center.

PHONOCARDIOGRAPHY The recording of heart sounds and murmurs, called phonocardiography, is an old technique that has been highly refined over the years. It is easy to use and quite safe and permits the doctor to listen to the heart in various positions or after the patient inhales certain substances which increase blood flow. An ECG lead marks the onset of each heartbeat, and the doctor places one or more microphones over different areas of the chest where sounds and murmurs are clearly heard. Often more than one pulse tracing can be recorded at the same time. Although phonocardiography rarely picks up sounds that cannot also be heard with a stethoscope, the technique permits the exact timing of heart sounds, and murmurs can be determined precisely. Sounds that may be misinterpreted when heard through a stethoscope can be properly identified from the phonocardiographic tracing. Moreover, the technique provide a permanent record which can be used for subsequent comparisons.

ECHOCARDIOGRAPHY A relatively new technique in cardiologic examination,

Microphones positioned on the chest pick up heart sounds, which are recorded then by the phonocardiograph into a permanent visual record. An electrocardiogram is simultaneously recorded as a timing reference.

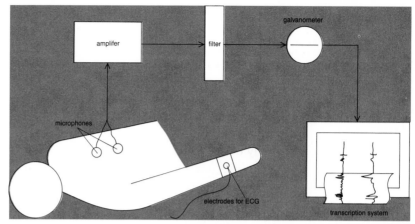

Phonocardiography

the ultrasound test called echocardiography is based on the principle of sonar. Sonar is used on ocean-going vessels to sound out the distance between the bottom of the ship and a solid structure, such as the floor of the ocean or a rock formation. When this technique is applied to the body, a microphone is positioned so that it sends out ultrasound waves which are reflected back into the microphone by the various structures inside the heart. The returning signals are caught electronically and proceed into a picture, or image. As the image is watched on a screen, movement of heart valves and chamber walls can be observed quite easily. The procedure, which is quite safe, uses an electrocardiographic lead tracing to mark each heartbeat. However, an adequate test may take as long as an hour because the various structures inside the heart must be found and visualized by the echo beam. The test provides valuable information on a number of heart problems, and in many instances a good echocardiographic test will answer questions that in the past could have been answered only by cardiac catheterization techniques.

CARDIAC CATHETERIZATION   The heart catheter test sometimes arouses anxiety among patients in spite of its safety and reliability. However, it is still the best test to get accurate information about heart function. It must be performed by a physician and requires expensive equipment and, almost always, hospitalization of the patient. In most instances, the patient experiences only slight discomfort, much of which is due to having to lie still for a long time. Injections of local anesthetics such as novocaine, using very small needles, are given to avoid pain from larger needles or from very small incisions required to get to a vein or artery just beneath the skin.

The principle of the heart catheter test is relatively simple. Long, narrow, sterilized tubes (catheters) are introduced into arteries and veins lying just under the skin near the elbow and frequently near the groin. In each individual case, the physician decides in advance which blood vessels are to be used, the kinds of catheters, and exactly which measurements are to be made. On the average, two or three catheters are required, and these are filled with the balanced salt water solution used for intravenous treatment. One end of the catheter is placed in a blood vessel, either by means of a needle or through a small incision. The other end is attached to precision instruments which accurately measure pressure and can be used to measure how much blood the heart is pumping per minute.

After the catheters are in place in the arm or groin blood vessels, the physician, wearing a sterile gown like those worn by surgeons, uses an image-amplifyng fluoroscope to watch the catheters as he very cautiously advances each one through the blood vessels toward the chest, into the large central vessels, and finally into the interior of the heart. Throughout this procedure, the electrocardiogram and the blood pressure at the tip of the catheter are constantly recorded to insure safety. Because the catheters follow the same route in which the blood flows, the patient need not fear that the tubes are being stuck through the chest or any other tissue.

Catheterization is rarely used to make a new diagnosis. Rather, it is used to confirm an already suspected condition and to measure the extent of the damage which that condition is causing. When the catheters are positioned in the interior of the heart, blood pressure can be measured in the heart chambers themselves. If there is a valve problem, the pressure difference across the diseased valve supplies an index of the severity of the disorder. Cardiac output—the amount of blood pumped by the heart—can also be measured. In one method, the difference in the amount of oxygen in the blood can be measured from two catheter tips while the patient breathes into a large bag so that oxygen intake can be measured. Another method is to inject a few drops of dye through one catheter and withdraw the dye from another in order to see how rapidly it gets to the tip of the second catheter. These measurements of the blood-pumping rate and the cardiac output are necessary for assessing the function of the heart.

After the measurements have been taken, the catheters are withdrawn, and bleeding at the point of entry, if any, is readily controlled by applying pressure. If an incision was made, as is often necessary, a few superficial stitches close the cut. The calculation of the measurements from a heart catheterization test may require a day or more for analyzing the data and preparing a report. This sort of delay should be expected, because a physician rarely is able to give a final report as soon as the test is finished.

CARDIAC ANGIOGRAPHY   A variation on catheterization is called angiography. In this technique, X-ray contrast dye is put into a blood vessel or heart chamber and X-ray pictures are taken. The dye clearly outlines the internal shape of the vessel or chamber in question. In cardiac angiography, an ounce or two of the contrast dye is introduced into a heart chamber through a catheter. Usually a mechanical injector is used, because it is almost impossible to inject the material fast enough by hand. The X-ray pictures may be made in one of two ways, each having an advantage in specific cases. In one method the image is recorded in a fluoroscopic device with a high-speed movie camera; the other method involves taking ordinary full-sized X rays rapidly with an automatic device. Both give detailed information about structural deformities inside the heart and are a valuable adjunct to cardiac catheterization.

Angiography of the coronary arteries—selective coronary arteriography —is being used more and more frequently, both alone and in association with cardiac catheterization. The catheter, however, is different from the kind used to enter heart chambers. It is maneuvered into the opening of the coronary arteries, just above the aortic valve. Then, with catheter in position, less than a third of an ounce of X-ray dye is injected by hand directly into the coronary arteries, and X-ray pictures are recorded. The procedure has become highly

PRINCIPLES

1. *A heart checkup begins with the doctor's interviewing the patient to gather information about age, occupation, habits, family medical history, past illnesses, and current complaints. A person with heart disease may have a single noticeable symptom, such as chest pain, shortness of breath, palpitations, swelling of the feet or ankles, fatigue, fainting, bluish discoloration of the skin, or blood in the sputum. In many cases, there are no obvious symptoms.*

2. *The physical examination includes checking blood pressure, pulse count, and breathing rate. The doctor feels pulses in the neck to evaluate circulation to the head, and in the groin, legs, and feet to test circulation to the legs. He thumps the chest and listens with a stethoscope to determine if the lungs are congested or if there is fluid in the lungs or between the lungs and the chest wall. He listens with the stethoscope to the sounds made by the opening and closing of the heart valves, and he checks the rhythm of the heartbeat. Pressing on the abdomen with his fingers, the doctor checks the size of the liver and the condition of the spleen, kidneys, and abdominal aorta. Feet and ankles are examined for any swelling, which may be a sign of cardiovascular disease.*

3. *Chest X rays provide important information about the size and shape*

*of the heart and the general condition
of the lungs. They also provide a
permanent record of all the structures
within the chest cavity.
Image-intensified fluoroscopy, an
X-ray technique, is sometimes used to
view the movements in the heart and
to identify abnormal calcification.*

4. *An electrocardiogram (ECG), a record
of the electric impulses within the
heart, provides information on heart
rate and how impulses travel through
the heart. It also reveals any scars on
the heart muscle, a sign of damaged
heart tissue.*

5. *Special tests required in unique
conditions may include use of one or
more of the following:*

*A stress test, in which an ECG is
taken during and after specific levels
of exercise, determines the heart's
exercise-tolerance level. It may also
disclose a disease condition that is not
evident at rest but becomes apparent
under stress.*

*Phonocardiography amplifies and
records heart sounds and permits an
exact timing of the sound as well as
accurate identification of vibrations
and murmurs.*

*Echocardiography, a new technique
in which ultrasound waves are
beamed into the heart, reflected back
on a recording device, and then
processed into an image, allows the
doctor to view movements of heart
valves and chamber walls and to
examine the condition of tissues.*

*Cardiac catheterization is done in a
hospital under local anesthesia. A
long, narrow tube (catheter) is
inserted in a blood vessel and guided
into the heart with the help of a
fluoroscope. Instruments measure the
blood flow and pressure in different
areas of the heart.*

*Cardiac angiography, which is similar
to catheterization, introduces a dye
into a blood vessel or chamber of the
heart. Moving X-ray pictures provide
information on the structure of the
vessels and are useful in identifying
deformities or obstructions in the
heart.*

refined and requires considerable skill, but it provides information about coronary artery problems and the causes of chest pain that simply cannot be found by any other method. There are a great many doctors who are competent to perform the test, and every day hundreds of persons throughout the United States undergo it—an indication of its value in cases of suspected coronary artery disease.

Angiographic techniques are applied to many structures besides the heart and coronary arteries. It can be used to outline virtually every major blood vessel system in the body. When angiography outside the heart is performed, the pictures are usually recorded on rapidly exposed full-size X rays, since high-speed cameras are less effective for blood vessels outside the heart.

Some patients may have an allergic reaction to the contrast dye. This can be predicted if you know that you are allergic to seafood or have previously shown an allergy to X-ray dyes. An allergy that appears for the first time during a test usually causes a few hives and itching which respond immediately to an antihistamine, and no problems are likely to develop. When doses of about two ounces of dye are used, the patient may, for a few moments, become uncomfortable, warm, and occasionally nauseated. These symptoms pass quickly and frequently do not recur with later tests.

It is very important to remember that special tests are required by only a few patients and should not be regarded as a routine part of a cardiac examination. Some of these tests are better suited for some cases than for others, and hardly any patient will require all the tests. In any event, all the tests described have been proved safe, and each provides important information which is not otherwise available.

In addition to the standard cardiac tests, some doctors like to have the results of certain simple screening tests normally done in a general physical checkup. These laboratory tests include a blood count to check for anemia or infection, a urine analysis as an initial survey of kidney function, and several blood chemistry tests, which might include a blood sugar test for hidden diabetes and a blood urea nitrogen test (BUN for short), which is a screening test for kidney problems. In recent years, it has become common practice to check blood lipids in most adult patients. Lipids are the various fatty substances in the blood, and two in particular, the levels of cholesterol and triglyceride, have been found to be related to the onset or progress of coronary disease. Before cholesterol and triglyceride tests, the patient is asked to fast for sixteen hours, which might therefore require a separate trip to a laboratory. Not infrequently, several members of a family have similar lipid problems, so the doctor may suggest that the test also be done on members of the patient's immediate family.

Careful examination by a personal physician during periodic checkups has proved to be the cornerstone of good comprehensive care for heart patients. Every person with a heart problem, no matter how mild, is strongly urged to participate in such a program. It is one of the most important steps you can take to safeguard your health.

8

HOW THE HEART FUNCTIONS

John T. Shepherd, M.D., D.S.C.

The human body is an intricate ecological system, a series of interrelated chemical, biological, and physical processes that sustain life in a wide range of environmental conditions. To understand how this complex system functions, it is helpful to look at its basic building block, the cell. The unicell, or single living unit, is the smallest independent form of living matter. Indeed, life on earth began in the single-celled organism, of which the most familiar is the amoeba. The single-celled organism draws in oxygen and such foodstuffs as glucose and vitamins, which are then physically and chemically transformed into more cellular material or into sources of energy. That process, called metabolism, enables the organism to live, grow, and reproduce itself. The organism also gives off waste products, just as an oil-burning furnace gives off its waste in a volatile or vapor form as smoke, or a wood- or coal-burning furnace leaves its nonvolatile waste as ashes. For the amoeba, the source of nutriments is the surrounding sea water in which it lives. Its waste products are eliminated directly into the environment, the volatile carbon-dioxide waste evaporating into the atmosphere and the nonvolatile waste dissolving in the sea.

Gradually, in the long evolution of life, more complex, multicellular organisms came into being. In these advanced life forms, groups of cells combined to form tissues and organs capable of specialized tasks beyond the capacity of the single cell. And as these more complicated functions evolved, a much vaster energy-producing and waste-disposal system was needed than the one that served the amoeba floating in the sea.

The organization of cells into more and more complex groups with more and more complex functions reached its most advanced stages in the higher vertebrates and particularly in man. Scientists estimate the number of cells in the adult human body in hundreds of billions, millions of which die and are replaced daily. Entire groups of cells (skin, bone, and connective tissue) exist mainly to protect or support other groups of cells. Within the framework of that support are the groups of specialized cells which form organs involved

The cell, the smallest form of living matter, is a highly complex unit composed mainly of water and several small organs called organelles. Each organelle is responsible for carrying out a specific function.

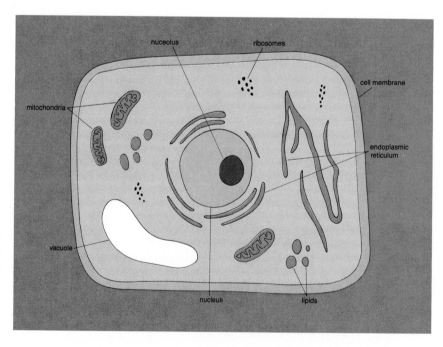

with communication (brain and spinal cord), digestion (stomach and small intestine), locomotion (skeletal muscles), respiration (lungs), and excretion (kidneys and large intestine). But no matter how diversified their functions, all cells have the same basic needs as the amoeba—a supply of nutrients and a means of eliminating waste products. And, as a reminder of the unicellular origin of life, each cell of the most complex multicellular organism is surrounded by a fluid which is remarkably similar to sea water.

The extracellular fluid is present in only minute amounts, but its composition cannot vary, except within narrow limits, without affecting the proper function of the cell. To maintain this internal environment in optimum condition, there must be a continuous stream of nutrients from the outside world and a continuous stream of waste products from the cells. The exchange is made possible by specialized tissues (lung, gut, and kidney) and a transport system (the cardiovascular system) that links the specialized tissues with the individual cells.

THE LIFE-SUSTAINING BLOODSTREAM

The circulatory system—the network of arteries, arterioles, capillaries, venules, and veins—transports blood from the heart to the cells and back again to the heart in a never-ending stream. If the full quantity of blood that courses through this closed system were weighed, it would be about 8 percent of the total body weight. In an average adult male weighing 154 pounds (70 kilograms) that is equal to approximately 11 pints (5.6 liters). Approximately half of that volume is made up of red and white cells, together with particles called platelets. The other half consists of a pale amber fluid known as plasma.

The red blood cells contain hemoglobin, a complex protein arranged around iron, which has the important role of taking up large quantities of oxygen as it passes through the lungs and then passing this oxygen to the body cells. As the blood in the lungs picks up oxygen, the hemoglobin becomes bright red (arterial blood). When the hemoglobin reaches its destination, the individual cell, it releases oxygen and picks up carbon dioxide, a waste product of metabolism. The color of the blood carrying carbon dioxide to the lungs for elimination from the body is a bluish red (venous blood). Hemoglobin has another important function; helping to maintain the acid balance of the blood. Each day the carbon dioxide resulting from cellular metabolism is equivalent to a little more than one-half gallon (2.6 liters) of concentrated hydrochloric acid. That high concentration of acid would injure the cells, so nature provides a neutralizing base, half of which comes from the food consumed each day and the remainder from the body's built-in buffering agents, one of which is hemoglobin.

In a healthy person the approximately 25 trillion red blood cells outnumber the white cells by about 700 to 1. Each red cell has a life span of three to four months, and an estimated 8 million of them are produced every second to replace an equal number of worn-out cells. The white cells vary in size and shape, but all share the essential function of ingesting and digesting invading bacteria. The platelets, named for their resemblance to tiny plates, are also part of the body's defense system. They trigger the blood-clotting process and thus prevent loss of blood through injury.

The plasma is a solution consisting of 90 percent water plus various salts, mainly sodium chloride, in concentrations similar to those in the extracellular fluid. Plasma also contains glucose, free fatty acids, cholesterol, and proteins.

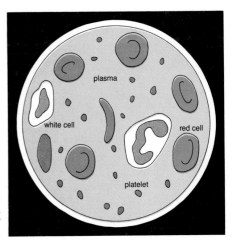

The composition of blood, showing red and white cells, together with platelets, suspended in plasma.

Plasma proteins, formed mainly in the liver, have several very complex functions. They transport molecules of iron, hormones, and lipids; act as antibodies in immune responses; join with sodium bicarbonate and other salts to buffer changes in the acidity or alkalinity of the blood. Plasma proteins provide a force which draws fluid from the intracellular space into the bloodstream—a mechanism called oncotic pressure which provides for the transport of waste products away from the body cells—and they also contribute an essential component to the chemical reactions leading to blood clotting.

STRUCTURE OF THE HEART   The continuous flow of blood throughout the circulatory system depends on the heart, a hollow, muscular organ divided into four chambers. The heart, the center of the cardiovascular system, is situated in the chest cavity between the two lungs. Its size varies with the size of the individual and is roughly the equivalent of two clenched fists. It weighs, in a fully developed adult, between 11 and 16 ounces (312-454 grams) and is conical in shape—wider at the top than at the bottom. The interior of the heart is divided into two pairs of compartments, the right atrium and right ventricle and the left atrium and left ventricle. The wall dividing the two sides of the heart is called the septum. Both atria are collecting chambers, into which blood flows and from which it

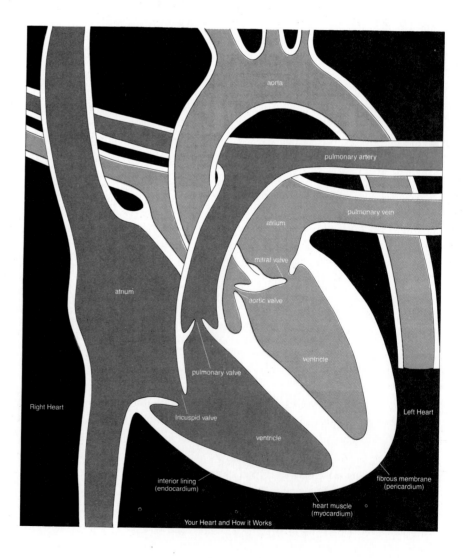

Your Heart and How it Works

is expelled into the two ventricles, which are both pumping chambers. The right atrium receives blood from the venous system and passes the blood depleted of oxygen to the right ventricle. The right ventricle then propels the blood through the large pulmonary artery leading to the lungs. The left atrium receives blood from the lungs, which is newly enriched with oxygen and ready to be pumped by the left ventricle to all parts of the body, including the heart itself. The oxygen-rich blood courses through the body via the arterial system.

When the ventricles contract, the blood that is being expelled is prevented from flowing back into the atria by means of two valves consisting of thin leaflets of tissue attached by thin tendons (chordae tendineae) to small muscles in the ventricular wall (papillary muscles). The papillary muscles contract with the ventricles, tightening the tendons and holding the valves firmly closed. The valve between the upper and lower chambers in the right side of the heart consists of three cusps; hence its name, tricuspid valve. The corresponding valve on the left side of the heart consists of two cusps in triangular shape, and because it resembles a bishop's headdress, it is called the mitral valve. The heart contains two other valves, the pulmonary valve and the aortic valve. The pulmonary valve lies at the junction of the pulmonary artery and the right ventricle, the aortic valve at the junction of the aorta and the left ventricle. These two valves are called semilunar valves (here, too, the name refers to the shape of the valve—in this case crescent-shaped). The pulmonary and aortic valves open during the ejection of blood from the ventricle but, because they are one-way valves, close to prevent backward flow when the heart muscle relaxes.

The heart itself, like every organ in the body, requires a steady supply of oxygen-enriched blood to perform. Blood for the heart is provided by the coronary arteries, which arise from the aorta in two branches that arch down over the top of the heart. When the heart is working at an increased level, the coronary vessels dilate, making more blood available to meet the increased oxygen requirements of the heart muscle.

The interior of the heart is lined with a smooth membrane, a single layer of cells called the endocardium. The same kind of membrane also lines the valves and the blood vessels, where it is called the endothelium. The lining prevents damage to the blood cells by reducing friction and by minimizing the danger of blood-clot formation either inside the heart (intracardiac) or inside the blood vessels themselves (intravascular). Between the endocardium and the outer layer of the heart (epicardium) is the muscular wall itself, the myocardium, consisting of muscle cells surrounded by connective tissue. This connective tissue is particularly abundant in the areas where the tricuspid and mitral valves are attached.

The many anatomical connections between muscle cells in the atria and the ventricles form the basis for the conduction of impulses from cell to cell. Near the entrance of the two veins that bring blood from the upper and lower parts of the body into the top of the right atrium (the superior and the inferior venae cavas) is a small bundle of highly specialized muscle fibers that generate impulses necessary for the coordinated contraction of the heart. This bundle is called the sinoatrial node, or pacemaker. The impulses from the sinoatrial node are collected and conveyed to the ventricles by another group of cells in the connective tissue between the left and right sides of the heart. This group is called the atrioventricular node, and from it other specialized muscle

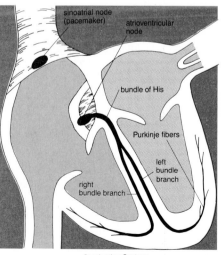

Conduction System

fibers, called the bundle of His after the German anatomist who discovered them, run from the upper to the lower chambers, splitting to left and right as they descend. The two main branches of the bundle of His connect with a network of smaller impulse-carrying fibers (Purkinje fibers), which run to all parts of the ventricles. It is by means of this intricate system of specialized fibers and cells that the heart receives the electrical impulses necessary to maintain a rhythmic, effective, and concerted beat.

The heart's intricate pumping, valve, and impulse-carrying system is protected by an outer fibrous double-layered membrane, called the pericardium, which surrounds the heart and the roots of the great blood-carrying vessels. The two layers of the pericardium are normally separated by a thin film of fluid.

THE CARDIAC CYCLE The four chambers of the heart are, in effect, a series of interreacting pumps whose function it is to renew the body's blood supply. When the ventricles relax, blood flows from the two venae cavas into the right atrium and from the pulmonary veins into the left atrium. During this first phase of the heart's pumping cycle, called diastole or period of relaxation, two of the heart's valves are open—the tricuspid, which allows blood to flow from right atrium to right ventricle, and the mitral, which allows blood to pass from left atrium to left ventricle. The blood flowing into these ventricles causes their volume to increase steadily because of the increased fluid pressures. The passage of blood from the atria is not a purely passive action, however, for both atria actually contract and force blood into the two ventricles.

The impulse to contract originates in the sinoatrial node. The impulse then travels to the atrioventricular node, and both ventricles now also contract as the impulses run swiftly along fixed routes through the remainder of the heart muscle. This phase of contraction of the ventricle muscle is called systole. The pumping stroke of the heart causes a rapid increase in pressure inside the ventricles, and that pressure in turn forces the tricuspid and mitral valves to shut, cutting off further flow of blood from the atria into the ventricles. The vibrations and turbulence that result from this activity are the first heart sounds a physician hears with a stethoscope.

That, in effect, is the beginning of the heart's rhythmic cycle. As the ventricles contract further, internal pressure mounts until it exceeds the pressure in the aorta and the pulmonary artery. With the difference in pressure, the aortic and pulmonary valves open, the ventricular walls shorten, and about

The heart's pumping cycle. In the diastole or relaxed period, blood flows through the open valves into the lower chambers, assisted by the contraction of the upper chambers (atrial systole). In the second phase of the cycle, the lower chambers contract (ventricular systole). The almost simultaneous nature of the pumping cycle is indicated by the time, given in fractions of a second.

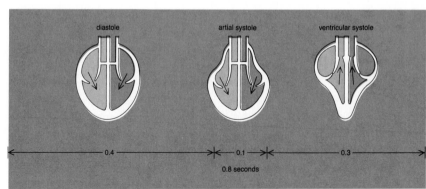

half of the blood in the ventricles is expelled into the aorta and the pulmonary artery. The amount of blood expelled by each ventricle is called the stroke volume; it is about 3 ounces (90–100 milliliters) when a person is at rest. The full amount of blood does not flow through the arteries all at once, however, since its passage is impeded at the terminal branches of the pulmonary artery and the aorta. As a consequence, the larger blood vessels become distended with blood during ventricular contractions.

When the ventricles relax (diastole), the backflow of blood from the aorta and the pulmonary artery causes the aortic and pulmonary valves to close. The closing of the valves gives rise to the second heart sound detected by a stethoscope, the familiar "lub, dub" sound. With muscular relaxation, the pressure in the ventricles drops below that in the atria, and the tricuspid and mitral valves open. The cardiac cycle is ready to begin again.

Since both sides of the heart are in series on the same circuit, both ventricles pump the same amount of blood per unit of time. The amount of blood that each ventricle pumps out in a minute is called the cardiac output; it is determined by the number of heartbeats in a minute multiplied by the amount of blood pumped out of the heart at each contraction (the stroke volume). When a normal adult is resting, each ventricle pumps out about 5 quarts (5.7 liters) of blood each minute—roughly 2,100 gallons (7,980 liters) a day. Over a biblical lifetime of three score and ten years, the heart pumps enough blood to fill about thirteen supertankers capable of carrying more than a million barrels each. But these calculations are only for the heart at rest—during strenuous exercise the heart's output can increase as much as five to six times that amount.

Even though both sides of the heart pump the same amount of blood per unit of time, they do not perform the same amount of work in that time. Because the lungs are close to the heart, much less energy is required to pump blood through the lungs than through the rest of the body. Moreover, the walls of the pulmonary vessels are thinner, and as a result the pressure generated by the right ventricle is about six times less than that generated by the left. The difference in the amount of work performed explains why the left ventricle is much larger and thicker than the right; in fact, the left ventricular wall is usually about three times thicker.

The two sides of the heart are able to pump the same amount of blood per stroke because the heart muscle cells contract more strongly the more they are stretched. If more blood enters the right ventricle, for example, the muscles of that ventricle stretch to accommodate the increased volume. The "stretch" then forces the muscle cells of the right ventricle to squeeze that much harder than normally, and much more blood is pumped into the pulmonary vessels. This in turn results in an increased flow of blood to the left side of the heart, which squeezes to expel more. This mechanism was described by the English physiologist Ernest Henry Starling (1866-1927) and his associates in 1914, and the principle they formulated is known as Starling's law of the heart. By this mechanism, the amount of blood ejected by both sides of the heart is balanced from beat to beat.

Describing the involved pumping process of the heart makes it sound like a long series of events, but in reality the single phase of systole and diastole is almost simultaneous, lasting less than a second. As the great English scientist William Harvey (1578-1657) observed, "Those two move-

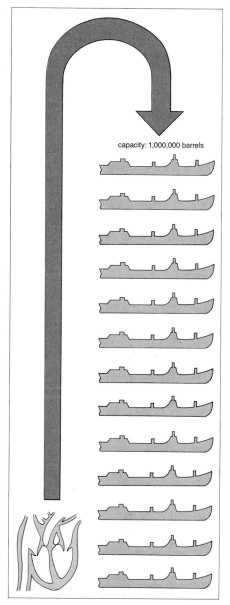

capacity: 1,000,000 barrels

The amount of blood the heart pumps in a minute multiplied by the amount of blood pumped with each contraction can reach the astounding volume depicted here. In the course of a life, the heart will have pumped enough blood to fill 13 supertankers, each with a capacity of 1 million barrels. As extraordinary as this figure is, it represents an average volume pumped by a heart at rest. Since the average person does more than "rest" in a lifetime, the volume of blood the heart pumps is actually many times that represented. During strenuous exercise--running, swimming, cross-country skiing, for example--the heart may pump as much as six times the volume it pumps when the body is at rest.

ments, one of the auricles [atria] and the other of the ventricles, occur successively, but so harmoniously and rhythmically that both [appear to] happen together and only one movement can be seen."

CIRCULATORY SYSTEM

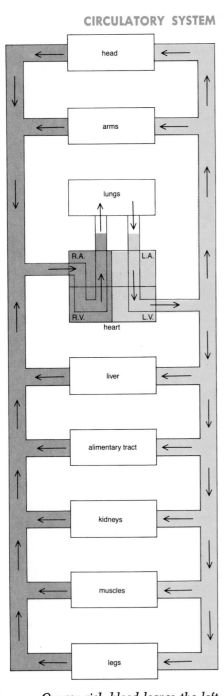

Oxygen-rich blood leaves the left ventricle via the aorta, which branches out into an intricate network of arteries carrying blood to all the organs of the body. Veins then carry the oxygen-depleted blood back to the heart, which pumps it through the lungs for a fresh supply of oxygen.

The heart is the center of the cardiovascular system, but the arteries, the channels through which oxygenated blood moves, also play a critical role. They are the supply lines to all the organs and tissues of the body and to the heart itself. Systemic circulation, the flow of blood through all parts of the body except the lungs, takes place in a great arch from the left ventricle, through the body, then back to the right atrium. Oxygenated blood leaves the left ventricle through the aortic valve into the aorta, the body's largest artery, which is about 1 inch in diameter. The heart's own blood supply is furnished by the coronary arteries, so called because they circle the heart like a crown. The left and right coronary arteries arise from the aorta, just beyond the aortic valve. Although coronary arteries are small (their diameter is about the same as that of a soda straw), they draw off about 4 percent of the cardiac output.

Immediately beyond the aortic valve, the aorta ascends from the left ventricle in an arch. Three major arteries—the innominate, the left common carotid, and the left subclavian—arise from the top of the arch. The innominate divides into two major vessels, the right common carotid artery and the right subclavian artery. The left and right common carotid arteries subdivide into a vast network to feed the cells of the neck and head, particularly the brain. The left and right subclavian arteries bring blood to the chest, the shoulders, and the arms.

The lower half of the body is supplied with oxygenated blood by the downward-turning aorta. Smaller arteries branch off from the segment above the diaphragm, called the thoracic aorta, to supply the chest. Below the diaphragm, the aorta is called the abdominal aorta, from which arteries fan out, each involved with the functioning of a specific organ: gastric arteries feed stomach tissue; hepatic arteries, the liver; renal arteries, the kidneys. Below the stomach the abdominal aorta splits into the right and left iliac arteries, which conduct blood to the pelvis and the legs. The femoral arteries are the major source of supply for the thighs, and the popliteal arteries provide for the circulation to the lower extremities.

The arteries divide into smaller branches, the arterioles, which act as adjustable faucets controlling the amount of blood delivered to each tissue. From each arteriole in turn, a network of fine tubes, the capillaries, reaches out to surround the tissue cells. Capillaries are so constructed that oxygen and nutritive materials can pass through them into the tissues, while at the same time carbon dioxide and other waste products exit from the tissues into the bloodstream. Capillaries converge to form larger vessels, the venules, which then feed into still larger collecting vessels, the veins. The system of veins parallels the great arterial tree, but in reverse order, returning the oxygen-poor blood to the heart. The venous system ends at the right atrium; here the superior vena cava deposits the blood it has carried from the upper part of the body, while the inferior vena cava does the same with blood from the lower part.

The walls of the blood vessels are composed of endothelium, muscle cells, and supporting tissue. All blood vessels have an endothelium, but the amounts of the other components vary according to the function the vessel performs. The aorta and the large arteries contain mainly connective tissue; the arterioles, mainly muscle cells; the veins and venules, a mixture of both; and the capillaries, only endothelium.

This network of arteries, arterioles, capillaries, venules, and veins comprises some 60,000 miles (96,540 kilometers) of tubing. Once the oxygen-depleted blood is deposited in the heart, a similar succession of vessels carries it through the lungs. With each contraction of the right ventricle, blood is propelled into the pulmonary artery, which soon subdivides into two branches, one to each lung. In the lungs, the arteries fan out into arterioles to reach all parts of the lungs. The arterioles end in clusters of capillaries that surround microscopic sacs filled with air. It is here that the exchange of carbon dioxide and oxygen takes place. The now oxygen-rich blood flows through a network of venules and veins which ultimately converge to form four pulmonary veins, two from each lung. The pulmonary veins enter the left atrium where, with the beginning of the cardiac cycle, the blood starts on its flow through the arteries.

To understand how the body's circulation is regulated, it is helpful to consider certain principles governing the flow of liquid through tubes and how these principles are related to the flow of blood through the body.

REGULATORS OF CIRCULATION

1. Liquid flows only from points of higher pressure to those of lower pressure.

2. Any tube resists the flow of fluid through it; the longer the length of the tube, the thicker the fluid (its viscosity), and the smaller the diameter, or bore, of the tube, the greater the resistance. In the human body, the length of the tubes (blood vessels) does not vary much, and the viscosity of the fluid (blood) remains relatively constant. Therefore, resistance is determined only by variations in the diameter of the blood vessels. If the diameter of the blood vessel decreases by half, the resistance offered by the blood vessel increases sixteenfold.

3. For a given resistance, the flow through a tube depends upon the pressure head; the greater the force at the point of origin, the larger the flow. Conversely, for a given pressure head, the flow is determined by the resistance; the higher the resistance, the lower the flow. The relationship of pressure, flow, and resistance is expressed mathematically as $P = F \times R$ (pressure equals flow multiplied by resistance). The body's blood pressure and the way in which it is naturally regulated observe this rule. In conditions where blood pressure tends to fall, the body compensates either by increasing the flow (cardiac output) through the system, or by increasing the resistance offered by the blood vessels. When the pressure tends to increase, the flow and the resistance are decreased. In this way the body maintains a constant blood pressure, and constancy is, in turn, the key to how the blood supply adapts to the individual needs of various kinds of tissues. Local alterations in the size of the arterioles determine blood flow in that particular area of the body, provided the pressure head remains constant.

4. Contraction of the heart transfers energy to the blood, but since the blood must overcome the resistance of the vessels it passes through, it loses part of the energy. Loss of energy decreases pressure, and the greatest drops

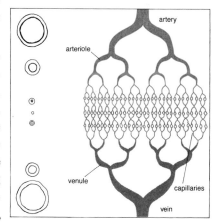

Large arteries divide into smaller and smaller branches until the smallest vessels, the capillaries, are reached. Capillaries converge to form larger vessels, venules, which converge into veins.

in pressure occur as the blood rushes through the small caliber arterioles.

5. The body's circulatory system is made up of a number of individual circuits (arteries, arterioles, capillaries, venules, veins), arranged in a parallel manner. As the diameter of the individual channel becomes smaller and smaller, the number of blood channels increases tremendously, from the aorta to the minute capillaries, and is greatest at the capillary level. As the capillaries converge to form venules and then veins, the total cross-sectional area of the vasculature decreases progressively, so that it is only slightly larger than that of the aorta and the venae cavas.

The fact that the total cross-sectional area is largest for the capillaries has important consequences for the exchanges occurring at that level. Since circulation is in a closed circuit, with the same amount of blood flowing through each section at each time, the velocity of flow becomes much less as the area increases, which it does at the capillary level. The velocity of blood flow is very high in the aorta, progressively decreases toward the periphery, and reaches its lowest level at the capillaries. The low velocity guarantees that there will be adequate time for the necessary exchanges with the extracellular fluid. From the capillaries, the blood accelerates as the total cross-sectional area decreases, reaching a final velocity in the venae cavas only slightly lower than that in the aorta.

6. Blood vessels are elastic tubes which expand with an increase in internal pressure (distending pressure) and shrink or recoil when the internal pressure decreases. The extent of the expansion is determined by two forces acting in opposite directions; pressure exerted by the heart on the blood (tending to dilate the vessels) and pressure exerted by the surrounding tissues (tending to compress the vessels). The blood vessels that supply the heart and skeletal muscles are subjected to wide variations in tissue pressure; each muscular contraction increases tissue pressure, thus compressing the blood vessels within the muscle. If the contraction is very strong, it can cause a complete halt of blood flow by offsetting the pressure generated by the heart. As long as the contractions alternate with relaxations (as with the heart's regular beating), the perfusion of the muscle cells with blood takes place between periods of increased tissue pressure. The increase in tissue pressure caused by rhythmically contracting skeletal muscles, together with the resulting compression of the blood vessels in the venous circulation, are important in returning venous blood to the heart against the force of gravity.

Role of the Blood Vessels The main goal of the blood vessels is to bring nourishment to the cells and to pick up waste products for removal to the outside of the body. To accomplish this goal, each component of the vascular system performs its own special function.

AORTA AND LARGE ARTERIES When the mitral and aortic valves open, the left ventricle suddenly expels a large volume of blood into the aorta and the large arteries. With the valve open, the pressure in both the ventricle and the aorta (systolic pressure) is equal. However, the aorta and the large arteries expand with each systole, because the resistance in the arterioles at the end of the arterial system does not allow the total amount of blood expelled by the heart to pass immediately into the capillaries. The distended aorta and arteries regain their original dimensions when the ventricle relaxes and the aortic and mitral valves close. The elastic recoil of the large arteries exerts pressure on the volume of blood, propelling it toward the periphery. The process maintains a relatively high pressure in the large blood vessels (diastolic pressure) at a time when the ventricles are relaxing. Thus the elastic property of the aorta and large arteries acts as a depulsator, transforming the intermittent flow generated by the contraction-relaxation cycle of the heart into a more steady flow in the capillaries.

ARTERIOLES   The arterioles are small in diameter, with a layer of muscle cells in their walls arranged so that the longitudinal axis of the cells follows the contour of the vessel. When the muscle cells contract, the diameter of the arteriole decreases; when they relax, it increases. Since the small diameter of the arterioles makes them the major determinant of vascular resistance, the moment-to-moment changes in diameter caused by the activity of the muscle cells have important consequences. The degree of opening of a given arteriole determines the amount of blood flowing through it, so the arteriole regulates the amount of blood going to a given capillary area.

The regulatory function of the arteriole can be compared to the action of a faucet; as long as the pressure head provided by the water tower (the heart) is constant (mean blood pressure), the amount of fluid flowing will depend on the degree of resistance offered by the faucet (arteriole). The critical question is how the degree of opening of the arterioles is established. The answer is related to the intrinsic activity of the arteriolar muscle cell. This activity is at its highest, and the diameter of the arteriole is at its narrowest, when the tissue being supplied with blood by the arteriole is at rest. When the tissue becomes active, the activity of the muscle cells lessens and the arteriole relaxes (increases in diameter). What inhibits the muscle cells of the arterioles is a decrease in oxygen concentration and the appearance of carbon-dioxide, hydrogen, and potassium ions, lactic acid, adenosine, and some other chemicals in the vicinity of the arterioles. In effect, the arterioles relax in proportion to the metabolic needs of the tissues they supply—active tissues mean "inactive" arterioles. While the tissue is active, the flow in the arteriole remains elevated, the muscle cells relaxed. When the activity ceases, the waste products are removed and a normal oxygen concentration is restored. At that point the intrinsic activity of the muscle cells again reduces the flow through the arteriole. The mechanism—as if it were a faucet that opened and closed with split-second timing—allows the organs of the body to receive an increased supply of oxygenated blood from the arterioles when it is needed. When, for example, the digestive organs begin to break down food, they receive extra blood supplies because the arterioles in that area of the body open.

CAPILLARIES   The capillaries, most of which consist of a thin layer of single endothelium cells, are so slender that ten of them bunched together are no thicker than a human hair. Red blood cells pass through each capillary one at a time in tandem, with plasma trapped between them. Between the cells forming the endothelium are small pores which allow water and waste products to pass from tissues to bloodstream. Larger entities, such as proteins, blood cells, and platelets, cannot pass through the pores and so remain in the capillaries.

The movement of fluid in and out of the capillaries is controlled by two opposing forces. Blood pressure within the capillary (hydrostatic pressure) tends to push water out of the vessel through the pores. That outward movement is counterbalanced by the attraction that plasma proteins exert on fluid outside the capillary (oncotic pressure). At the point where the smallest arterioles merge into the capillaries hydrostatic force is greater than oncotic attraction, and therefore water loaded with nutrients and oxygen leaves the capillaries for the extracellular fluid. As the blood moves along the capillary network, the proteins become more concentrated because of a loss of water. Thus a decrease in hydrostatic pressure is accompanied by an increase in oncotic pressure. When oncotic pressure exceeds hydrostatic, most of the extracellular fluid loaded with waste products and carbon dioxide is taken up at the side of the capillaries that merges into the venules. These capillary exchanges insure a continuous washing of the extracellular space. The fluid remaining in the extracellular space, called lymph, is eventually returned to the circulatory system via the lymphatic system.

The total area of the capillary walls in a human body is about 60 to 70 thousand square feet (roughly the area of one and a half football fields). The exchanges that take place throughout this vast area are not uniform, however; they vary according to the function of the organ involved. In the lungs, the hydrostatic pressure which drives fluid out of the capillaries into the air sac is about half the oncotic pressure exerted by plasma proteins. More fluid is retained in the capillaries of the lungs, therefore, and the air sacs are kept "dry," allowing the interchange of gases between air and blood to proceed without interference.

In the kidneys, however, the hydrostatic pressure inside the capillaries is about three times the oncotic pressure. Under these special conditions, great quantities of fluid are driven from the capillaries into a vast number of small tubes (tubules). Here waste products are extracted, but most of the water is returned to the bloodstream, as are essential elements such as glucose and sodium. Each kidney has roughly 1 million of these intricate screening mechanisms (which are called nephrons), the tiny clusters of capillaries and tubules that perform this cleansing function. Every twenty-four hours approximately 45 gallons (170 liters) of plasma pass through the filtering system, with about 99 percent reabsorbed and returned to the bloodstream. The remainder, only a little more than 1 quart (1.5 liters) of fluid and waste (urine), passes from the nephrons to the bladder for excretion.

LYMPHATICS The fluid that does not re-enter the capillaries after the exchange of nutrients and waste products is drained off and returned to the heart by way of the lymphatic circulation. All the lymphatic vessels in the body converge in one major vessel, the thoracic duct, which ends in one of the major branches of the superior vena cava. The lymph fluid is sucked into the vein by the rapid flow of venous blood. Lymphatics are equipped with swellings containing white blood cells, an essential factor in the body's defense against infection.

VEINS About 75 percent of the body's blood supply is contained in the veins, the reservoir controlling the return of the blood to the heart. Although the total blood volume remains constant, the distribution of blood within the system changes as the metabolic activity of various organs creates different levels of need. With muscular exercise, for example, the arterioles throughout the active muscle mass become widely dilated, increasing the total capacity of the vascular system. If the increased capacity was not immediately compensated for by decreased capacity in another part of the system, there would be a drop in the level of blood returning to the heart while the dilated arterioles were being filled. And that would be happening just when the cardiac output must be not only maintained but also increased markedly. Any rapid increase in cardiac output demands a sudden surge of blood toward the heart from the only available reservoir, the venous system. The veins are able to make such rapid moment-to-moment changes in capacity because their walls consist mainly of elastic tissue and muscle fiber. These cells have the power to contract actively, causing the surge of blood to the heart. To effect this, the contraction of the venous system must be coordinated by the body's nervous system.

The fact that man has evolved into an upright position subjects the veins in his limbs to a greater force of gravity than they would receive if he was a four-footed creature. To prevent backflow of blood to the periphery from sudden changes in hydrostatic pressure, valves have developed along strategic points in many of the larger veins of the human body, particularly those of the legs. The movement of blood toward the heart is greatly facilitated by the massaging action of the skeletal muscles, especially in the legs. This "muscle pump" is important during exercise performed when the body is upright, because both the muscles in the legs and the heart itself then require more oxygenated blood. In running, for instance, the very action of the leg muscles squeezing against their veins helps move some of the blood back to the heart, where it is reoxygenated to nourish the heart and legs during the period of exercise.

PULMONARY VASCULATURE Like the systemic vascular tree, this consists of a sequence of arteries, arterioles, capillaries, venules, and veins. There are, how-

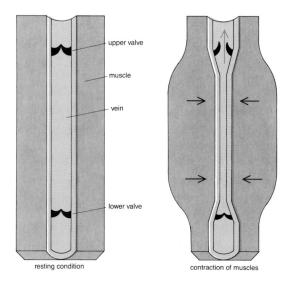

upper valve

muscle

vein

lower valve

resting condition

contraction of muscles

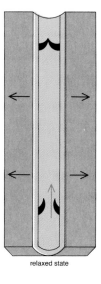

relaxed state

Contracting muscles compress the vein, forcing blood into an area of less pressure. Internal valves in the larger veins open to allow blood to flow toward the heart and close to prevent it from flowing backward.

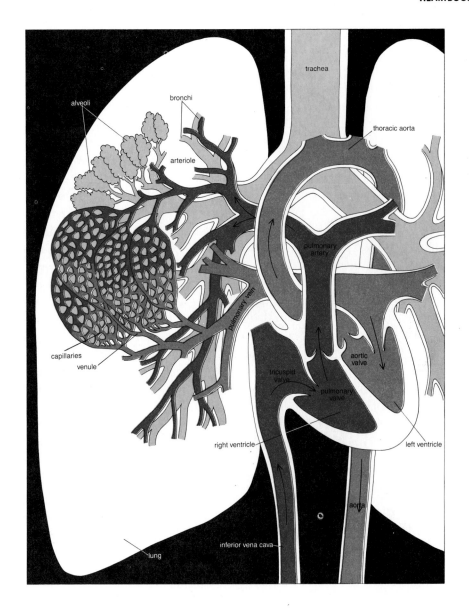

ever, some important differences between the two parts of the body's circula-tion. Because pulmonary arterioles are much wider than systemic ones, they offer much less resistance to the flow of blood. Less pressure is therefore needed to drive blood through the lungs, and pressure in the pulmonary artery is about six times lower than in the aorta. The low pressure also ex-plains why no fluid passes from the capillaries in the lungs into the air sacs. These sacs, or alveoli, increase in number from about 25 million at birth to several hundred million in the fully developed lungs. The total surface area of the alveoli is about 870 square feet (80 square meters), of which nearly 90 percent is covered with pulmonary capillaries. That means that the actual size of the area where lung capillaries and alveoli meet—the internal place of contact between the body and the air from outside it—is forty times greater than that of the more obvious place of contact, the skin.

Since both capillaries and alveoli have very thin walls, the large area of contact between them makes possible an effective diffusion of oxygen from the higher concentration in inhaled air to the lower concentration in the venous blood. In the same way, carbon dioxide diffuses easily from the venous blood to the air in the alveoli that is to be exhaled. The muscle cells in the arterioles of the lungs are sensitive to changes in the oxygen concentration in the alveoli. Unlike arterioles of other systems, those in the lungs contract when the oxygen concentration decreases. If some of the alveoli do not receive fresh air, the arterioles subserving the capillaries surrounding them will constrict so that only the ventilated alveoli are in contact with the blood. Without this safeguard, some of the venous blood going through the lungs would not be exposed to fresh air, and the total oxygen content of the blood leaving the lungs would be below normal.

It is helpful to consider the regulation of the body's circulatory system in terms of the concept of homeostasis—that is, the effort a system makes to maintain a steady internal environment despite multiple and varied demands made on it. Consider the myriad activities a human being can engage in: eating, drinking, making love, bearing children, writing books, laying bricks, shoveling snow, playing tennis. Each of these acts initiates a series of internal processes involving some parts of the body and not others and activating certain cells in certain ways. Homeostasis means that no matter what the activity, the body will attempt to compensate for the changing external and internal conditions, trying to maintain a constant environment while satisfying the requirements of the cells.

CARDIOVASCULAR CONTROL CENTERS

The cardiovascular system is, in effect, the body's major environmental control, being at once the source of power to keep the system operating, the means of delivering power where and when it is needed (in the form of oxygenated blood and blood sugars), a temperature-control mechanism regulating both heating and cooling processes, and the vehicle by which the waste products of all this activity are quickly and efficiently removed from the entire system. To perform so many complicated functions, the cardiovascular system utilizes a battery of sensors and monitoring devices which can either trigger corrective action or relay information on which other systems—the brain, for example—will act to restore equilibrium to the environment.

In order to meet the metabolic needs of the body tissues, blood pressure must remain constant. Any change in blood flow in a specific, localized area must be balanced either by compensatory increases in resistance to flow in other areas or by adaptation of total blood flow throughout the system. The balance is achieved by a series of monitors within the cardiovascular system. As the monitors constantly measure blood pressure, they relay the information into a central integration unit in the brain, where it is analyzed and compared with other data from other monitors. The brain units then send "commands" to the heart and blood vessels in the form of nerve impulses containing information on what adjustments are necessary. Chemical substances (hormones) are also secreted into the bloodstream to modulate the activity of the muscle cells of the heart and blood vessels, thereby supporting the nervous system in its monitoring function.

The Nervous System

Blood pressure is regulated primarily by the brain stem, where different groups of nerve cells (neurons) are specialized to control the activity of the heart (the cardiac centers) and of the blood vessels (the vasomotor center). The cardiac centers are in turn divided into a cardiac-activating center and a

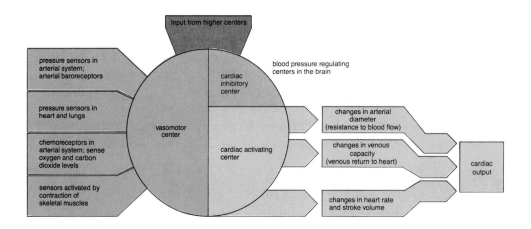

cardiac-inhibitory center, and the interaction of the two controls heart function. The vasomotor center governs the caliber (diameter) of the blood vessels by increases or decreases in its own activity.

Commands from the cardiac-activating center and the vasomotor center are conveyed by the sympathetic nerves. These nerves, distributed throughout the body and the vascular system, terminate in the immediate vicinity of the muscle cells in the heart and the blood vessels, although they do not actually touch cells or vessels. Contact between a nerve and a muscle cell is made through a chemical substance, norepinephrine (called a neurotransmitter), which is released from the activated nerve ending. The norepinephrine attaches itself to the membrane of the muscle cell and activates it. In the heart, the norepinephrine stimulates the cells of the sinoatrial node, the heart rate then increases, and the heart contracts more forcefully as the norepinephrine acts on the other heart muscle cells. At the same time the blood vessels, particularly the arterioles and the veins, constrict. Thus, the cardiac-activating and vasomotor centers unite to augment blood pressure by enhancing the return of venous blood, cardiac output, and peripheral resistance.

The brain's other cardiac control center, the cardiac-inhibitory center, operates in a different fashion. Commands from the inhibitory center are sent to the sinoatrial node only and are carried there by the vagus nerves. At the vagal nerve ending a different chemical substance, acetylcholine, is liberated by nerve impulses, and it attaches itself to the membranes of the sinoatrial node cells. Acetylcholine reduces the activity of these cells, and the heart slows. The inhibitory process is usually paralleled by decreased activity in the cardiac-activating and vasomotor centers, with the result that blood pressure falls.

The brain stem centers are informed by a major pressure sensor system located in the aorta and in the carotid arteries supplying the brain. The system consists of specialized cells, called stretch receptors, within the blood vessel wall. The cells are so arranged that they stretch as the pressure within the blood vessel rises, and the stretching causes them to send a nerve impulse or signal to the brain. When the cells are not stretched, the number of impulses decreases, which is what happens when the pressure in the aorta and the carotid arteries falls. When blood pressure rises in the aorta and carotid arteries, the stretching of the cells inhibits the cardiac-activating and vasomotor centers and at the same time stimulates the cardiac-inhibitory center.

This control system, which constantly alters the activity of the brain stem centers, normally maintains blood pressure within very narrow limits.

The brain also receives information from a second set of stretch receptors located in the heart and lungs. These receptors monitor the fullness of the vascular system, transmitting information on the volume of blood within the heart and lungs. Signals from these receptors lead to adjustments within the cardiovascular system, including the venous reservoir, via the sympathetic nerves. Longer-term adjustments in the total volume of blood in the system are brought about by the release of hormones from the brain into the bloodstream. The hormones permit the kidneys either to expel more fluid if the blood volume increases or to retain more if the volume decreases.

In addition to the pressure-sensing mechanism, there is another set of cells called chemoreceptors, which constantly "taste" the chemical composition of arterial blood. These cells are also situated in the aorta and the carotid arteries. That both chemoreceptors and stretch receptors are located in the same site is significant—the composition of blood to the brain is continuously monitored at the same time that the pressure head to the brain is being registered. If, for example, the chemoreceptor cells note a decrease in oxygen in the blood or an increase in concentration of carbon dioxide ions and hydrogen ions, they send impulses to the respiratory center. Respiration then increases, in order to bring more oxygen to the blood as it passes through the lungs and to eliminate more carbon dioxide. Simultaneously, the circulatory system adjusts to constrict the venous reservoir, more blood is directed to the lungs to be purified, and arterial blood pressure increases. As a result, body tissues continue to receive an adequate amount of blood while changes are being made.

Other important sensors, located in the skeletal muscles, are activated by the contraction of muscles during exercise. These sensors send signals to the respiratory, cardiac, and vasomotor centers which help the body's circulation and ventilation systems adapt to the demands of exercise.

The higher centers of the brain can also influence the brain stem and thus modulate the nervous activity of the heart and blood vessels. In the midbrain, for instance, there is a temperature-regulating center capable of responding to the temperature of the blood supplied to it. Thermosensitive cells in this center can respond to a blood-temperature drop of even a fraction of a degree and quickly initiate a series of heat-conservation actions, including constriction of blood vessels in the skin. Thermosensitive cells can also detect and respond to equally minute increases in blood temperature. The common experience of excessive perspiration during emotional stress is also a result of the activity of the higher centers of the brain modulating the activity of the sweat glands. At the same time, there is an increase in cardiac output and in blood flow to the skeletal muscles. These responses prepare the body for "flight or fight." The higher centers also help regulate circulation and respiration during exercise.

Altogether, the various sensors continuously monitor the performance of the cardiovascular and respiratory systems. The information they supply to brain centers is essential for the relaying of proper signals to the heart and blood vessels. On the basis of these signals, adjustments are made in the circulation so that it can respond to any stress. Such a strenuous physical exercise as diving from a high board provides a good example of body systems under stress and making appropriate adjustments. Holding one's breath cuts off the supply of oxygen entering the blood. Circulation is immediately adjusted so that the oxygen stored in the blood is delivered preferentially to the brain and the heart muscle. The cardiovascular system becomes for the moment a "heart-brain circuit," delivering almost all the oxygen reserve in the blood and lungs to these vitally important tissues. The signal to make this adjustment means increased activity of the vagus nerves on the sinoatrial node, causing an immediate slowing of the heart (bradycardia). Increased activity of the sympathetic nerves results in a powerful constriction of the blood vessels; the flow of blood to the peripheral tissues, including the muscles being exercised in the dive, therefore virtually stops, and the muscles no longer draw oxygen from the blood. Skeletal muscles can continue to contract for some time in the absence of oxygen, but the oxygen debt incurred during the exercise must be paid back later.

Despite a greatly reduced cardiac output during the dive, blood pressure is maintained by the severe constriction of the peripheral blood vessels. The blood vessels of the brain do not constrict, however, since their nerve supply is sparse. On the contrary, brain blood vessels actually dilate in response to the accumulation of carbon dioxide in the blood in the absence of breathing. Thus, blood flow to the brain is maintained while the slowing of the heart's activity greatly reduces its need for oxygen.

All these adjustments take place while the diver is under water; when he surfaces and begins to breathe again the changes are quickly reversed. There is a rush of oxygen-rich blood to the heart, together with a cessation of the inhibitory effects of the vagus and sympathetic nerves on the heart and dilatation of the blood vessels. The resulting large blood flow to all the tissues repays the oxygen debt. The surfacing diver gulps in great gasps of air to repay the oxygen debt as quickly as possible.

One of the benefits of strenuous exercise carried on over a long period of time is the development of a larger heart with stronger muscles. The cardiac muscle of athletes is often so developed that a rate of less than sixty beats a minute satisfies their bodies at rest, leaving a tremendous reserve of muscle strength for the time when power and endurance are needed. The larger heart of an athlete is not the same as the enlarged heart developed by a victim of heart disease, however. In disease, the heart grows larger when it attempts to compensate for a deficiency such as narrowing of the aortic valve (aortic stenosis), in which the left ventricle enlarges because of the excessive work load placed on it. Although the over-all size of the heart is greater, the enlarged area in this condition is not well irrigated with blood, the cells of the muscle fiber are weaker, and the efficiency of the heart is reduced.

The Endocrine System   The action of the nervous system on the circulation is augmented when necessary by hormones secreted into the bloodstream from specialized cells (endocrine glands). Among the many hormones that can affect the function of the heart and blood vessels, the most important are adrenal catecholamines and angiotensin II.

ADRENAL CATECHOLAMINES   There is an adrenal gland located just above each kidney. These glands consist of a central group of cells, the medulla, surrounded by a layer of different cells, the cortex. The medulla produces two substances called catecholamines, norepinephrine and epinephrine. The norepinephrine secreted by the medulla increases the rate of the heart beat and the strength of heart muscle contraction and at the same time causes constriction of the muscle cells in the blood vessel walls. The epinephrine causes relaxation of blood vessels in the skeletal muscles, which augments the blood flow to the muscles during exercise.

The cells of the adrenal medulla are controlled by the sympathetic nerves; each increase in the number of impulses from these nerves increases the secretion of the catecholamines. The cells of the adrenal medulla can, in fact, be considered sympathetic neurons that liberate their neurotransmitter into the bloodstream. Increased secretion from the medulla is part of any reaction involving an increased activity of the vasomotor and cardiac-activating centers, sustaining and prolonging the immediate cardiovascular changes caused by augmented sympathetic nerve activity.

ANGIOTENSIN II Cells located in the walls of kidney arterioles produce a chemical substance, renin, which is converted into angiotensin II. This very active product increases the formation of aldosterone (one of the hormones produced by the adrenal cortex), which in turn causes greater reabsorption of sodium and water from the kidneys and a subsequent increase in blood volume. Because angiotensin II allows the nerve cells of the sympathetic system to work more efficiently, the vasomotor and cardiac-activating centers can send more impulses to the periphery, and the sympathetic neurons can release more norepinephrine per impulse. Angiotensin II also acts more directly to cause muscle cells in the walls of the arterioles to contract; the result of all this activity is an increase in arteriolar resistance.

Normally, the amount of renin released, and thus of angiotensin II formed, depends on the pressure in the renal arterioles and the ionic composition of the body fluids. Too little sodium leads to more angiotesin II (and therefore more aldosterone), allowing the kidneys to recover more sodium from the urine. A drop in pressure in the kidney arterioles where renin is formed will result in an increased amount of renin secreted into the bloodstream. The angiotensin II that is then formed will cause an increase in blood pressure because of the way the substance affects sympathetic nerves and arterioles. The renin–angiotensin II system, in parallel operation with the arterial stretch receptors, is like a hormonal feedback control designed to maintain blood pressure. It follows that when the system overproduces at abnormally high levels, as happens in certain cases of hypertension, blood pressure will increase above normal levels (see Hypertension, chapter 10).

ADAPTATION TO STRESS

The cardiovascular system is under least stress when the body is at rest in a horizontal position in a relaxed, comfortable environment. The amount of blood then pumped out by each ventricle ranges from 5 to 8 quarts (4.8 to 7.6 liters) a minute, and the heart rate is between fifty-five and eighty beats a minute. These figures are for healthy adults; the variations depend on such factors as age, physical fitness, length of time since eating, and degree of mental and physical calm. The change from resting in a horizontal position to standing upright in a relaxed posture causes about 2 pints (0.9 liters) of blood to be displaced from the upper part of the body into the lower abdomen and the legs. Thus the force of gravity decreases the volume of blood in the heart and the lungs by about 20 percent. The force of blood expanding the heart chambers during their filling is lessened, and therefore the amount of blood pumped out is also reduced. But since the need of body tissues and organs for oxygen is unaffected by body position, oxygen continues to be extracted from the blood as it passes through the capillaries. Even though cardiac output is decreased by the upright position, arterial blood pressure does not fall, because a series of reflexes are set in motion through the carotid and aortic stretch receptors and the receptors within the heart and the lungs. These receptors inform the centers in the brain that regulate the diameter of blood vessels (vasomotor centers) of the shift in blood volume. The vasomotor centers then increase the activity of the sympathetic nerves to the heart and blood vessels, causing the heart rate to increase and the arterioles in the kidneys, intestines, and skeletal muscles to constrict. At the same time, the veins in the liver and intestines constrict to minimize the volume of blood they contain. Because arterial blood pressure equals cardiac output, multiplied by peripheral resistance, blood pressure is maintained as the decrease in output is offset by the increase in resistance—that is, by the constriction of the arterioles in various parts of the circulatory system.

Exercise During rhythmic exercise the working muscles require a large increase in oxygen to get the energy for their contractions. The supply of extra oxygen is achieved by dilation of the arterioles in the muscles, thereby increasing the blood flow, together with a simultaneous increase in cardiac output. The rate and depth of breathing also increase, providing for an accelerated exchange of oxygen and carbon dioxide in the lungs. These complex changes are brought about by a closely coordinated series of events, beginning with local metabolic changes in the active muscles, which, by some as yet unknown chemistry, adjust the diameter of the muscle arterioles.

Coronary blood vessels supplying the heart muscle react in the same way. As skeletal muscles contract they squeeze on the blood within them, speeding up its return through the venous system to the heart. The sympathetic nervous system to the heart is activated, and the restraint which the vagus nerves usually exercise on the sinoatrial node is suspended. The heart rate quickens and the chambers contract more forcefully. Since during exercise most of the blood from the left ventricle must go to the brain, the heart muscle itself, and the active skeletal muscles, the sympathetic nerves begin to reduce blood flow in other parts of the body, such as the kidneys, the intestines, and inactive muscles. The veins in the intestines and liver constrict, making more blood available to fill the heart and expand its chambers.

Exercise activates the reflexes that produce the changes in the activity of the nerves to the heart and blood vessels, as well as the deepening and quickening of respiration. Science has not yet pinpointed the precise role of each reflex, but it seems likely that all contribute. The carotid and aortic stretch receptors, in conjunction with those in the heart and lungs, work to stabilize blood pressure by increasing the force and frequency of the heartbeat and by constricting the vessels in internal organs and inactive muscles as the muscle blood vessels dilate. The chemoreceptors probably augment respiration and adjust the circulation if the oxygen, carbon-dioxide, or acid content of the blood changes. Receptors in the skeletal muscles, which are activated when the muscles contract, are able to boost respiration and reinforce the sympathetic outflow to the heart and the blood vessels.

Much is yet to be learned about the complex series of events by which heart rate, cardiac output, and ventilation increase in proportion to the severity of exercise—that is, in proportion to the increased oxygen demands of the active muscles. According to one theory, more of the adjustments arise directly from the higher centers of the brain (the motor cortex) than from peripheral receptors. The motor cortex sends impulses to the skeletal muscles, causing them to contract, and the force of the contraction relates to the frequency of such impulses. Signals are sent at the same time to the respiratory, cardiac, and vasomotor centers in the brain stem. Thus the brain instructs the muscles and adjusts the cardiovascular and respiratory systems to deal with a specific amount of muscular work.

The body's response differs according to whether rhythmic exercise is conducted in an upright position or a horizontal position. In an upright position, the amount of blood pumped out by the heart is about 2 quarts (1.9 liters) less per minute than it is for the same exercise in a horizontal position. Since total oxygen needs are identical for either position, more oxygen is extracted from the blood by the tissues during upright-position exercise. With maximal effort, however, the difference in output disappears. The reason for the smaller output when upright is that the reflexes activated by standing upright are reinforced by the reflexes activated by the exercise; thus there is an even greater reduction of blood flow to the kidneys, the intestines, and the muscles not involved in the exercise.

ISOTONIC AND ISOMETRIC EXERCISE   The rhythmic contraction of the skeletal muscles in such forms of exercise as jogging, bicycling, and swimming is called isotonic exercise. A sustained contraction of the skeletal muscles, such as weight lifting requires, is known as isometric exercise. The two types of exercise have different effects on the cardiovascular system and on breathing. Isotonic exercise is accompanied by changes in cardiac output, heart rate, and ventilation in proportion to the body's need for oxygen. At the same time, the arterial blood pressure is so adjusted that there is no major change in it. In isometric exercise, by contrast, the increase in cardiac output, heart rate, and breathing is disproportionate to the increased oxygen requirements, and the arterial blood pressure increases markedly. Medical research indicates that the sustained contraction of even a few muscles may cause excessive activity in the sympathetic nerves going to the heart and blood vessels. The excessive activity cannot be overcome by the action of the carotid and aortic stretch receptors. Isometric exercises are therefore much more taxing on the cardiovascular system than are isotonic exercises, especially for people who have cardiovascular diseases or who are otherwise incapacitated. Anyone with a cardiovascular problem would be wiser to enter rehabilitation programs that stress walking, jogging, swimming, or bicycle riding rather than weight lifting or other isometric exercises.

Healthy young men can exercise continuously for up to eight hours without excessive fatigue, providing their heart rate does not exceed 120 beats a minute. They can also exercise for longer than four continuous hours with a heart rate of 140 beats a minute, and for longer than two hours at a rate of 160. Although the maximum heart rate is about 180 beats a minute, this can

PRINCIPLES

1. *To maintain the billions of cells that make up the human body, there must be a continuous stream of nutrients from the outside world and a continuous removal of waste products from the cells. The cardiovascular system is in effect the transportation link between such specialized tissues as the lungs, gut, and kidneys and the individual cells. Blood from the heart to the cells and back to the heart is carried by the network of arteries, arterioles, capillaries, venules, and veins that is known collectively as the circulatory system. Red blood cells pick up oxygen as they pass through the lungs, then pass this oxygen to the individual cells. The red cells then pick up carbon dioxide, a waste product, for eventual release through the lungs.*

2. *The continuous flow of blood through the circulatory system depends on the heart, a hollow, four-chambered muscular organ situated in the chest cavity between the two lungs. The heart has two collecting chambers (atria) and two pumping chambers (ventricles). Four valves in the chambers prevent any backward flow of blood during the cycle of receiving and pumping out blood. Blood for the heart itself is circulated through the coronary arteries.*

3. *The cardiac cycle consists of the relaxation (diastole) and the contraction (systole) of the ventricles. During diastole, blood flows into the ventricles; during systole, blood is pumped out of the ventricles. The two aspects of the pumping process occur almost simultaneously, lasting less than a second.*

4. *Oxygen-rich blood leaves the heart via the aorta, the body's largest*

be sustained for only short periods of strenuous exercise. In the average healthy man, the maximum cardiac output is from 21 to 26 quarts (20 to 25 liters) of blood a minute. In well-trained athletes, the cardiac output can go up to 31 quarts (30 liters), or four to six times the resting level, but only for short periods.

Above the age of thirty, however, there is a gradual decrease in both the heart rate and in oxygen consumption during maximal exercise. The decrease continues with increasing age, with systolic pressure rising from 110 at the age of fifteen to about 160 at sixty-five years of age. The increase, roughly 1 millimeter a year, probably reflects a gradual decrease in the capacity of the arteries to expand. Diastolic pressure increases from 70 at fifteen years of age to about 90 at sixty-five, or slightly less than one-half millimeter a year. Systolic and diastolic pressures also vary according to sex; they are lower in women under fifty but higher in those over fifty than they are in men of the same age groups.

Cardiac output is no greater than normal shortly after eating a meal, but as digestion proceeds the heart rate and cardiac output increase to provide more blood to the intestines, reaching a maximum about three hours after eating. By this time, the heart rate may have increased 15 beats a minute and the cardiac output about a third. Exercise undertaken at this time places additional demands on the cardiovascular system.

Exercise also places major stress on the cardiovascular system of an excessively overweight person. Even at rest, the volume of blood pumped out of the heart is slightly higher in an obese person than that in an average-weight person, because blood volume increases in proportion to the excess fatty tissues. During exercise, oxygen consumption and breathing rate are twice as great in the excessively overweight as in the average-weight person performing the same activity.

VARIATIONS IN TEMPERATURE   Internal body temperature is determined by the balance between heat production and heat loss and is normally maintained at the traditional 98.6° F (37° C). Body heat is continuously produced by metabolism in organs such as the heart, liver, and muscles. At rest, sufficient heat is generated to raise internal temperature at the rate of a little less than 2° F (1° C) an hour. The rate would increase five times during moderate physical activity if no means were available for its dissipation. But some heat is lost from the respiratory tract when the air breathed in is warmed, and some is lost by evaporation. The major loss of heat, however, is by radiation from the skin, by conduction from the blood to surrounding objects, and by evaporation of sweat. The body's thermoregulatory mechanism can quickly adjust alterations in blood flow through the skin and in sweating. Shivering, the involuntary contraction of skeletal muscles to maintain or increase body temperature, is one example of the body's rapid adjustment to a changing environment.

During exercise in hot temperature, the heart must supply a large volume of blood to the skin (to dissipate body heat) and to the active muscles (for their metabolic needs). To accommodate those needs, blood flow to the kidneys and intestines decreases more severely than it does during exercise in a comfortable environment. The ultimate check on a person's capacity for exercise, therefore, is the ability of the heart to supply the oxygen demands of the tissues and the flow of blood to the skin needed for heat regulation. If the heart cannot supply the blood flow needed to dissipate heat, body temperature rises and heat stroke may follow. However, most untrained persons exercising in less than tropical heat will usually be stopped by fatigue well before the cardiovascular system ceases to be able to cope with the demands of tissues and the build-up of heat. In a cold environment, blood vessels close to the skin constrict, reducing arterial flow near the surface. Because smaller amounts of oxygenated blood are being pumped to these vessels, the skin may develop a bluish tint. Exercise on a cold day helps to maintain the body's normal internal temperature because of the heat generated by the contracting muscles.

artery, then flows to all the organs of the body through a system of arteries and smaller vessels (arterioles), from which in turn radiate even smaller vessels (capillaries). Veins returning blood to the heart begin at the capillaries, graduating from the smallest in diameter (venules) to the largest, the vena cavas, which deposit the oxygen-depleted blood in the right atrium.

Emotions

Poetry and song have always referred to the effect of love on the beat of the heart, and folklore is not misleading on this point. Most people have experienced a cardiovascular response to a loved one, to put the matter clinically; most have also probably felt a less pleasant response to the appearance of a summons-bearing policeman or an irate employer.

The cardiovascular response depends on the intensity and duration of the stimulus. Generally speaking, however, under emotional stress, the heart rate, cardiac output, and arterial pressure all increase. Blood flow through the muscles also increases, even in the absence of movement, while that through the kidneys and intestines decreases. Some of these changes are the result of a sudden release of epinephrine from the adrenal medulla into the circulating blood, causing vessels in the skeletal muscles to dilate and those in the kidneys and intestines to constrict. Intense fear and anger are known to increase the heart rate by as much as thirty to forty beats a minute, increase the cardiac output by about 2 quarts (1.9 liters) a minute, and elevate blood pressure as much as 10 millimeters.

5. As the diameter of the individual blood vessels decreases, their number increases, being greatest at the level of the capillaries. Since the circulation is a closed system, the velocity of flow is least at the capillary level, guaranteeing that there will be adequate time for necessary exchange of nutrients.

6. In addition to the systemic circulatory system, there is a pulmonary circulatory system consisting of a sequence of arteries, arterioles, capillaries, venules, and veins. This system's significant differences guarantee that the venous blood going through the lungs is

Pregnancy

During pregnancy the resting heart rate increases gradually until the thirtieth week and then declines toward the end of the pregnancy. The maximum increase in a normal pregnancy is only ten beats a minute, however. In the absence of complications, blood volume gradually increases up to the thirtieth week, reaching a maximum of 25 to 30 percent above normal. The same figures apply to cardiac output.

exposed to fresh air and that the blood returned to the heart is sufficiently oxygenated.

7. Because the cardiovascular system is the major environmental control center in the body, it utilizes a

Prolonged Immobility

Standing still for long periods, especially in a warm environment, can cause a brief loss of consciousness (vasodepressor syncope, or the simple faint). Although fainting may also be a response to pain or stressful emotion, it is more often a result of immobility, prolonged confinement in bed, fatigue, or sometimes a recent loss of blood. The usual sequence of events is pallor, sweating, yawning, nausea, followed by slowing of the heart and loss of consciousness. The symptoms reflect a diminished supply of oxygen to the brain, the result of a sudden decrease in arterial blood pressure. The decrease is the result of relaxation of arterioles in the skeletal muscles and the slowing of the heart. With the slowing of the heart, less blood is pumped out at a time when the muscle arterioles are relaxed. The situation is different from that during exer-

battery of sensors and monitoring devices to trigger corrective action or relay information to other body systems. Thus monitors within the cardiovascular system measure blood pressure and send this data to the brain, which then determines necessary adjustments.

8. The primary regulator of blood pressure is the brain stem, in which groups of specialized nerve cells control the activity of the heart (cardiac-activating and cardiac-inhibitory centers) and another nerve-cell group regulates the diameter of blood vessels (vasomotor center). Blood pressure is augmented when the sympathetic nervous system carries commands from the cardiac-activating center to increase the heart's activity and from the vasomotor center to constrict arterioles and veins. Blood pressure is decreased when the vagus nerves convey commands from the cardiac-inhibitory center to the sinoatrial node, slowing heart activity.

9. When blood pressure rises sensors in the aorta and carotid arteries send impulses to the brain which inhibit the cardiac-activating center and the vasomotor center and simultaneously stimulate the cardiac-inhibitory center.

10. Sensors in the heart and lungs monitor the volume of blood in the vascular system. Messages sent by these receptors lead to adjustments in the circulatory system via sympathetic nerves. Other sensors monitor the oxygen content of blood and lead to changes in the respiratory system. These various monitoring cells supply the brain with the essential data for adjusting the circulation so that it can respond to any stress.

11. Hormones secreted by specialized cells in the endocrine glands augment the nervous system's activity in regulating circulation when necessary. Increased secretions of the specialized cells in the medulla of the adrenal gland sustain and prolong the activity resulting from stimulation of the cardiac-activating and vasomotor centers. A chemical substance produced in the walls of the kidneys increases the blood volume by causing greater reabsorption of salt and water from the kidneys. It also acts directly on the muscle cells in arteriole walls, causing them to contract and thereby increasing their resistance.

cise, when the relaxation of vessels in the active muscles is accompanied by an increase in cardiac output in order to maintain blood pressure.

The precise sensors in the body or in the brain that actually trigger a faint have not yet been identified. The abrupt dilation of the vessels in the muscles may be due to a sudden decrease in the activity of the sympathetic fibers leading to the muscle arterioles, or perhaps to activation of other fibers leading to muscle vessels, causing them to dilate. Recovery takes place when the person lies flat.

The cardiovascular system is obviously an enormously complex piece of machinery, not the least of whose virtues is its hardiness. It is difficult to name a device of such intricacy and magnitude which can operate for so many years and with so prodigious an output. Although the system is equipped with a number of backup and emergency arrangements, it is as likely to break down as is any complex mechanical system. But the cardiovascular system shares another characteristic of complex machinery; prevention of breakdown is generally more effective and less costly than repairs.

9

SYMPTOMS OF CARDIOVASCULAR DISEASE

Robert A. O'Rourke, M.D.

All living creatures depend on their senses to advise them of danger, and they are constantly on the alert for warning signals. Animals in the wild live or die as a result of their ability to react to sounds, smells, sights, and changes of temperature. Human beings have implemented their natural survival mechanisms with mechanical devices to alert them to threats. A pilot of an airplane is warned by the sound of a bell that his craft is in danger of stalling out. The driver of a car realizes that something is amiss when the oil-pressure gauge suddenly glows red. A whiff of smoke will trigger an alarm system in a home or other building in the event of fire. Should an individual ignore these warnings, he does so at peril of his safety.

In medicine, the word for warning signal is "symptom," which is of Greek derivation. In its root form the word means an occurrence that accompanies something else. In matters of health a symptom is a manifestation of some underlying disease, an ache or pain that accompanies an injury or a malfunction. In some instances the symptom itself must be treated, as in the case of a fever, although doctors also attempt to control the infection that produced the fever. In other illnesses, the symptom itself does not concern the doctor; the cause is his principal target. In cardiovascular disease there are symptoms that in themselves must be treated along with the underlying disease and there are instances where the symptom is relatively unimportant and the source is the object of the physician's attention. In our mechanized society, the evaluation of warning signals is important; a buzzing alarm may have only responded to a nearby cigarette and is no cause for further action. On the other hand, a very real fire may be sending smoke to the alarm. So it is with medical symptoms. Some are inconsequential, but to ignore others is to place life and well-being in jeopardy.

Since the 1950s considerable advances have been made in the diagnosis and treatment of a number of cardiovascular diseases. The most notable of these are the special intensive-care units for treating patients with heart attack; the improved surgical procedures for congenital, coronary-artery, and valvular heart diseases; and the more recent improved emergency medical services. Yet the death rate from cardiac disease remains alarmingly high. The inevitable conclusion, therefore, is that improved diagnostic and therapeutic techniques depend for their success on early diagnosis of symptoms and prompt medical or surgical intervention. Fortunately, there are enough early warning signals of cardiovascular disease to alert the individual and the physician to potential danger. A quick, effective response to symptoms could save many of the approximately 60 percent of heart attack victims who die before emergency medical care can be obtained.

CHEST PAIN
Angina Pectoris
The most frequent initial symptom of coronary heart disease is discomfort in the chest, caused by a decrease in the blood supply to the heart muscle. The discomfort, when of short duration, is called angina pectoris (literally, chest pain), and results from a disparity between oxygen supply and demand. When coronary arteries are narrowed by fatty deposits on their inner lining (a condition called atherosclerosis) the supply of oxygen-rich blood is inadequate to the needs of the working muscle. The oxygen insufficiency sets off a chemical reaction which irritates nerve fibers and results in chest pain. Characteristically, pain is felt when the demand for oxygen is increased by exercise, emotional upset, or even after a heavy meal. Blood flow through

partially narrowed arteries may be adequate when the body is at rest, but in-adequate to the heart muscle's need for additional oxygen in circumstances that increase heart rate and blood pressure.

Most people with angina pectoris describe their discomfort as a pressing or squeezing sensation that lasts only a few minutes. The discomfort is located in the center of the chest and affects an area about the size of a clenched fist. Sometimes it spreads to the shoulders, down both arms, into the neck or jaw, and through to the back. On rare occasions the pain or pressure is more pro-nounced in the neck, jaw, left or right arm, shoulder, elbow, or wrist, back, or upper part of the abdomen. Generally lasting no longer than one to three minutes, the sensation disappears when the effort which provoked it is dis-continued. Consequently, most patients with angina pectoris learn to slow the pace of their physical activity. However, pain or discomfort that resembles angina pectoris should not be ignored. It indicates the need for a complete medical examination, including diagnostic tests, to determine whether the oxygen supply to the heart is adequate. Early diagnosis of angina, with appropriate medical or surgical treatment, decreases the frequency of symp-toms and may reduce the possibility of a subsequent heart attack.

Unlike the discomfort of angina pectoris, the pain of a heart attack is often severe, lasts longer (usually more than thirty minutes), and is relatively constant, not being relieved by rest. Victims describe the pain as "heavy," "squeezing," "crushing," and even as the worst they have ever experienced, and many report a sense of "impending doom" or imminent death. In most instances, the pain is located in the central portion of the chest and the upper abdomen, but it also spreads to the arms in about one out of four cases. Less commonly the back, jaw, and neck are also affected. When pain is felt in the upper portion of the abdomen and is accompanied by nausea, with or without vomiting, heart attack may be mistakenly diagnosed as acute indigestion. These symptoms occur when the lower surface of the heart, just above the diaphragm, is experiencing a drastic loss in blood flow.

Chest pain and other symptoms of heart attack may begin during a pe-riod of exertion, but they also occur when the person is at rest or even asleep. As in angina pectoris, the symptoms result from an insufficient supply of oxygen to the contracting heart muscle because of reduced blood flow in the coronary arteries. When the shortage is so great and lasts so long that the heart muscle is destroyed and cardiac cells die, the patient suffers a myo-cardial infarction—that is, a heart attack. The difference between a heart attack and angina pectoris, then, is in the duration and severity of the episode of inadequate blood supply. In angina, the period of inadequate oxygen is brief and causes no permanent injury. In a heart attack, the possibility of death and the degree of disability after recovery are directly related to the amount of heart muscle tissue actually destroyed by a prolonged interruption in blood supply (see Coronary Artery Disease, chapter 11).

Warning symptoms are common during the week or two preceding a heart attack, usually in the form of vague chest pain or typical angina pec-toris. Then, and often without any obvious precipitating cause, the chest pains do not pass quickly. Untreated, they can last for hours, varying in intensity from an uncomfortable feeling of pressure to extreme agony. The severity of the discomfort, however, is not an absolute indication of the extent

Pain of Heart Attack

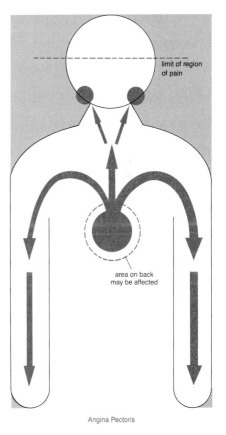

limit of region of pain

area on back may be affected

Angina Pectoris

Pain radiating from the center of the chest during a period of exertion signals an inadequate oxygen supply to the contracting heart muscle.

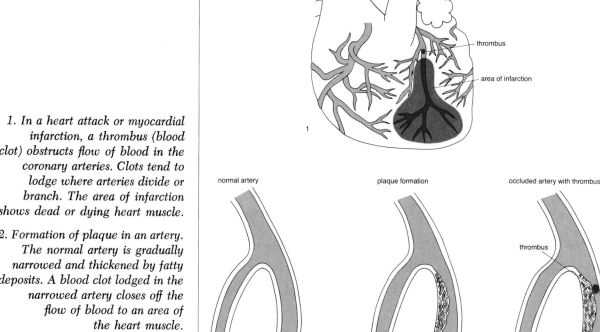

1. In a heart attack or myocardial infarction, a thrombus (blood clot) obstructs flow of blood in the coronary arteries. Clots tend to lodge where arteries divide or branch. The area of infarction shows dead or dying heart muscle.

2. Formation of plaque in an artery. The normal artery is gradually narrowed and thickened by fatty deposits. A blood clot lodged in the narrowed artery closes off the flow of blood to an area of the heart muscle.

of heart damage. In fact, 10 to 20 percent of patients have no history of prolonged chest discomfort, even though an electrocardiogram shows evidence of a heart attack.

Symptoms of impending heart attack constitute a medical emergency and require immediate attention. If the patient's physician cannot be reached, an ambulance or emergency medical service should be contacted and the patient taken to the nearest medical facility equipped to handle cardiac emergencies. Since the heart-attack patient often has severe and potentially fatal disturbances in heart rhythm in the hours immediately following the attack, the medical facility must be equipped with staff and monitoring machinery capable of detecting and coping with such problems.

Pain from Other Causes Although it is important to be alert to the symptoms of a heart attack, it is equally important to recognize that not all chest discomfort is indicative of coronary insufficiency and potential coronary attack. Chest pain can come from disease of other organs in the chest cavity besides the heart (lungs and esophagus, for example) and from diseases of the bony structure of the chest and spine. It may be due to inflammation of the muscles of the chest wall or to increased tension or emotional stress. And it may also reflect disease in abdominal organs which have a similar nerve supply (stomach ulcer, for example).

Pains originating in the muscles or bones in the chest wall, the shoulders, or the arms can be easily distinguished from those signaling heart disease. In bone or muscle damage, there is localized tenderness, and the pain is clearly related to movement. Deep breathing, turning or twisting the chest, or moving the shoulder and arm will elicit and duplicate the pain. Unlike anginal pain, which normally disappears in a few minutes, muscular aches may last many hours. The pains from injured bones, on the other hand, are sharp or have a "sticking" quality. A feeling of tightness, probably due to associated spasm of the chest muscles, often accompanies pain that originates in the chest wall, shoulders, or arms. The result is the characteristic "morning stiffness" associated with many skeletal disorders. Chest wall pain that is recent and follows an injury, a strain, or unusual activity involving the pectoral muscles is easily differentiated from the chest pain of coronary artery disease. The cause—sports, housework, or other physical effort—has produced the effect.

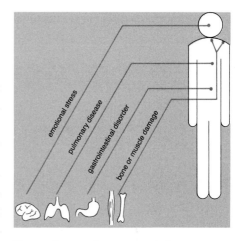

Noncardiovascular causes of chest pain

Anxiety is a common cause of chest discomfort in people with no evidence of cardiac disease. The distressful sensation usually localizes below the nipple of a breast. It rarely radiates to other areas, does not occur during effort, and is not aggravated by breathing. The distress is associated with other signs of anxiety: periodic deep-sighing respiration, rapid deep breaths (hyperventilation), fast heart rate, fatigue, and a fear of enclosed places, where the patient imagines a shortage of air to breathe. Anxiety pains may come as a series of short stabs lasting for a split second, or as a dull ache that may endure for hours or days. They may have no organic cause, and yet they can be disabling as well as emotionally disturbing.

Since the discomfort associated with anxiety and the pressing sensation of angina pectoris may and frequently do coexist, great skill and care are needed to distinguish between them. The pain of anxiety is real, probably developed through unconscious and prolonged muscular activity, as in repeated grimacing and rapid clenching of the fist. It can be intensified by hyperventilation, which causes painful contraction of the chest wall muscles. Such pains are clearly distinguishable from angina, however, because they last a long time, are associated with fatigue or tension but not with exertion, and do not limit the person's capacity for exercise.

Pain in the lower leg, foot, or toes during activity is a common symptom when the arteries supplying these parts of the body are narrowed by fatty deposits (atheromata) and the supply of blood to working muscles is reduced. The characteristic feature of lower extremity pain (intermittent claudication), is that it occurs when muscles are active and is promptly relieved when they are at rest. The pain is usually brought on by walking and may be located in the foot, calf, thigh, or buttock, depending on the site of arterial blockage. The pain, described as a cramp, an ache, a charley horse, numbness, or weakness, subsides when the person stands still for a few minutes. Then when walking is resumed for about the same distance, it will reappear. If the arteries are seriously blocked, however, pain will be felt even at rest, and the inadequate blood supply makes the skin cold and pale. The symptoms of intermittent claudication, which is described in greater detail in Peripheral Arterial Disease, chapter 14, are warnings of possible arterial blockage and should be reported to a doctor.

PAIN IN THE LOWER EXTREMITIES

HEADACHE Pain, in the form of a headache, can be a sign of elevated blood pressure (hypertension), although most people with this disease have no symptoms at all. An aching or throbbing pain at the back of the head or base of the skull is present when the person wakes up in the morning and subsides after several hours without medication or treatment. Other symptoms sometimes associated with hypertension are dizziness, susceptibility to fatigue, and recurrent nose bleeds. Although there are many causes of headache, anyone with a recurring early morning headache should have a blood pressure reading as part of a general medical examination.

SHORTNESS OF BREATH Shortness of breath (dyspnea) does not specifically indicate heart disease, since many conditions force increased efforts in breathing. Chronic lung disease, obesity, anemia, pregnancy, and anxiety are all associated with shortness of breath following exertion. Of these, anxiety is perhaps the cause most frequently confused with heart disease, since chest pains are a common symptom. In addition, many anxious people complain that they cannot draw a "satisfying breath" or their breath "doesn't go down far enough." These symptoms are similar to those of cardiac patients, but the anxiety itself **may** cause the symptoms. The deep sighing which is characteristic of anxiety attacks interrupts normal breathing patterns, and prolonged periods of rapid breathing can bring on numbness of the arms, hands, and lips.

Excessive shortness of breath after mild to moderate exercise is, however, a common complaint of patients with lung congestion, in which the functioning of the lower left chamber of the heart (left ventricle) is impaired. When the ventricle cannot contract sufficiently to pump blood out through the aorta, the blood backs up in the left atrium and the veins draining the lungs (pulmonary veins). Pressure increases in these structures, and large amounts of fluid pass from the vascular system into the lung tissue.

Pressure also builds up when the valve regulating the flow of blood from the lungs into the left ventricle (the mitral valve) is obstructed. Then the vascular system of the lungs becomes saturated with blood, and the excessive fluid in lung tissue reduces both the ability of the lungs to expand and their capacity to absorb oxygen. The respiratory muscles are required to work much harder to inflate the lungs, and this effort is felt as shortness of breath or labored breathing.

When shortness of breath is the result of failure of the left side of the heart, symptoms at first appear only during exercise. This may simply represent an aggravation of normal breathlessness during exertion. But as heart function continues to deteriorate, the breathlessness comes on with less and less strenuous activity, until the patient suffers even when at rest. The chief difference between respiratory distress during exertion in normal and in cardiac cases is the amount of activity needed to produce the symptom. Shortness of breath while a person is lying down generally indicates more advanced failure of the left side of the heart, although for inactive persons it may be the first symptom of congestive heart failure. (See Congestive Heart Failure, chapter 13.) The volume of blood that returns to the heart and lungs when the body is prone is greater than that when the body is erect. The increase in volume is due to a change in gravitational forces, which become equal when the legs and trunk are on the same level, and a healthy heart is able to cope with it. For the person with heart failure, however, the augmented blood volume adds to the work load of the malfunctioning heart and congested lungs. A patient who has difficulty breathing while lying down can get relief by sleeping with the head propped up on several pillows or by sitting erect. However, as heart failure and lung congestion progress, shortness of breath can become so severe that the patient cannot lie down at all but must spend the entire night sitting bolt upright—in front of an open window if weather permits.

Paroxysmal or intermittent respiratory distress is an attack of severe shortness of breath at night, which usually awakens one from sleep and is accompanied by coughing and wheezing and sometimes by a feeling of suffocation. When the cause is heart disease, the condition is called cardiac asthma. The fluid that was retained in the abdomen and the lower extremities during the day is redistributed in the first hours of sleep, and the added volume in the blood vessels of the lungs leads to increased congestion. The symptoms are sometimes, but not always, relieved by sitting up for an hour or longer.

When wheezing and shortness of breath are a long-standing complaint—from childhood, for example—bronchial asthma, or lung disease, is likely to be the cause. But when an adult over forty begins to have recurrent wheezing and breathlessness, along with other symptoms of heart disease, heart failure is to be suspected and there is reason to seek medical attention. Coughing, particularly when it produces blood-streaked sputum, is also symptomatic of failure of the left side of the heart. The sputum may become grossly bloody if a distended vein in the lungs ruptures. The distention of the vein may be due to high pressure in the left atrium that builds up when the mitral valve is obstructed. Congestion in the lungs' vascular system also increases markedly when there is impairment in the function of the left ventricle. The resultant accumulation of fluid in the lungs causes chronic coughing. In children, a chronic cough, with or without evidence of recurrent respiratory infections, is an important symptom of congenital heart disease. A cardiac defect, referred to as a "hole" in the heart, causes shunting of blood from the left to the right chambers, and results in a marked increase in blood flow to the lungs (se Congenital Heart Defects, chapter 16).

AWARENESS OF THE HEARTBEAT

Under normal circumstances, the rhythmic beating of the heart goes on without our being conscious of it. Many individuals, however, have heart rhythm abnormalities or disturbances which bring the usually silent process vividly to attention. They are aware of "skipped" beats, a fluttering in the chest called "palpitations," and the feeling that the heart "pounds," "stops," "starts up," "jumps," or "races." The type and severity of such symptoms are not directly related to the seriousness of the heart disease, if indeed any exists. Nor are such symptoms always related to a particular type of rhythm disturbance. Many individuals who have marked rhythm disorders feel no unusual sensations in their chest, while others feel abnormal beats but show no evidence of heart disease. Many presumably healthy people are aware of a forceful, regular heartbeat. In short, a person may perceive "abnormalities" in the heartbeat when the heart rate and rhythm are entirely normal, or when the regular cadence of the heart is interrupted by a chance abnormal contraction, an intermittent rapid beat, or an extreme slowing of the heart rate.

Awareness of the heartbeat is a common, if unpleasant, subjective phenomenon which is not characteristic of any particular cardiac or noncardiac disease. It is more often a manifestation of anxiety and emotional stress than a symptom of a physical disorder, but it can play an important role in the over-all health of an individual. The clear association between heart rhythms and the function of the heart generates apprehension and anxiety, which in turn can result in increased activity of the nervous system and an increase in the heart rate and the vigor of the heart's contraction. When, as occasionally happens, the final result is an increased severity of the rhythm disturbance, the anxious person is caught in a vicious circle.

Palpitations following strenuous physical activity or emotional upset are fairly common and generally reflect normal heart activity. Forceful and regular palpitations are usually caused by an increase in the volume of blood that is being ejected from the left ventricle into the aorta. And it is normal for most people to feel their hearts pounding after vigorous activity. However, this awareness of the heartbeat is also a symptom of cardiac slowing, which may result from the sudden development of a heart block or a change in rhythm. It is not safe, therefore, to conclude that overactivity is the cause of palpitations. For the anxious patient who does not have heart disease a chest X ray and electrocardiograms taken while the symptom is being felt and when the patient is at rest can provide reassurance. In other circumstances, identification of the abnormal cardiac rhythm responsible for the symptoms enables the physician to begin appropriate treatment.

FLUID RETENTION AND SWELLING

When the heart fails to pump adequate amounts of blood to the body, salt and water are retained, resulting in swelling (edema) of the lower extremities, weight gain, and an enlarged abdomen. The patient may notice pitting of the skin when pressure is applied, particularly over the lower extremities. However, as much as ten to fifteen pounds may be gained before other symptoms of water and salt retention are noticeable.

Abnormal accumulation of fluid is the result of many conditions besides heart disease, and symptoms vary greatly. Depending on the primary cause, edema may be localized or generally distributed over the body. Generalized fluid retention is most apparent in facial puffiness and prolonged indentation of the skin when pressure has been applied. Clothing suddenly feels too tight, especially at the waist, or a ring no longer comes easily off a finger. In cases of heart failure, the legs are often affected, with one leg sometimes swelling more than the other. The edema may shift from the lower extremities to the lower back when the patient is confined to bed. When the right ventricle fails to empty normally and pressure in the veins increases, excess fluid accumulates in the abdominal cavity, increasing its girth (ascites). Ascites is not a specific indication of cardiac disease; it may also also be due to severe liver and kidney diseases. The condition usually does not manifest itself until after swelling of the legs has occurred.

LOSS OF CONSCIOUSNESS

Loss of consciousness (syncope) may be transitory or prolonged, depending on a number of causes ranging from disease to injury. Syncope is the medical term for temporary loss of consciousness, a sudden onset of unconsciousness as blood flow and oxygen supply to the brain become inadequate. It is difficult, however, to distinguish between syncope and episodic faintness, lightheadedness or giddiness, and reduced alertness, because the difference is basically quantitative. Faintness refers to a lack of strength, with sensations of impending loss of consciousness. Syncope literally means a "cutting short" —that a cessation, or pause in consciousness, has occurred. It is, therefore, synonymous with "faint," describing a generalized weakness of muscles, with an inability to stand upright and an impairment of consciousness.

A syncopal attack usually develops rapidly, although probably not with the same absolute suddenness of an epileptic seizure. At the onset of the attack, the person is almost always standing or sitting upright and is usually warned by a sense of feeling poorly, of giddiness and confusion and occasionally of nausea. The victim yawns or gasps and sees spots before his eyes, or his vision may dim. There is a striking pallor or ashen-gray color to the face, and cold perspiration bathes the face and body. Because these distinct symptoms precede loss of consciousness, the victim is often able to protect himself as he falls, and injuries are uncommon. Complete loss of consciousness can sometimes be averted if the victim can lie down promptly at the onset of the symptoms.

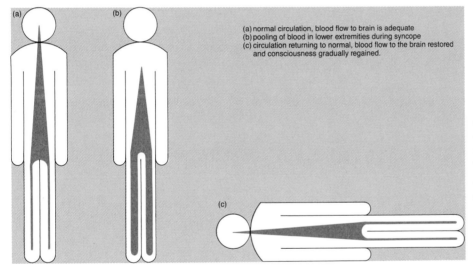

(a) normal circulation, blood flow to brain is adequate
(b) pooling of blood in lower extremities during syncope
(c) circulation returning to normal, blood flow to the brain restored and consciousness gradually regained.

Syncope or fainting results from the sudden reduction of blood flow and oxygen supply to the brain. When the victim lies down, normal blood flow to the brain is restored and consciousness returns.

The depth and duration of unconsciousness vary. Sometimes the victim is completely oblivious to his surroundings and unable to respond; at other times unconsciousness is not total. Usually the victim lies motionless with skeletal muscles relaxed, although in exceptional cases a few muscle jerks in the limbs and face occur shortly after the beginning of unconsciousness. Generalized convulsions are never a part of syncope, and bladder and rectal sphincter control are usually maintained. The pulse is feeble and cannot be felt, blood pressure is low, and breathing almost imperceptible. The reduction in vital functions and powers simulates death, and the victim may remain in this suspended state for seconds, minutes, or even as long as half an hour.

Once the victim of syncope is in a horizontal position, gravity no longer hinders the flow of blood to the brain. The strength of the pulse improves, color returns to the face, breathing becomes quicker and deeper, and consciousness is regained. The patient begins to become aware of things about him but feels intense physical weakness and may even faint again if he attempts to get up too soon. Headache, drowsiness, and mental confusion, the aftermaths of convulsion, do not follow a syncopal attack.

The list of conditions that cause weakness, faintness, and loss of consciousness is long and varied. But the most common causes of syncope can be reduced to a few simple mechanisms which result in a reduction of blood flow and oxygen to the brain. Cardiac syncope stems from a sudden reduction in cardiac output, most commonly as a result of fluctuation in the rhythm of the heartbeat (cardiac arrhythmia). In normal circumstances, slow heart rates (40 to 60 beats a minute) and fast rates (100 to 175 beats a minute) do not reduce cerebral blood flow, especially when a person is lying down. Changes in pulse rates outside these limits, however, impair cerebral blood flow and mental function. The most common form of cardiac arrhythmia that leads to fainting and syncopal episodes is complete heart block, with a low ventricular pacemaker and a heart rate of less than 40 beats a minute (see Arrhythmias, chapter 12). Cardiac syncope may also result from an acute heart attack, particularly when the cardiac damage is associated with a low blood pressure (90/60). Narrowing or obstruction of the aortic valve (aortic stenosis) sets the stage for a syncopal attack following exertion, because the flow of arterial blood that should occur during exercise is restricted.

Syncope is also a symptom of cerebral vascular disease and may be caused by partial or complete blocking (occlusion) of the large arteries in the neck. Disease conditions involving the arteries that supply blood to the brain include narrowing of the artery by atherosclerosis, occlusion of an artery by a blood clot, rupture of an artery with hemorrhage into the brain tissue, or disease in cerebral blood flow as a result of a drop in arterial blood pressure.

Most victims of stroke—that is, decreased cerebral function from impaired blood supply—have one or more short-lived warning symptoms, which are called transient ischemic attacks. The symptoms which herald the oncoming vascular catastrophe include numbness or weakness in one or more of the extremities, confusion, dizziness, impaired vision in one or both visual fields, blindness in one eye, loss of speech, slurred speech, or headache (see Stroke, chapter 19).

FATIGUE AND WEAKNESS

Before the use of modern diuretic agents, which promote excretion of salt and water, cardiac patients who retained fluid and suffered from lung congestion complained most often of shortness of breath. Today, the common complaint is of fatigue and weakness. Although the actual physiological mechanism linking heart failure with fatigue is not known, fatigue is thought to be the result of an inadequate amount of blood ejected by the heart with each beat. Thus the heart fails in its primary task of nourishing all the tissues and organs of the body, including the skeletal muscles. This failure may result in general body fatigue. Since fatigue, unlike labored breathing or swollen ankles, cannot be observed by the physician and may even be underestimated by the patient, it is possible for it to be ignored as a possible symptom of heart failure. Despite the fact that fatigue has many causes, it may actually be as closely related to low cardiac output—and heart failure—as shortness of breath is to congestion of the lungs.

When a patient complains of heaviness of limbs on exertion, of weakness and lack of vigor, and of generalized tiredness and exhaustion, the practical problem is to distinguish symptoms of cardiac failure from symptoms of anxiety or other kinds of mental stress which cause the same symptoms. The diagnosis is made easier, however, by the clear association of fatigue due to cardiac failure with effort and physical exertion. In addition, this kind of fatigue is always accompanied by genuine signs of congestive heart failure.

Cyanosis is the medical term for the bluish tint of the skin and mucous membranes (of the mouth and nose, for example), that results from a decreased supply of oxygen in the small blood vessels in these areas. Oxygen is carried in the blood by hemoglobin; hemoglobin is bright red when saturated with oxygen, but blue or purple when not saturated. When the amount of nonsaturated hemoglobin exceeds 5 grams per 100 centimeters of blood, the skin takes on a bluish tint.

Cyanosis can be of two types, central and peripheral. In the central type, there is inadequate oxygen in the arterial blood and both the mucous membranes and the skin are affected by bluish discoloration. Central cyanosis is one of the most frequent first signs of a congenital heart defect in infants ("blue babies"). It may also be an early sign of disease of the lungs, central nervous system, or metabolic system, as well as of abnormal hemoglobin in the bloodstream (see Congenital Heart Defects, chapter 16).

Peripheral cyanosis, which is usually limited to the hands and feet, is the result of a slowing of blood flow to the extremities, and to the removal by the tissues of a greater than normal amount of oxygen from arterial blood. This happens when the arterial vessels are constricted and blood flow is diminished from exposure to frigid temperature, shock, congestive heart failure, or peripheral vascular disease. In these conditions, the mucous membranes of the oral cavity or those beneath the tongue are rarely affected. The most common cause of peripheral cyanosis is exposure to cold air or water. It is a normal, transient response to an environmental stimulus. But when cardiac output is low, as in severe congestive heart failure and shock, constriction of the small arteries in the skin is a compensatory mechanism to divert the blood to more vital areas. Intense cyanosis, associated with cold extremities, may result. In such episodes, cyanosis results even though the arterial blood is saturated with oxygen. The reduction in blood flow through the skin and reduced oxygen tension at the venous end of the capillary bed are responsible for the cyanosis.

Prompt recognition of the symptoms of cardiovascular disease by an individual can be a life-saving technique in the very literal sense of that phrase. It is a technique, moreover, that everyone can and should acquire. Too often medical help is sought only when the symptoms are so acute and so severe that the person is already incapacitated. Many psychological factors enter into the reluctance to acknowledge symptoms of a serious disease and to report them promptly. Very often, people refuse to believe that a cardiac condition actually exists and needs medical attention, and many are reluctant to inconvenience their doctors, even those they have consulted for a long time. It is better to err on the side of overcaution, however, than to ignore symptoms

BLUENESS OF THE SKIN

PRINCIPLES

1. *Chest pain is the most common symptom of cardiovascular disease. Chest pain due to heart disease is caused by an insufficient amount of oxygentated blood flowing through the coronary arteries (angina pectoris) or by the injury and death of cardiac muscle tissue due to stoppage in supply of oxygenated blood (myocardial infarction or heart attack).*

2. *Angina pains, while possibly severe, are usually temporary, occurring after physical exertion, during emotion stress, or after heavy meals. The more severe pain of a heart attack lasts longer and may spread through the left shoulder and arm, up the neck and to the jaw and even to the back.*

3. *Angina attacks are sometimes relieved with cessation of activity but this is not the case with heart attack pain.*

4. *Chest pain may also be due to injury or disease of the muscles and bones of the chest or abdomen. Such pains, unlike those related to cardiovascular disease, increase with deep breathing or movement of the chest. Anxiety can cause a type of chest pain that*

SUMMARY

is distinguished from cardiac disease by its long duration, its connection with emotional upset, and its limited effect on ability to work or exert oneself physically.

5. *Pains in the feet and legs on walking (intermittent claudication) can be a sign of narrowing of blood vessels in the lower abdomen and legs.*

6. *High blood pressure occasionally causes headaches and dizziness, recurrent nose bleeds and fatigue after mild effort. Hypertension is a major threat to health and should be treated by a physician.*

7. *Shortness of breath (dyspnea) may be due to fluid retention in the lungs as a result of impaired pumping of the heart; it may also be due to lung disease, pregnancy, anemia, and other conditions. If the cardiac condition worsens, shortness of breath may occur with very little or no exertion and even at rest.*

8. *Awareness of the beat of the heart in the form of skipped beats, flutters in the chest (palpitations), and rapid spurts may be indicative of cardiovascular disease but may also be inconsequential. Anxiety may cause these symptoms.*

9. *Fluid retention (edema), usually noticeable as swelling in the abdomen or extremities, may be caused by other diseases, but is often a sign that the heart is failing to pump strongly enough.*

10. *Loss of consciousness (syncope) may be due to failure of the heart to beat regularly or strongly enough to supply the brain with blood, or it may be due to narrowing of the arteries that lead to the head and brain. The dramatic symptoms of syncope are usually relieved within a brief time by lying down. Continued attacks may be warning signals of possible stroke.*

11. *Faintness and fatigue in the absence of prolonged effort or a triggering incident may be due to cardiac disease.*

12. *Blueness of the skin (cyanosis) is due to a decrease in the supply of oxygenated blood to the surface blood vessels. Cyanosis may also result when the flow of blood to the vessels near the skin surface is diverted to supply deeper organs. It is a common symptom in newborn babies with congenital heart defects (blue babies).*

which may be early warnings of serious malfunction. An informed person can monitor, and to some extent, evaluate, some of the more prominent symptoms of cardiovascular diseases and report them to a doctor who can ascertain the cause. The life-saving potential of such knowledge is well worth the effort involved in acquiring it.

10

HYPERTENSION

Harriet P. Dustan, M.D.

Hypertension, defined in simple terms, means that the blood circulates through the arteries at a pressure which is higher than normal. Pressure in the arteries is determined by a number of factors, beginning with the contraction of the heart itself, the source of the energy that makes blood circulate through the body. Each time the heart contracts, 2 to 3 ounces (59 to 89 milliliters) of blood are ejected into the arterial system, creating a sudden surge of pressure. This is called the pressure pulse, the steady beat the physician records when he takes the pulse or calculates the heart rate.

Because there are two distinct aspects of every heartbeat—contraction (systole) and relaxation (diastole)—there are two aspects of the pressure pulse. Systolic pressure is the level to which pressure rises with each heart contraction; diastolic pressure is the level to which pressure falls when the heart relaxes. Systolic pressure is determined by the amount of blood the heart pumps with each stroke, by the speed with which the heart contracts, and by the elasticity of the large arteries close to the heart, particularly the aorta, which receives most directly the energy of each heart contraction. Diastolic pressure, on the other hand, is determined by the resistance to the flow of blood from the arteries into the capillaries, where the exchange of gases and nutrients vital to body cells and tissues takes place. The resistance is actually created by the arterial system's smallest vessels, the arterioles, which control the blood flow and the pressure from arteries to capillaries.

With each contraction of the heart the arterial system is filled suddenly, and between beats it empties in a complicated process whereby blood flows out through millions of minute arterioles. Obviously, then, if the arterioles become narrowed, the resistance to the flow of blood into the capillaries will increase and pressure in the arteries will rise. That is exactly what happens in most cases of hypertension; diastolic arterial pressure rises as the resistance to outflow from the arteries increases. And when diastolic pressure rises, systolic pressure also rises in order to keep blood circulating.

Systolic hypertension is often seen alone, however, particularly in the later years of life. Arteries lose some of their elasticity and become stiffer with age, and because the aorta is one of the determinants of systolic pressure, the loss of flexibility results in an increase in pressure. At younger ages, the more flexible aorta is able to absorb some of the energy of each cardiac contraction by stretching and thus "dampening" the pressure. When the heart then relaxes, the aorta relaxes as well, releasing the energy it has absorbed. The released energy is transformed into the pressure that keeps blood flowing into the capillaries. Another factor that contributes to systolic hypertension in the elderly is the presence of atherosclerosis, adding to the rigidity of the arteries. When the heart contracts, the rigid aorta cannot absorb the pressure, and systolic pressure becomes elevated.

BLOOD PRESSURE MEASUREMENT

Blood pressure can be measured either directly or indirectly—that is, either inside or outside the body. In the direct, internal method, a small catheter is inserted into an artery. The catheter is connected to a device which is able to transform the blood pressure into an electronic signal. The signal is then amplified and converted into a permanent record.

The indirect method, which is not as precise and does not produce a permanent record, has the advantage of being simple to perform and easily learned by the patient, who may have to make daily or weekly pressure

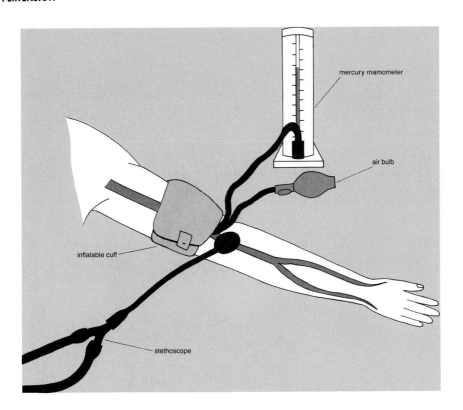

readings. The instrument used in the indirect method is called a sphyg-momanometer (*sphygmos*, Greek for pulse, and *metron*, Greek for a measure). It consists of an inflatable cuff which wraps around the upper arm above the elbow, a rubber bulb to inflate the cuff, and a device to measure the levels of pressure, which are recorded in terms of millimeters of mercury. A stethoscope is used to listen for certain characteristic sounds within the artery. When the cuff is securely placed on the arm, air is pumped into it, compressing the main artery of the arm until the blood flow is momentarily interrupted. The mercury level is highest at this point, indicating air-pressure measurement in the cuff. Air is gradually let out of the cuff, and as the air pressure drops, the person taking the measurement listens with the stethoscope to the artery just below the cuff. Blood again begins to flow through the artery, creating a distinct sound. As soon as this sound is heard, the pressure is noted. This is the systolic pressure, the highest pressure of the heartbeat and the highest pressure within the artery. The diastolic pressure is then determined by continuing to let air out of the cuff. As the cuff deflates, allowing blood to flow freely through the artery, the distinct sound disappears. The pressure at the moment of disappearance, that is, when there is the least amount of pressure in the artery, is the diastolic pressure. The pressure is recorded by two numbers (for example, normal pressure, 120/80), the first being the systolic reading and the second the diastolic reading. A pressure reading of 196/74 would indicate systolic hypertension; 188/132 would indicate both systolic and diastolic hypertension.

Hypertension is an important public health problem in all industrialized societies because it is so widespread and because it leads to disability and in many cases to premature death. In the United States alone, hypertension afflicts

EFFECTS OF HYPERTENSION

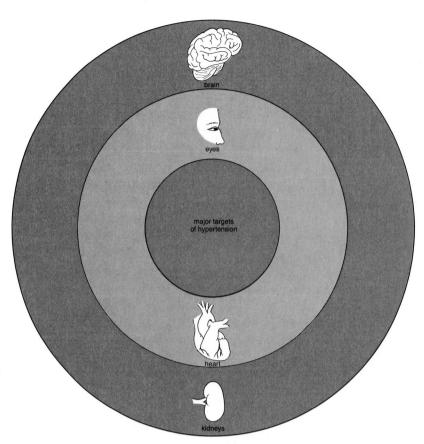

Untreated hypertension can cause stroke, eye damage, heart attack, heart failure, and kidney failure.

from 10 to 15 percent of the adult population, and there are comparable statistics from other nations with similar economic and cultural patterns. Hypertension creates a major risk of heart attacks and strokes and is implicated in a variety of kidney disorders. A number of statistical studies show that even mild degrees of hypertension are associated with shortened life span; thus even pressure levels regarded as within a "normal" range may be threats to life.

Evidence available at the present time indicates that diseases of the arteries and the arterioles are the result of high pressure within these blood vessels. It is now accepted medical opinion that high intra-arterial pressure is a threat to health, not because it is dangerous in itself but because it injures arteries and arterioles. Fortunately, sufficient evidence has been gathered to support the conclusion that when blood pressure levels are reduced to normal or near normal, the consequences of some of the associated vascular diseases are either eliminated or substantially diminished.

Since hypertension occurs within the arterial circulation, it is the arteries and arterioles, rather than the veins, that are affected. The two main types of diseases, arteriolar sclerosis and atherosclerosis, have their own characteristics and create particular problems for the hypertensive patient. Arteriolar sclerosis results in structural changes in the walls of the arteries, particularly the arterioles. These changes can occur anywhere in the body. Atherosclerosis, on the other hand, affects the aorta and the large arteries.

The structural changes in arteriolar sclerosis result in an increased thickness of the arteriolar wall and a narrowing of the internal dimension of the vessel (the lumen). In addition to the structural changes, there is a functional change due to contraction of the smooth muscle of the arteriole, which narrows the vessel (vasoconstriction). The end result of both changes is an increased resistance to blood flow.

As the arterioles progressively narrow, the heart is forced to provide more and more energy to circulate the blood through them. One way the heart is able to produce more energy is by increasing the size of the heart muscle itself. But because the added muscle must be kept supplied with blood, a still greater burden is placed on the already overworked heart. As the resistance to blood flow becomes greater, the heart can no longer meet the ever-increasing workload, and heart failure is the final consequence. Heart failure was, in fact, the most common cause of death among hypertensive patients before antihypertensive drugs were widely available. Today heart failure can be prevented by treatment of the underlying hypertension. Even when an untreated condition progresses to heart failure, it can be controlled if drugs are administered to reduce blood pressure.

The kidneys are particularly susceptible to the damaging effects of hypertension. These highly vascular organs receive about 20 percent of the cardiac output, a rate made necessary by the kidneys' function of ridding the bloodstream of waste products. Because in hypertension blood vessels narrow and thicken, blood flow decreases at times to such an extent that normal function is impossible, and kidney failure results. In terms of the over-all number of cases of hypertension, this is a relatively infrequent complication. It is, however, much more frequent in the small group of individuals who have what is termed "malignant" hypertension.

Malignant hypertension bears no relationship to cancer, but it rapidly leads to death if it is not treated. A severe, destructive arteriolar disease, malignant hypertension affects the kidneys particularly, resulting in kidney failure. This form of hypertension also damages arterioles in the eyes, causing red blood cells and plasma to leak out of the vessels. The hemorrhages that form in the retina reduce vision, sometimes to the point of blindness. In some cases, the nerve head at the center of the retina swells as a result of increased pressure within the head—a condition called papilledema or choked disk.

Hypertensive encephalopathy is common in the more severe form of hypertension. In this condition, blood flow to the brain is decreased because of severe shrinkage of the interior of the blood vessels. Symptoms include severe headache, nausea, vomiting, restlessness, and coma. Malignant hypertension often results in heart failure, but this condition, as well as encephalopathy, can be effectively and efficiently treated by rapid reduction of blood pressure by drugs or other means.

Eye Changes in Hypertension

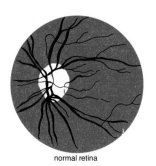 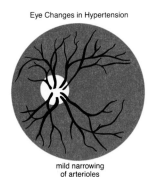 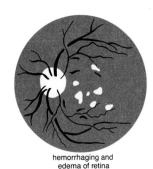

normal retina

mild narrowing of arterioles

hemorrhaging and edema of retina

The small arteries in the eye, the only blood vessels which can be viewed directly, reveal damage caused by hypertension. In advanced cases, red blood cells and plasma leak out of the arterioles, reducing vision and sometimes destroying it completely.

Hemorrhagic strokes, which result from the rupture of blisterlike formations (aneurysms) in small arteries within the brain, are a frequent complication of hypertension. These strokes are different from strokes caused by blood clots (thrombotic strokes), which are the result of atherosclerosis. Aneurysms of the type found in hemorrhagic strokes are unique to the brain. They occur normally in elderly persons but are few in number. In hypertensive patients, however, the number of aneurysms is greater and they develop at much earlier ages. The ruptured aneurysm bleeds directly into the brain, injuring or destroying tissues. This type of hemorrhage is called intracerebral hemorrhage, or hematoma.

Atherosclerosis, which also accompanies hypertension, affects the aorta and other large and medium-sized arteries. Atherosclerotic plaques in the blood vessels grow slowly over many years, progressively narrowing the arteries. Symptoms of the disease depend on which organ the affected artery supplies; if the blockage is in an artery to the brain, the result is a stroke; if it is in the heart, angina pectoris or a heart attack may follow; if in the legs, pains or cramps (intermittent claudication) occur while walking, and ultimately gangrene may result from lack of blood circulation. Atherosclerosis occurs to a greater or less extent with aging (although evidence suggests this is not true for every culture on a worldwide basis), and the disease develops at an earlier age in those with hypertension. There is now ample evidence that hypertension accelerates the development of atherosclerosis.

FACTORS AFFECTING HYPERTENSION

An individual can be "at risk" for hypertension because of factors that are avoidable (overweight) or unavoidable (age and family inheritance). Each plays a different role in an individual case, and no single factor in itself seems to be the primary determinant of who actually does develop hypertension.

OBESITY   The relation of this major risk factor to hypertension in Western, industrialized societies has been demonstrated repeatedly. Although not all hypertensives are obese, nor are all individuals with normal pressure thin, there is more obesity among groups of hypertensives than among groups with normal pressures. In one community study of young persons with mild hypertension, the only feature common to those who subsequently developed more severe hypertension or complications of hypertension was rapid weight gain. The development of obesity apparently contributes directly to hypertension and its complications. There is also a great deal of evidence indicating that reduction of weight is accompanied by reduction in arterial pressure in hypertensive obese patients.

AGE   This is a major unavoidable risk factor. Generally speaking, hypertension appears in the third or fourth decade of life. In unusual instances it develops in children, and when this happens before the age of twelve, the disease almost certainly indicates the presence of an abnormality of the adrenal glands or the kidneys. When systolic hypertension develops in elderly persons, it usually starts after the age of fifty and becomes progressively higher with advancing age. Diastolic hypertension, however, almost never occurs after the fifty-year mark without some underlying cause. Anyone more than fifty years old who has had normal pressure throughout life has a very good chance of never developing diastolic hypertension, although systolic hypertension may,

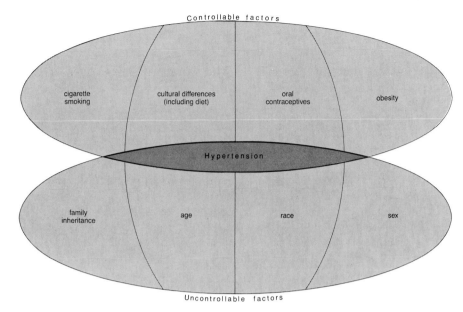

Controllable factors

cigarette smoking   cultural differences (including diet)   oral contraceptives   obesity

Hypertension

family inheritance   age   race   sex

Uncontrollable factors

Each risk factor plays a different role in each individual. No single factor alone determines who will suffer hypertension.

of course, develop with age. When a person with no history of diastolic hypertension develops the disease in later life, it is a signal to look for previously unsuspected and underlying causes.

RACE   Another unavoidable risk factor is race; studies have shown that black males are more likely than white males to have hypertension and have the disease in a more serious form.

INHERITANCE   This seems to be a factor in predisposing a person to hypertension, and one type of hypertension is believed to be genetically determined. The inheritance is polygenic—that is, a number of genes are involved. The subject of genetic inheritance is complex, but in simple terms, research indicates that hypertension develops more frequently when one of the parents is hypertensive, and when both are hypertensive, the likelihood of their offspring's developing hypertension is even greater.

CULTURAL DIFFERENCES   Diet and eating patterns, and other cultural factors, play a significant role in the incidence of hypertension. In general, hypertension is an abnormality that affects populations in highly structured, industrialized, "developed" societies. In these cultures, blood pressure levels rise with age, but in many nonindustrialized cultures this does not occur. Exact reasons for these differences among cultures are still subject to speculation, although some authorities suggest that the differences are related to the high consumption of salt and frequent occurrence of gross overweight in industrialized nations.

SEX DIFFERENCE   The incidence of hypertension does not seem to be directly related to sex. The disease occurs with about equal frequency in men and women, although men tend to suffer complications of hypertension at an earlier age than women do.

ORAL CONTRACEPTIVES   Although it is not a frequent complication, hypertension affects about 10 percent of women who take oral contraceptives. In rare instances the contraceptive agents have been associated with malignant hypertension and stroke. Fortunately, in most cases the high blood pressure can be returned to normal by stopping the medication.

CAUSES OF HYPERTENSION Hypertension, like fever, is a symptom of an underlying problem. Although many factors may be involved, the basic problem in hypertension, as far as it is understood, is an exaggeration of some normal biologic mechanism. Hypertension, therefore, can be viewed as a "disease of regulation," in which one or more of the factors known to control arterial pressure become deranged, while at the same time other factors fail to compensate for these derangements. Moreover, there is no evidence that any outside agents, such as bacteria or viruses, cause the condition.

The factors controlling arterial pressure directly are blood flow (the output of the heart), resistance to that flow, the flexibility of the aorta, and blood volume. Several other body systems affect these factors; the autonomic nervous system, the part of the central nervous system that regulates involuntary bodily functions such as heartbeat, breathing, and digestion; the salt stores of the body, a hormone system from the kidneys (the renal pressor system); and aldosterone, a hormone from the adrenal gland which determines the salt and water balance of the body. These systems are all interrelated, and in hypertension the relationships are disturbed.

Since hypertension is an expression of altered relationships in the factors that determine arterial pressure, in certain instances the causes of hypertension have actually been identified.

RENAL HYPERTENSION Two types of abnormality of the kidneys cause hypertension. One type is associated with narrowing of one or more of the main arteries directly carrying blood to the kidneys. This condition is called renovascular hypertension. The second type is associated with renal parenchymal diseases, the diseases related to inflammation, infection, and changes in the structure and function of the kidneys. In renovascular hypertension there is increased production of the kidney hormone, renin, because the artery supplying one or both kidneys is narrowed. Although renal parenchymal disease is often accompanied by hypertension, the mechanism is different from that in renovascular hypertension. The first step is some deficiency of salt and water excretion, the next is constriction of small blood vessels, and then the blood pressure rises.

ADRENAL HYPERTENSION Tumors of the adrenal glands, either in the central portion of the gland, the medulla, or the surrounding portion, the cortex, also cause hypertension. The results are different in each case, because the medulla and the cortex produce very different hormones. The medulla forms chemical substances called catecholamines, one of which, norepinephrine, is also found in sympathetic nerves. The cortex produces a variety of steroid hormones, but aldosterone is the most significant in terms of hypertension. A tumor of the adrenal medulla, pheochromocytoma, causes hypertension through excessive production of catecholamines. Because this mimics the action of the sympathetic nervous system, the heart rate is often fast, cardiac output is elevated, and resistance to blood flow increased. Blood volume is usually low, and renin

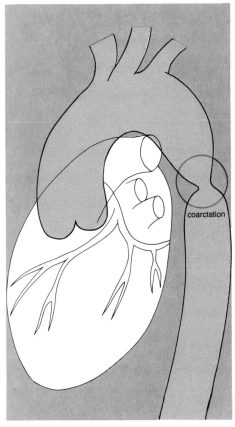

Coarctation of the aorta

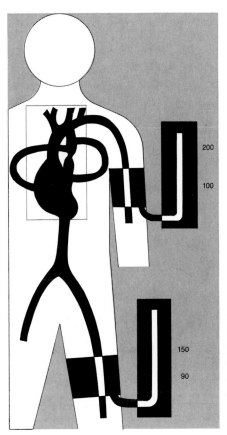

The pinched aorta is abnormally narrow and small. When the heart forces a normal amount of blood through this opening, the pressure above the narrowing is elevated but that below it is lowered.

release slightly increased. The most significant kind of tumor of the cortex in causing hypertension is one that produces aldosterone, because this situation leads to salt and water retention.

COARCTATION OF THE AORTA A congenital defect in which there is a marked narrowing or pinching of the aorta results in systolic hypertension, because the heart ejects a normal volume of blood into an abnormally small aortic "container." Blood pressure in arteries above the narrowing is elevated, but it is very low in arteries below the pinched area. The other factors that determine arterial pressure do not seem to be involved.

ESSENTIAL HYPERTENSION This term is used to designate hypertension of unknown cause. It is the most frequently encountered type, accounting for about 90 percent of all hypertension. Further knowledge is necessary for precise definition of the causes of essential hypertension, but fortunately drug treatment is effective in reducing arterial pressure to normal or near normal levels.

The first drugs with long-term effectiveness in the treatment of hypertension were introduced in the early 1950s, and a wide variety of such drugs has since become available. When the drugs were first used, it soon became clear that malignant hypertension could be controlled by a reduction in arterial pressure, and the condition was no longer considered "malignant." Many years of study were required, however, before it was evident that these drugs could benefit patients with less severe forms of hypertension. The evidence finally became

TREATMENT OF HYPERTENSION AND ITS COMPLICATIONS

available in 1967 and 1970, through two studies conducted by the Veterans Administration on middle-aged men. The 1967 study was of a group with a pretreatment diastolic pressure between 115 and 129. The 1970 study involved a group whose diastolic pressure was between 90 and 114. Both studies convincingly demonstrated that the development of heart failure, kidney damage, visual complications, and hemorrhagic stroke was sharply reduced when hypertension was treated. Although the occurrence of heart attacks did not seem diminished by treatment, this does not mean that treatment of hypertension does not affect the progress of atherosclerosis in coronary arteries. Since atherosclerosis develops over many years, the men in both studies had had the disease for a long period before the hypertension was treated. The studies, moreover, covered a relatively short period—two to four years. It seems likely that if treatment of hypertension is to lessen the progress of coronary atherosclerosis, it must start during the early years of the development of hypertension.

Antihypertensive Drugs Drugs are by far the most widely applicable form of treatment for hypertension. The three types in use are diuretics, sympatholytics, and vasodilators.

DIURETICS Drugs that increase the flow of urine are effective in about half of all cases of hypertension. There are many diuretics, most of them related to the parent compound chlorothiazide, the first one produced. They vary in potency and duration of action, but the strongest are most useful when the patient's kidney function is reduced. One drawback of all chlorothiazide type drugs is that, used over long periods of time, they cause a fall in the level of potassium in the blood. This is potentially dangerous in patients who are taking digitalis.

Two non-chlorothiazide drugs which do not affect potassium levels are now in use; spironolactone, which blocks the effect of aldosterone on the kidneys; and triamterene, which works through another mechanism. Neither of these is a particularly potent diuretic by itself, but each is effective when combined with a chlorothiazide. Spironolactone is particularly useful for patients with increased aldosterone production (primary aldosteronism), but its usefulness is limited because of side effects, as a synthetic steroid hormone it can cause breast enlargement in men and women, impotence in men, and menstrual irregularity in women.

To be an effective antihypertensive drug, a diuretic must first increase the urinary excretion of salt and water and in long-term use prevent fluid from reaccumulating. Diuretic treatment is not only effective in itself, it can also intensify the blood-pressure-lowering effects of other drugs. For example, the effectiveness of sympatholytic drugs is often counteracted by their fluid-retention effect. The addition of a diuretic overcomes this liability.

SYMPATHOLYTIC DRUGS So named because they decrease the activity of the sympathetic nervous system, these drugs do so in various ways. Some act on the brain centers that control blood pressure. Others affect only the sympathetic nerve endings so that the electrical impulses from the brain have diminished effectiveness. Still others act on both the brain and the peripheral nerves, and a final group acts directly on the heart and blood vessels.

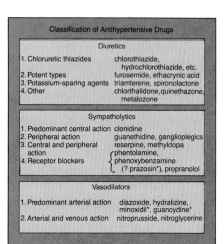

Classification of Antihypertensive Drugs

Diuretics

1. Chloruretic thiazides	chlorothiazide, hydrochlorothiazide, etc.
2. Potent types	furosemide, ethacrynic acid
3. Potassium-sparing agents	triamterene, spironolactone
4. Other	chlorthalidone, quinethazone, metalozone

Sympatholytics

1. Predominant central action	clonidine
2. Peripheral action	guanethidine, ganglioplegics
3. Central and peripheral action	reserpine, methyldopa
4. Receptor blockers	phentolamine, phenoxybenzamine (? prazosin*), propranolol

Vasodilators

1. Predominant arterial action	diazoxide, hydralizine, minoxidil*, guancydine*
2. Arterial and venous action	nitroprusside, nitroglycerine

These drugs are effective in many types of hypertension, although they are not particularly beneficial in salt-and-water-dependent types. They also have the potential for causing fluid retention, and this, for reasons unknown, causes arterial pressure to rise. The addition of a diuretic reestablishes good blood pressure control.

VASODILATORS These drugs relax arteriolar smooth muscles, dilating the arterioles, which allows the blood to flow more easily and reduces blood pressure. The most potent ones are given intravenously, to treat the crises of hypertension. One type can be taken by mouth but generally is not very effective in the severe forms of hypertension. At present vasodilator therapy does not offer as wide a variety of drugs as are found in the diuretic and sympatholytic categories. Vasodilators may also produce unpleasant side effects, such as palpitations, rapid heart rate, and fluid retention. These can be controlled by other drugs.

PRINCIPLES

1. *Hypertension means that the blood circulates through the arteries at a pressure which is higher than normal. In most cases of hypertension, the arterioles, the smallest of the arteries, have become narrowed, causing a*

Surgery

Surgical treatment is possible for a few specific types of hypertension, including coarctation of the aorta, renovascular hypertension, and tumors of the adrenal medulla and cortex. In cases of coarctation, the narrowed segment of the aorta is removed and the two ends are sutured together, or the defective segment is replaced with a Dacron graft.

resistance to the flow of blood into the capillaries and a rise in pressure within the arteries.

In renovascular hypertension, several surgical procedures are possible to normalize blood supply through the arteries leading to the kidneys. If the area of narrowing is sharply localized, it can sometimes be removed, or a Dacron graft or a segment of a vein can be inserted to bypass the narrowed area, thus establishing a normal arterial pressure–blood flow relationship in the affected kidney. If only one kidney is affected and neither of these procedures can be used, the kidney can be removed. Tumors of the adrenal medulla and cortex can also be removed by surgery.

2. *Blood pressure can be measured directly, by the insertion of a small catheter into an artery, or indirectly, by measurements taken with a sphygmomanometer, an instrument consisting of an inflatable cuff, a rubber bulb to inflate it, and a device to measure the levels of pressure, which are recorded in terms of millimeters of mercury. The doctor*

Long-Term Therapy

Since most hypertension cannot be cured, it must be kept under control by medication taken regularly. At one time it was thought that keeping blood pressure at lowered levels for a long period of time (several months to a few years) would allow body mechanisms to "reset" so that blood pressure would remain normal when the medication was discontinued. Now we know that this is not the case and that the only way to avoid the complications of hypertension is to continue treatment month after month, year after year.

measuring blood pressure listens with a stethoscope for certain characteristic sounds within the artery as the cuff is inflated and then gradually emptied of air.

Long-term treatment poses problems for many people. If drugs have side effects, these are difficult to tolerate and much patience and persistence is required to continue treatment. Also, since most hypertension causes no symptoms, it is difficult to appreciate the benefit of treatment. If one feels well, the value of therapy is not apparent. The need for protection from the complications of hypertension—strokes, heart failure, kidney failure, and heart attacks —does not seem urgent to someone who has never suffered from any of these. Yet the long-term benefits are real, as evidenced by the striking decrease in deaths from hypertension that have occurred in the last twenty years. It is the responsibility of the physician to help patients understand why treatment

3. *Hypertension, which afflicts from 10 to 15 percent of the adult population in this country, creates a major risk of heart attacks and strokes and is implicated in a variety of kidney disorders. Heart failure, the most common cause of death among hypertensive patients before the use of anti-hypertensive drugs, can be prevented by treatment of the underlying hypertension. Malignant hypertension can result in kidney*

failure and significant damage to the arterioles in the eyes and perhaps even blindness.

4. *The avoidable risk factors for hypertension are obesity, diet and eating patterns, and the taking of oral contraceptives. Unavoidable risk factors include age, race, family inheritance, and sex differences.*

5. *Hypertension is called a "disease of regulation," in which one or more of the factors known to control arterial pressure become deranged, while other factors fail to compensate for these derangements.*

PREVENTION OF HYPERTENSION

6. *Drugs are the most widely applicable form of treatment for hypertension. These include diuretics, or drugs that increase the flow of urine; sympatholytic drugs, or those that decrease the activity of the sympathetic nervous system; and vasodilators, or drugs that relax arteriolar smooth muscles, dilating the arterioles and allowing the blood to flow more easily, thus reducing blood pressure.*

7. *Surgical treatment is possible for a few specific types of hypertension, including coarctation of the aorta, renovascular hypertension, and tumors of the adrenal medulla and cortex.*

8. *Most cases of hypertension cannot be cured, but they can be kept under control with regular medication. The striking decrease in deaths from hypertension in the last twenty years testifies to the effectiveness of long-term drug therapy for hypertension.*

9. *Although little is known about the causes of most kinds of hypertension, and therefore about its prevention, obesity seems clearly to be a contributing factor. Current research findings do not indicate what proportion of hypertension is caused by excess intake of salt. It may, however, be wise to reduce intake of salty foods and use salt sparingly.*

is important and to work out treatment programs that are not only effective but also as simple as possible.

For many people with hypertension, measurement of blood pressure at home is not only easy but a good way to judge the success of treatment. True, it is one more thing that has to be done to help take care of one's problem, and that is a disadvantage. However, it is very often worth the trouble.

Many sphygmomanometers have been especially designed so that the average person can measure his own pressure. The instruments are easy to use; the technique of measurement is very simple and can be learned quickly. Pressure should be measured once or twice a day at times that are most convenient and least disruptive of the daily routine—in the morning just after waking up and in the evening at bedtime are particularly good times. It is advisable to keep a record of the pressures because it helps the physician in adjusting treatment.

Although very little is known about the causes of most kinds of hypertension, and therefore about its prevention, evidence concerning obesity as a risk factor is so compelling that there seems a strong likelihood that a substantial proportion of hypertension cases could be prevented. Studies indicate that (1) obesity is more common in hypertensive people than in those with normal blood pressure, (2) primitive populations who do not gain weight as they age have very little hypertension, (3) weight gain in early adult life is a potent risk factor for subsequent development of hypertension, and (4) weight reduction of obese hypertensive patients, rather regularly, reduces blood pressure. This evidence is an adequate basis for weight control; young people who are not obese should be careful not to gain weight as they grow older; obese young people should lose weight; and for obese patients weight reduction should be as much a part of treatment programs as antihypertensive drugs.

A high salt intake is widely believed to cause hypertension. This belief is based on the absence of hypertension among primitive people who eat little salt (and who also are not fat) and on the ease with which hypertension can be produced in laboratory animals by a high salt intake. We do know that certain types of human hypertension are salt dependent, and we also know that diuretic drugs and low salt diets are effective treatment for many hypertensive patients. However, we do not know what proportion of hypertension is caused by salt excess. Until more information is available, there is no justification for recommending rigid salt-restrictive diets. However, since most people's usual intake probably exceeds their body needs, it may be wise to reduce intake of salty foods and add salt to foods sparingly.

11

CORONARY ARTERY DISEASE

Elliot Rapaport, M.D.

The heart pumps about 5 to 6 quarts (5 to 6 liters) of blood each minute and may increase its output to more than 20 quarts (20 liters) during exercise. Carrying out this work requires a continually available, adequate supply of energy to the heart muscle, which is provided by the nutrients and oxygen carried in the blood. Nutrients may be stored within the heart for later use, but oxygen cannot be stored. The heart muscle therefore cannot tolerate interruption of its blood supply for long periods.

Blood is transported to the heart muscle by the left and right coronary arteries, the first arteries to arise from the aorta as it leaves the heart. The left coronary artery divides soon after its point of origin into the anterior descending branch and the circumflex branch. The anterior descending artery courses down the front of the heart in a groove between the two ventricles. Normally, it passes to the very apex of the heart, supplying a large part of the wall (septum) between the two ventricles and most of the front wall of

The right heart receives blood from the body and pumps it through the pulmonary artery to the lungs where the blood gets rid of carbon dioxide and picks up a fresh supply of oxygen. The left heart receives oxygen-rich blood from the lungs via the pulmonary veins and pumps it through the aorta to the body.

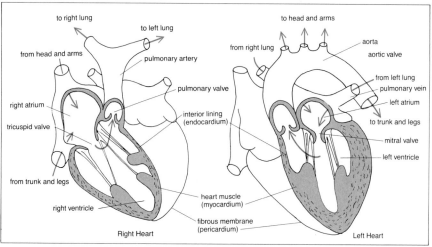

How the Human Heart Works

Coronary circulation. The two main coronary arteries descend from the aorta, then divide and subdivide, girdling the entire heart in the manner of a crown.

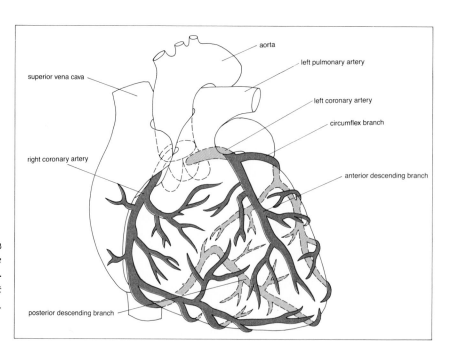

the left ventricle. The other branch, the circumflex coronary artery, courses in a groove between the left atrium and the left ventricle. It runs down the back of the left ventricle, primarily supplying this area with blood. The right coronary artery has its origin at the right side of the aorta and runs in the groove between the right atrium and the right ventricle, supplying blood to the right ventricle and parts of the back of the left ventricle.

Approximately 5 percent of the total blood flow from the heart goes through the coronary circulation each minute. The oyxgen needs of the heart are only minimally met by this amount of blood flow, however, so that the heart muscle extracts more oxygen from the blood than does any other tissue in the body. If the heart rate speeds up, if the heart has to pump against elevated blood pressure, or if the heart's output increases, more oxygen is required, and this requirement is met by increased blood flow to the heart muscle itself. Thus, as the work of the heart increases under stress, the coronary circulation must deliver more blood per unit of time. Normally, this presents no problem, but if the coronary arteries are significantly diseased or obstructed, this may not be accomplished. An imbalance will then exist between the amount of oxygen needed by the heart muscle to carry on its work and the amount of oxygen delivered to it by the coronary circulation.

Any imbalance between oxygen demand and delivery leads to alterations in the metabolism of the heart muscle cells, with the production of certain byproducts (metabolites) that result in the sensation of chest discomfort. When this imbalance is transient—that is, when acute stressful situations, either emotional or physical, result in a sudden increase in oxygen demand unmet by the circulation—the chest discomfort is also transient, lasting only minutes before disappearing as the person recovers from the stress. This transient chest discomfort is usually felt under the breastbone as a heavy ache, sometimes radiating up into the neck and left shoulder and down the left arm. The term "angina pectoris" is used to describe this clinical picture. If there is an acute decrease in oxygen delivery at rest, such as that resulting from the adherence of a blood clot to an atherosclerotic plaque, a portion of the heart muscle may become infarcted or die. When this happens, prolonged, often severe chest discomfort is usually felt under the breastbone, radiating down the left arm and lasting from twenty or thirty minutes up to several hours. The term "acute myocardial infarction" is applied to this clinical situation.

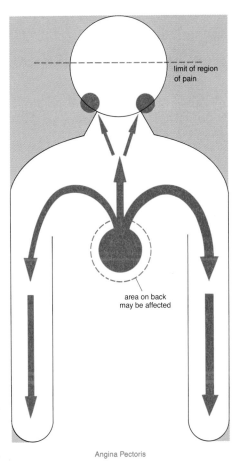

Angina Pectoris

Area in color shows the most common radiations of pain resulting from inadequate oxygen supply to the working heart muscle.

CORONARY ARTERY DISEASE

Coronary artery disease is almost always the result of atherosclerosis—hardening of the arteries. Coronary atherosclerosis primarily results from the accumulation of fatty deposits in the walls of coronary arteries, which leads to the formation of fibrous tissue in the vessel wall. Coronary artery disease is the most common type of heart disease and the leading cause of death in the United States as well as many other countries. In the United States alone, an estimated two-thirds of a million persons die each year from coronary artery disease.

The exact sequence of events which ultimately leads to severe obstruction of coronary arteries by atheromatous plaques is unknown. Most authorities believe that the process is lifelong, beginning in childhood or early adulthood. Fatty materials, principally cholesterol, move from the blood-

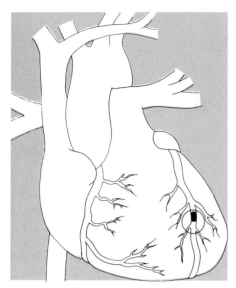

Atherosclerotic deposit in the wall of a coronary artery narrows the opening through which blood flows, reducing the supply of oxygen to the heart muscle. A blood clot trapped in the narrow opening may completely obstruct the flow and thus deprive the tissue of vital oxygen.

stream directly into the lining of the blood vessel and are usually deposited near the beginning of the artery, particularly at the point where it branches. In the coronary circulation, these lesions occur in the large vessels and are rarely seen once the branches of the coronary vessels dip into the muscle of the heart prior to branching into capillaries. The fatty deposits cause a reaction within the vessel wall, and scarlike, fibrous tissue may build up around the deposit, forming a plaque which may become calcified. Generally, the plaque does not cover the entire circumference of the vessel but only part of it, protruding into the lumen (the opening) and progressively narrowing it until in some cases total obstruction or occlusion takes place. Significant interference with the blood flow does not occur until well over half the vessel is occluded by a plaque. Coronary artery disease may be present, therefore, without evidence of coronary heart disease.

Coronary heart disease or symptoms of disturbed myocardial function resulting from interference in the blood flow occasionally take place when only one vessel is obstructed. More commonly, however, by the time a patient develops angina pectoris or has an acute heart attack or myocardial infarction, two or three major vessels are affected by one or more atherosclerotic plaques (atheromata). At times, an acute myocardial infarction may result when a coronary atheroma leads to the secondary formation of a blood clot (thrombus) which totally occludes or blocks the vessel. Blood platelets (cellular components involved in blood coagulation) tend to stick to atherosclerotic plaques, and the aggregation of these platelets may lead to the formation of a blood clot which completely occludes the vessel. When this happens, an acute heart attack may ensue. However, an acute heart attack may also occur without the presence of a recent thrombus if the plaque occludes a large segment of the vessel.

Incidence of Coronary Artery Disease

Coronary artery disease is much more common among males than among females, affecting ten times as many males as females under the age of forty-five. The sex preference falls off rapidly between the ages of forty-five and sixty, although males in this group have about twice as many heart attacks as do females. In the very elderly, the incidence is about the same for both sexes.

Although the basic cause of coronary artery disease is unknown, scientists have identified a number of factors which are associated with a distinct increase in the likelihood that a person will develop a heart attack later in life. These factors, which correlate with the presence of coronary heart disease, are spoken of as "risk factors." Some risk factors are unavoidable, such as racial and genetic susceptibility, prevalence in males, and increased likelihood of having a heart attack as aging occurs. A number of known risk factors are, however, susceptible to modification. Particularly important among these are high blood pressure, cigarette smoking, and elevated serum cholesterol. Approximately 50 percent of those who have heart attacks are persons who have one or more of these three risk factors. Recent studies show that modification of some of these risk factors may decrease, in part, the original susceptibility to a future heart attack or stroke. A prudent approach, therefore, appears to be elimination or attenuation of these risk factors whenever they are identified. Specifically, it is important to insure that patients with high blood pressure take medication to keep their blood pressure in normal range even when no symptoms of hypertension are evident. Furthermore, anyone with abnormal levels of lipids or fats in the blood should be on an appropriate diet and possibly a drug regimen to reduce serum lipids, particularly cholesterol and triglycerides. Finally, cigarette smoking should be eliminated.

A number of studies of the incidence of coronary heart disease among large population groups have been conducted in recent decades. The results of these studies indicate that patients who have angina pectoris as a new complaint will succumb at an average rate of 4 percent a year. (It must be remembered that this is an average figure and clearly may not be applicable to any single patient.) Follow-up studies of patients who have undergone coronary arteriography, an X-ray technique for viewing arteries, show that mortality is particularly related to the extent of coronary artery disease and the degree to which the functioning of the left ventricle is impaired. For example, on the basis of follow-up studies it has been projected that well over 90 percent of patients with a single significant lesion in the descending coronary artery will be alive after five years, whereas approximately half the patients with severe disease of three vessels will not be alive after the same period. If coronary artery disease so damages the heart muscle as to result in heart failure, there is approximately a one-in-four to one-in-three chance the patient will die within one year. However, the statistics relating survival to the findings of coronary arteriography were compiled from uncontrolled, retrospective studies and reflect a period when medical management of coronary heart disease had not progressed greatly. Many of the patients included in these studies had had no medical treatments and were simply followed without specific treatment. It is possible, therefore, that survival statistics compiled in the coming years for patients who have received medical treatment but have not undergone surgery will be somewhat better than past studies indicate.

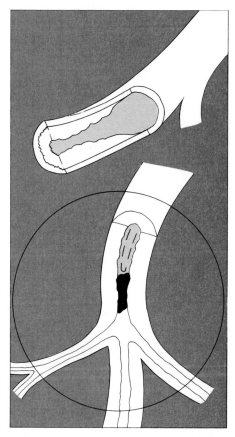

The survival rate for patients who have recovered from a heart attack is similar after the first year to that of patients with angina pectoris. The risk of death during the first year after a heart attack is roughly 8 to 13 percent and thereafter falls to an average of 4 percent per year.

Symptoms

The clinical picture resulting from coronary artery disease varies considerably. If the location and degree of coronary atheromata do not seriously block the blood flow, the patient may be entirely free of symptoms. However, unrecognized coronary artery disease can lead to sudden death; the most common finding at postmortem examination of patients who die suddenly is extensive coronary artery disease. If coronary circulation is adequate to meet the needs of the heart during periods of relatively normal activity but becomes inadequate when the work of the heart demands increased flow, angina pectoris may result. If the coronary circulation is suddenly unable to meet the demands of the contracting heart because of a sudden irreversible or only partly reversible decrease in blood flow to a portion of the heart wall, an acute myocardial infarction may occur. Finally, in some cases, coronary artery disease presents a clinical picture which is somewhere between that of angina pectoris and acute myocardial infarction. This may be thought of as an intermediate syndrome or unstable state in which the patient hovers between the death of some of the heart muscle or infarction and muscle ischemia resulting from a transient decrease in blood flow. The term "unstable angina" has recently been applied to this condition. Patients with unstable angina exhibit prolonged chest pain (up to twenty or thirty minutes), which may be unrelated to exercise or if produced by exercise, requires little stress to provoke it. These patients should be hospitalized at once in a coronary care unit and treated acutely with drugs designed to improve myocardial blood flow and decrease the work of the heart. In those cases in which the symptoms of unstable angina do not subside relatively promptly, emergency arteriography is usually performed. If the condition is anatomically amenable to bypass surgery, emergency coronary vein bypass graft surgery is carried out.

MYOCARDIAL INFARCTION

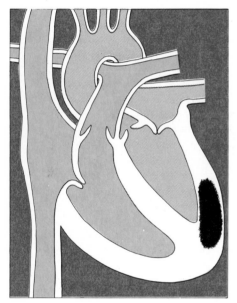

Patients with severe myocardial infarction usually experience severe, crushing pain under the breastbone (substernal), which may be confined to the chest or may radiate into the left shoulder and down the left arm or down both arms. Sometimes the pain extends into the neck or jaw. The pain has been likened to the sensation of having an elephant step on the chest or of having the chest squeezed in a vise. This crushing pain is generally unaffected by movement, position, or other physical efforts, and frequently morphine is required for relief. The pain is often associated with some shortness of breath and marked sweating. The patient also may experience some nausea and, on occasion, even vomiting. The pain usually persists for several hours unless it is relieved by narcotics.

When a large part of the heart muscle has been damaged, the result may be failure of the heart's pumping action. This condition manifests itself either by symptoms of cardiopulmonary congestion, such as acute shortness of breath, an inability to lie flat because of difficulty in breathing, and coughing up blood-tinged sputum, or by an inadequate supply of blood to the peripheral tissues of the body resulting in cold, clammy skin, drowsiness or mental confusion, a fall in urine output, low blood pressure, and ultimately clear-cut shock.

Treatment

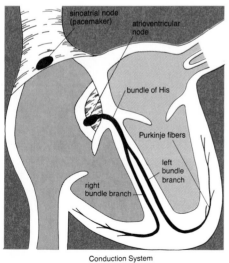

Conduction System

Electrical impulses produced by the heart's natural pacemaker cause the heart to beat.

The overwhelming majority of patients who have acute myocardial infarctions do not have such extensive destruction of heart muscle that severe impairment of over-all heart function results. Once the pain has been relieved by morphine and the patient is placed on bed rest in a coronary care unit, no other treatment may be required. Patients are often allowed to sit quietly in a chair beside their bed several times a day. The greatest risk to these patients is a sudden, unexpected occurrence of a disturbance in heart rhythm (see Arrhythmias, chapter 12). Life-threatening arrhythmias are looked for by nurses and physicians in the coronary care unit through continuous electrocardiographic monitoring. In most cases, irregularities in heart rhythm that may precede life-threatening arrhythmias can be managed through the use of such drugs as lidocaine. This drug and others like it are administered intravenously to suppress evidence of heart irregularity.

In some cases, a heart attack affects the conduction system or specialized tissue that conducts the electrical discharge from the heart's pacemaker to the walls of the heart muscle, where it results in contractions. When the damage involves critical areas of the conduction system or the pacemaker itself, the heart rate may be so slowed that the blood flow from the heart becomes inadequate or it may be a prelude to total cessation of the heartbeat. In this emergency, the physician may insert a slender, flexible tube called a catheter through a vein and lead it into the right ventricle while viewing the heart through a fluoroscope. The catheter has a special metal tip through which an electrical impulse can be transmitted from an external pacemaker, stimulating the heart to contract at a rate determined by the physician. This temporary transvenous pacemaker may be used for hours or days to keep the heartbeat under control while the conduction system recovers from the swelling and inflammation produced by the surrounding damage.

Susceptibility to a fatal disturbance in the heart rhythm is most acute in the first several days after a myocardial infarction, and the patient is therefore usually kept in a coronary care unit where facilities are available for immediate emergency treatment. Once the critical period has passed, the patient is transferred to the general hospital area. Some hospitals have an intermediate coronary care area where the patient's heart rhythm can be monitored, even though the patient is not under constant supervision.

The majority of patients who die from an acute myocardial infarction succumb within the first two hours after the onset of their attack; most of these deaths are the result of electrical instability leading to heart rhythms inconsistent with life. These unstable rhythms can be stabilized successfully by the administration of drugs, temporary pacemakers, and possibly electric shocks to the chest wall if the patient is in the hospital. The importance of early recognition of a heart attack therefore cannot be overemphasized, because early hospitalization is imperative. Patients who have coronary artery disease should be aware of the more common symptoms of a heart attack so that if such symptoms occur, they will call their physician or get to an emergency care facility immediately. Even if the patient is uncertain of the significance of his symptoms, he should always err on the side of assuming the worst and contact his physician.

An increasing number of communities have developed emergency care systems which, in response to a telephone conversation, send mobile coronary care units to the side of the patient suspected of having a heart attack or dispatch paramedics or an ambulance with trained emergency medical technicians. These technicians and paramedics are trained in cardiopulmonary resuscitation and may also be authorized to perform electrical defibrillation from a portable unit carried in the ambulance. Many mobile emergency units have equipment for transmitting the patient's electrocardiogram to a central monitoring station from which a physician or nurse can instruct the paramedics on appropriate drugs and other measures to be taken while the patient is in transit.

Persons who have apparently collapsed and died unexpectedly have been successfully revived by individuals trained in cardiopulmonary resuscitation who instituted appropriate rhythmical sequences of chest compression and mouth-to-mouth ventilation within three or four minutes. This maintenance of the circulation and respiration can keep a patient alive without permanent brain damage until such time as an ambulance, staffed with trained personnel and appropriately equipped, can reach the scene and take over. In communities with highly trained citizen populations and rescue personnel stationed in such a manner that they can reach a collapsed victim within less than five minutes anywhere in the city, as many as one out of two patients who have apparently died may be resuscitated. Of these, about half eventually leave the hospital without serious permanent damage.

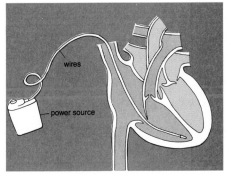

Artificial Pacemaker

Electrical impulses flow through very small wires at a pace to match the heart's natural conduction system.

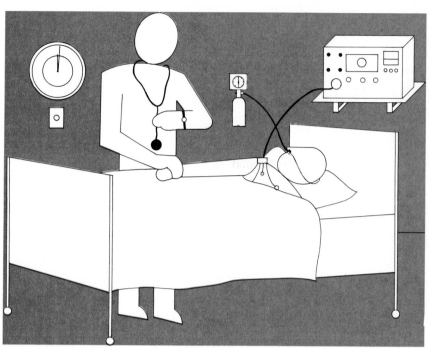

Coronary Care Unit

Most patients with an acute myocardial infarction who reach the hospital recover from their attack. Less than 15 percent of patients die after they are hospitalized, and the majority of these are likely to be the very elderly or patients who have had prior heart attacks and have considerable residual damage. The average patient can be transferred off the coronary care facility after several days and is gradually able to walk about during the second week of the attack. If the heart attack has been uncomplicated, most patients can return home somewhere between the second and third weeks after the attack.

Diagnosis The diagnosis of acute myocardial infarction is based primarily on three sets of criteria. The first of these is the clinical presentation, including the characteristic symptoms already described, and also findings from physical examination which suggest impaired heart functioning. The latter includes disturbances in heart rhythm, soft heart sounds, the presence of a third heart sound indicating disturbed function of the left ventricle, the presence of a fourth heart sound reflecting a change in the stiffness of the heart following a heart attack, and the presence of crackling sounds over the lung bases heard with a stethoscope as the patient breathes and due to accumulation of fluid in the lungs from acute heart failure. Fever and some fall in blood pressure may also be present.

The second criterion is that provided by electrocardiograms. Acute myocardial infarction produces a series of abnormalities which can be seen on the electrocardiogram over the course of several days. This is the single most reliable and specific criterion needed to diagnose the presence of an acute heart attack. Furthermore, the electrocardiogram will demonstrate which portion of the heart wall is being injured or destroyed as a result of the lack of adequate blood flow and some measure of the extent of the damage. The electrocardiogram may also reveal evidence of prior damage to another part of the heart wall from a previous heart attack. The electrocardiogram also identifies the exact nature of any irregularities in heart rhythm if these are present.

The third criterion is the appearance of abnormalities in certain enzymes found in the bloodstream. These enzymes are cellular enzymes which are involved in metabolic functions within the heart and which escape from the heart cell into the bloodstream when the cell dies. In acute myocardial infarction, there will be an abnormal rise in the activity of these enzymes in the blood, readily detected through analysis of blood samples from the patient during the first several days of the attack. The enzyme activities most commonly analyzed today are serum glutamic oxalacetic transaminase, lactic dehydrogenase, and creatine phosphokinase.

Generally at least two of the three criteria enumerated above must be met before most doctors are willing to make an unequivocal diagnosis of an acute myocardial infarction.

Once a patient who has suffered a myocardial infarction is sent home, he **After the Attack** should gradually increase his degree of activity and exercise until he is again fully active, approximately six weeks to two months after his attack. After another month or so, most patients are able to resume work, although some adjustments in work responsibilities may be desirable, depending on the amount of heart damage sustained, the general condition of the patient, the nature of the work, and the physical and emotional stress required by the job.

Patients with angina pectoris are often free of symptoms during most of the **ANGINA PECTORIS** day. However, when they are under physical or emotional stress they may reach a point where the part of the heart muscle supplied by a severely obstructed coronary vessel may transiently fail to receive adequate blood flow to meet its needs. During this period patients will note a chest discomfort similar in distribution to that observed in patients with acute myocardial infarction, except that the discomfort lasts only seconds to minutes if the patient stops the activity in which he is engaged or if he places a nitroglycerin tablet under his tongue.

Drugs used to treat coronary heart disease affect the balance between myo- **Medical Management** cardial oxygen supply and demand in two ways: (1) by changing the supply or (2) by changing the demand. Coronary vasodilating drugs improve the blood flow, thus supplying more oxygen to the contracting heart muscle. Drugs that decrease the oxygen demand work either by decreasing the systemic resistance (and therefore the arterial blood pressure) or by decreasing the volume of the heart by reducing the amount of blood returning to it. Both mechanisms result in less demand for oxygen when the heart contracts. A nitroglycerin tablet placed under the tongue is rapidly absorbed. The drug reduces the oxygen requirements of the heart by decreasing heart size and improves the collateral blood flow by dilating the vessels that go to the area of the heart muscle that is receiving inadequate nourishment. Patients who have frequent attacks of angina during the day may be given longer-acting nitrates which are placed under the tongue. The effects of these preparations may last for several hours at a time. In addition, nitroglycerin paste can be applied to the skin of the chest in a specific amount, and this will be absorbed slowly. This is particularly appropriate at night so that the patient does not have to awaken to take medication.

In recent years, another drug, propanolol, has been shown to be highly useful in treating angina pectoris. Propranolol helps the patient with angina pectoris in two major ways. First, because the drug has an effect on the sympathetic nerves that help to regulate the heart rate, patients who take propanolol have a slower heart rate, which means the amount of oxygen used by the heart per minute is decreased. Second, the drug tends to decrease the speed with which the heart fiber contracts, and this too tends to decrease the amount of oxygen needed. Both effects are beneficial to the angina patient by reducing oxygen requirements of the heart muscle.

Other medical measures usually undertaken in the treatment of angina include reduction of obesity, gradual physical reconditioning ranging from walking on a level surface for increasing distances to supervised exercise rehabilitation programs, and intervention directed against identifiable risk factors. When adequate medical treatment, including the use of long-acting nitrates and propranolol, remains ineffective in suppressing attacks of angina pectoris and the patient is severely restricted in his work and daily activities, cardiac surgery may be considered.

Symptoms The chest discomfort experienced during an episode of angina pectoris is characteristically located underneath the breastbone. However the pain may be felt in the upper part of the abdomen, the left chest, or the neck, although this happens infrequently and usually is accompanied by pain underneath the breastbone. The chest pain may radiate up into the left shoulder and down the left arm. The discomfort usually lasts only seconds or minutes and almost never lasts longer then fifteen or twenty minutes. The patient often experiences a feeling of impending doom and learns almost immediately to stop whatever activity is provoking the attack in order to achieve relief. Placing a nitroglycerin tablet under the tongue makes the pain disappear more rapidly —relief of symptoms occurs within seconds or one or two minutes. Many patients with angina pectoris report that the discomfort is particularly severe in the morning, when walking against a brisk wind, when walking or exercising after a heavy meal, during periods of emotional stress, occasionally while smoking or immediately after smoking a cigarette, and during sexual intercourse. There may also be some shortness of breath, but the chest discomfort is usually what forces the patient to stop his activity. The frequency of episodes varies widely, not only from patient to patient but also from time to time in the same individual. Several weeks or even months may go by without an episode of angina, particularly for the patient under medical care who is taking medication and has learned to avoid the kinds of severe exercise that are likely to provoke chest discomfort. At other times, however, a patient may have as many as ten to twenty attacks a day. When angina occurs in the presence of adequate medical treatment, it generally implies inadequate control and suggests that further therapeutic measures should be undertaken. Specifically, it suggests that the patient should be considered for possible coronary vein bypass graft surgery.

The diagnosis of angina pectoris is primarily based on the history of typical attacks as described by the patient. Unlike the electrocardiogram readings in acute myocardial infarction, those in angina pectoris may be normal, particularly if the patient is free of pain when tested. For this reason, stress testing while recording the electrocardiogram is useful in confirming the diagnosis. Exercise is performed on a treadmill designed to increase the heart rate gradually until it reaches as high as 90 percent of the patient's maximum rate. During the course of this progressive increase in exercise load, the patient's electrocardiogram is carefully monitored for evidence of myocardial ischemia (diminished blood supply), which would be an indication of a positive test. At the same time, the patient is observed for evidence of disturbances in heart rhythm, a significant drop in blood pressure, and chest pain typical of angina pectoris. Approximately two out of three patients with angina pectoris will have the diagnosis confirmed by an exercise stress test.

Recently, a new technique called radionuclide imaging has been combined with stress testing to help confirm the presence of ischemic areas of the heart muscle as well as to show the areas that may be receiving inadequate blood flow. In these tests, a minute or trace dose of a radioactive compound is injected while the patient is exercising. This radioisotope is carried in the bloodstream and diffuses into the heart muscle. Proportionately less of the isotope will reach those portions of the heart muscle that have an acute impairment of blood flow. At the end of the exercise, a radioactive detecting unit is placed over the patient's heart; the radioactivity from the areas of impaired blood flow will be less than that emitted from the other areas. This can be demonstrated pictorially.

Surgery has become increasingly employed in recent years for patients with coronary artery disease. In particular, coronary vein bypass graft surgery has been shown to be very useful for patients with angina pectoris. This operation consists of taking a section of the saphenous vein from the patient's own leg and sewing it onto the aorta and one or more branches of the coronary artery, bypassing the areas that are obstructed by coronary artery disease. Such operations require prior identification of the areas of the coronary artery which are totally or almost totally obstructed, so that the surgeon may know where to place the graft in order to bypass the area.

The areas of obstruction in the coronary circulation are identified by coronary arteriography, a procedure in which catheters are introduced through a peripheral artery into the aorta and passed under fluoroscopic control to the base of the heart where each of the coronary arteries are individually cannulated. When the tip of the catheter reaches the mouth of the artery, an iodinated dye is injected. The dye outlines the arteries as high speed X-ray movies of the fluoroscopic image are recorded so that the course of the dye as it passes down the artery can be studied later. When this is done, in several projections, the areas of obstruction in the coronary arteries on both the right and the left sides of the heart can be readily identified. The technique is useful not only in identifying the locations where bypass grafts are to be placed but also in determining whether surgical intervention is warranted. Surgical intervention is generally reserved for patients who have responded

Diagnosis

PRINCIPLES

1. *The work of the body requires a continual supply of oxygen, which cannot be stored as other nutrients are. More oxygen is extracted from the blood as it circulates through the heart muscle than from any other organ or tissue. A shortage of oxygen in the cells of the heart muscle can produce the acute discomfort in the chest known as angina pectoris. A sharp decrease in the delivery of oxygen, if prolonged, may lead to a heart attack, clinically known as an "acute myocardial infarction."*

2. *Blood is transported to the heart muscle by the left and right coronary arteries, the first to arise from the aorta as it leaves the heart. Approximately 5 percent of the total blood flow from the heart goes through the coronary circulation each minute. Obstructions in the circulation through the coronary arteries are thus a leading cause of the imbalance in the supply of oxygen that can lead to angina or a heart attack.*

Surgical Treatment

3. *Coronary artery disease, the most common type of heart disease and the leading cause of death in the United States, is almost always the result of atherosclerosis, the clinical name for hardening of the arteries. Atherosclerosis begins with the accumulation of fatty deposits in the walls of the arteries, leading to the formation of fibrous tissue in the vessel wall.*

4. *Although the basic cause of coronary artery disease is unknown, scientists have identified a number of risk factors that appear to correlate with the likelihood of heart attacks in later life. These include high blood pressure (hypertension), cigarette smoking, and high levels of cholesterol in the bloodstream. Medication can bring down blood pressure, and the amount of cholesterol in the bloodstream can be*

controlled by attention to diet. Coronary artery disease affects ten times as many males as females under the age of forty-five. Among older persons, the difference falls off rapidly; the incidence among the very elderly is about the same for both sexes.

Unstable Angina

5. *Symptoms of acute myocardial infarction include severe pain under the breastbone, sometimes radiating into the left shoulder and down the left arm or along both arms. Often the pain is accompanied by acute shortness of breath. A series of abnormalities can be seen on the electrocardiogram, which is the most reliable criterion for diagnosing a heart attack. A third criterion is the appearance in the bloodstream of abnormal cellular enzymes which have escaped from the heart cells, and which can be detected through analysis of blood samples.*

6. *The mortality among those patients who reach the hospital following a heart attack is less than 15 percent. Ordinarily, a patient recovering from an uncomplicated heart attack will be able to go home somewhere between two and three weeks after the attack, and be fully active within anywhere from six weeks to two months.*

7. *The medical management of coronary heart disease includes two kinds of drugs: 1. those that improve the blood flow by dilating the arteries, and 2. those that decrease the demand for oxygen, such as nitroglycerin and propanolol.*

8. *Surgery has become increasingly common in recent years for treating patients with coronary artery disease. In particular, coronary vein bypass graft surgery has been shown to be very useful for patients with angina pectoris. Although it has yet to be proved that coronary surgery actually prolongs the life of the patient, there is little doubt that it relieves the painful symptoms of the disease, and it has been shown to increase the patient's tolerance for exercise.*

poorly to medical management and continue to have frequent attacks of angina pectoris which interfere with a reasonably normal existence. Although it has yet to be proved that coronary surgery actually prolongs life in coronary artery disease, there is little doubt that it either improves or totally relieves the symptoms of angina pectoris in the overwhelming majority of patients. It has also been shown to increase the patient's exercise tolerance.

Unstable angina generally represents a condition more serious than chronic stable angina pectoris. The term "unstable" indicates that the patient is in a changing situation, which may be a prelude to an acute myocardial infarction or a return to a more stable pattern. There are a number of subsets of unstable angina recognized clinically. The onset of angina pectoris for the first time may be considered a form of unstable angina for the first six to eight weeks, as are periods of marked increase in the frequency or severity of pre-existing angina. One form of unstable angina, called variant or Prinzmetal's angina, is characterized by attacks that occur at night while the patient is resting or asleep and by unusual changes in the electrocardiogram readings; ST segment elevation rather than depression during the period of chest pain. The term "variant angina" implies these unusual features, and anatomically this form of angina has been shown to be associated with spasm of the coronary arteries. These spasms may (but do not necessarily) occur in the presence of associated coronary artery atheromatous disease.

Another manifestation of unstable angina is sudden, severe coronary-type chest pain which may last for several hours but does not demonstrate the usual serial electrocardiographic changes or the serial blood enzyme changes of myocardial infarction. The most serious form of unstable angina, however, is crescendo angina. In this form of angina, the patient has frequent attacks of chest pain, sometimes for prolonged periods, which occur following minimal exertion or even at rest. These patients are hovering between recurring ischemia and myocardial infarction, and little is needed to tip the balance in favor of the latter. These patients should be hospitalized immediately in a coronary care unit and treated as if they were having a heart attack, with medical treatment designed to decrease the oxygen needs of the heart muscle. If the attacks do not subside within twenty-four to forty-eight hours, coronary arteriography should be performed with a view toward immediate coronary vein bypass graft surgery.

The last few decades have witnessed remarkable advances in the understanding of coronary heart disease, and yet the disease still presents a very great challenge to the medical profession. The physician is often taxed to establish an accurate diagnosis, handle the problem in such a way that the patient's life-style is altered as little as possible, and at the same time insure that the patient understands the nature of the illness and how it must be managed.

12

ARRHYTHMIAS

Nancy C. Flowers, M.D.,
Daniel E. McMartin, M.D.

Poet Robert Frost was once asked why young children who have never before been exposed to poetry or music nevertheless respond to these arts. He speculated that it was the regular rhythms in poetry and music that captured the attention of youngsters. Frost remarked that rhythm might very well be the earliest sensation in the person's experience. Before birth a fetus may feel the steady beat of the mother's heart. The moment infants emerge from the womb they develop an awareness of the periodic thumping of their own hearts.

The poet's perception may be debatable, but the rhythm of the human heart is a vital and constant feature of that organ. The regular contractions and relaxations of the heart muscle produce a smooth-flowing "river of life"— oxygenated, nutrition-rich blood to feed the cells and then participate in the process that cleanses the body of wastes.

An orchestra generally depends on an underlying rhythm to blend its components into musical sounds, to produce melody and harmony. There may be sections of a piece of music that are played faster or slower according to the directions of the composer. But an irregular rhythm will reduce the assembled sounds of an orchestra to a jumble of noise.

The rhythm of the heart may also speed up or slow down in response to demands of the over-all needs of the body and its organs. This is normal and is an example of the way the body copes with the added work load or with emotional ups and downs. Indeed, sometimes in anticipation of extra physical effort, a signal goes to the heart, which sets it to a faster beat in preparation for the coming task—an experience common to athletes just before they start an event. However, there are conditions that produce departures from a regular beat in terms of both rate and pattern. These irregularities may be only momentary or they may last a few minutes, and they represent a temporary discord. In some instances, the heartbeat is steady, but the rate is slower or faster than normal, outside the usual range for the heart. This type of abnormality may also threaten the continued harmonious performance of the body.

Physicians have a term to describe the various kinds of irregular beats; they call them arrhythmias. To understand the consequences of arrhythmias, whether serious or inconsequential, it is necessary to know how the heart comes to beat as it does.

The heart muscle, the myocardium, surrounds a cavity which is divided by muscular walls and by valves into the right atruim and right ventricle and the left atrium and left ventricle. The beating of the heart pumps a forward flow of blood; the valves prevent the blood from flowing backward. The rate at which the heart beats is controlled by two separate links with the brain; the sympathetic link results in speeding, and the parasympathetic link results in slowing down. The contractions and relaxations of the heart muscle are maintained at a steady, regular pace by the activity of special cells within the heart muscle. These special cells, called pacemaker cells, actually originate the electrical impulse that causes the heart to beat; flow of current is transmitted by means of a system of interlocking cells through the atria and the ventricles, resulting in a uniform and rhythmic contraction—the heartbeat.

Disturbances in rhythm can come from many causes and can involve the pacemaker cells themselves or parts of the conduction system in the atria and ventricles. These abnormal heart rhythms (arrhythmias) vary in seriousness from very minor disturbances of short duration to extremely serious abnormal

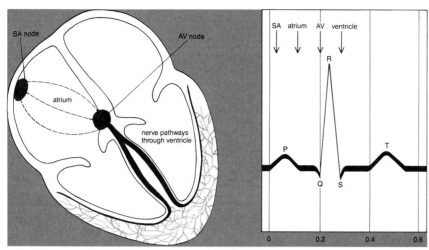

The Heart's Natural Pacemaker

rhythms which, if not checked, can result in complete disruption of heart rhythm and, ultimately, death.

The heart's natural pacemaker is located in an area relatively high on the right side of the heart, in the right atrium. It is here, in what is called the sinoatrial or sinus node, that the electrical impulses which stimulate the heart muscle to contract are originated. The ability to originate impulses, a characteristic called automaticity, is a property of the sinus node as well as of certain other cells which, together with special fibers that transmit current, make up the conduction system in the heart.

CONDUCTION OF IMPULSES

Another part of the conduction system is called the atrioventricular node (AV node). This group of cells is located in the lower anterior wall of the right atrium, at the juncture of the right atrium and the right ventricle and near the tricuspid valve. After the impulse leaves the sinus node, it spreads throughout the atria and then passes through the atrioventricular (AV) node. The AV node connects to a group of conducting fibers called the bundle of His, which soon divides into a left and right branch. The impulses then travel to the ventricles through a special conduction pathway which runs along the partition (septum) dividing the two ventricles. When the apex of the heart is reached, the electrical wave then moves up to the base of the ventricles. The smaller fibers that spread into the walls of the heart muscle are called the Purkinje fibers.

In essence, then, the heart's specialized cells and fibers originate and pass on electrical impulses which finally result in contraction, which is followed by relaxation. The ventricles receive blood, and then pump it into the circulatory system, the right ventricle delivering blood to the lungs, and the left to the rest of the body.

Although the chemical and electrical changes involved in conduction take place on the microscopic, cellular level, science has devised a way to make them recognizable by the naked eye. Because the voltage variations initiated by the pacemaker cells produce electrical fields that reach the surface of the body, they can be picked up by electrodes positioned at specific locations on the chest and the limbs. This electrical activity is recorded on a strip of paper,

ELECTROCARDIOGRAPHY

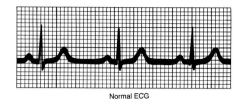

Normal ECG

the electrocardiogram (ECG), which is a standard feature of most medical examinations. This is a graphically visualized record of the combined electrical activity of all the cells of the heart. The waves of electrical activity are designated by letters—P, QRS, T, and U waves. The letters are not abbreviations of specific terms; they were arbitrarily chosen to represent the sequence of activation and recovery.

Electrocardiograms are printed by a heated stylus on specially waxed paper or more often by an ink stylus, divided to represent time intervals and voltage. Each horizontal block division of 1 millimeter represents 0.04 second; each vertical block of 1 millimeter represents $\frac{1}{10}$ of a millivolt. Each square of five blocks is marked with a darker line; five of these larger squares, read horizontally, represent 1 second in time; two of the larger squares, read vertically, represent 1 millivolt. The first wave on the graph paper, the P wave, represents the voltage change associated with the electrical impulse spreading throughout the atria. The second wave complex, the QRS, represents the voltage change as seen on the skin resulting from movement of the impulse through the ventricles. Ventricular contraction begins near the end of the QRS. (The impulses of the sinus node, the AV node, the bundle of His, and the Purkinje fibers are not usually visible in the standard electrocardiogram.) Repolarization of the ventricles is indicated by the T wave. The ST segment occurs after depolarization and before repolarization. Relaxation occurs near the end of the T wave. The U wave is only occasionally seen, often in patients with a potassium deficiency. The fraction of a second in which each depolarization and repolarization of the heart muscle takes place can be accurately estimated from readings on the electrocardiographic tracing. In normal readings, the PR interval is less than 0.21 second and more than 0.11 second. The QRS complex ranges in adults from about 0.075 second to somewhat less than 0.12 second.

Every normal heartbeat displays basically the same general electrocardiographic form, and any deviation from the normal rhythm can be readily detected. Not all deviations are signs of heart disease or defects; individual rhythms vary considerably, and many irregular rhythms represent no threat to health. Nevertheless, an abnormal sequence of waves may reveal serious rhythm disturbances which may require treatment. The standard electrocardiogram is merely a brief sampling of cardiac rhythm, taken at rest under more or less favorable conditions. Because many arrhythmias are present for only brief periods, often during or after physical activity; a new kind of electrocardiographic recording process has been developed. Instead of the large piece of equipment used in a doctor's office, a small, portable device carried by the patient records the heart's rhythm as the person goes about his daily activity. The record is preserved on a magnetic tape and then reviewed by a computer. The result is a continuous record of the heart's rhythm for up to twenty-four hours.

Continuous monitoring of the heart's activity is critically important in the several days immediately following a heart attack. A bedside monitor and a television-like screen that displays a nonstop record of the heart beat alert specially trained nurses to shifts in the tempo of the damaged heart, and immediate, often lifesaving methods are put into operation.

The electrocardiogram not only is helpful in detecting cardiac rhythm disturbances but is useful in diagnosing heart attack (myocardial infarction),

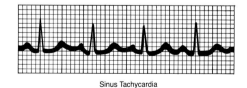

Sinus Tachycardia

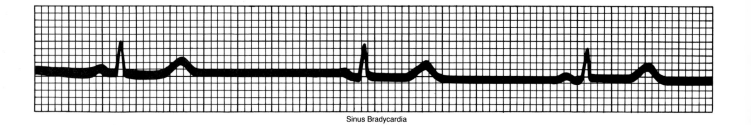
Sinus Bradycardia

acute pericarditis (inflammation of the membrane surrounding the heart), and fainting or weak spells due to disturbances of cardiac rhythm. It can predict an enlarged heart and certain disturbances of the body chemistry as well as other disease states.

The value of the electrocardiogram is enhanced by complete absence of risk or discomfort for the patient and the relative ease with which it can be interpreted. It can be recorded not only by doctors but also by nurses, technicians, and even students.

SINUS RHYTHM DISTURBANCES

At rest, a normal heart beats between about 60 and 100 times a minute. A heart rate slower than 60 beats a minute is called bradycardia (literally, slow heart); a heart rate faster than 100 beats a minute is called tachycardia (fast heart). Bradycardia does not in itself indicate an abnormality in the heart or in the conduction system. Sinus bradycardia may be present when the heartbeat mechanism—the sinus node and the conduction system—is functioning well; in fact, it often indicates a more efficient heart. Many well-trained athletes have bradycardia. They have actually trained their hearts to beat more slowly and eject a greater volume of blood with each beat. Sinus bradycardia has also been observed during sleep in many persons with normal hearts. In older people, however, severe sinus bradycardia may indicate a disease within the sinus node or in the conduction pathway. The condition is rare, but if it exists, the impulse for cardiac contraction may originate from cells outside the sinus node. When the impulse comes from other sites, there may intermittently be fast beats alternating with slow beats. The abnormality has been called the tachycardia-bradycardia syndrome, a manifestation of the "sick sinus syndrome." This usually produces no symptoms and requires no therapy. If, however, the patient suffers dizziness or loss of consciousness, an artificial pacemaker may have to be inserted to stabilize the heart rhythm.

Sinus tachycardia also can occur with a normal heartbeat mechanism and normal conduction. Because the heart is beating more than 100 times a minute, this condition results in increased blood flow—the normal response of the heart to exercise, anxiety, excitement, stress, nervousness, or fright. In itself sinus tachycardia requires no therapy except when a severe attack occurs or when the condition exists together with other cardiovascular problems, but it may be the response of the heart to an underlying disease—for example, anemia, infection, and many others.

ATRIAL RHYTHM DISTURBANCES

The sinus rhythm in a normal heart may, on occasion, be interrupted by impulses that originate in atrial cells outside the sinus node. This happens because other cells in the atrium acquire a pacemaker function and are thus able to initiate an impulse, which then moves along the conduction system and produces a premature beat. The atrial premature beats do not necessarily indicate heart disease; studies show that heavy users of alcohol, coffee, and tobacco are among those who are likely to have atrial premature beats, and the condition usually disappears when the stimulants are no longer used.

In many cases, atrial premature beats present no disturbing symptoms; such cases usually require no treatment. But when the condition is combined with frequent episodes of palpitation and fluttering in the chest, rapid heartbeat, dizziness, or shortness of breath, treatment with such drugs as digitalis, quinidine, or propranolol may be necessary. Treatment may also be required when premature beats accompany rheumatic heart disease or when severe lung disease causes a drop in oxygen levels in the blood. In the latter case, the condition improves or disappears when the lung disease is treated.

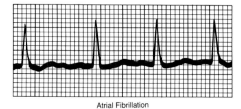

Atrial Fibrillation

Atrial fibrillation, an irregularity in which the muscles of the atrium contract erratically and without coordinated and organized rhythm, may be a more serious condition. It can take place when the normal sinus node function is impaired, when the blood oxygen level falls, or when other factors irritate the cells and fibers of the heart, making them more excitable. In the very fast chaotic atrial activity characteristic of this condition, the AV node is bombarded with frequent impulses. No organized atrial P wave is visible on an electrocardiogram. Because the AV node recovers more slowly than the atrium, and with very fast rates may conduct impulses to the ventricle more slowly, the ventricle receives only a fraction of these impulses and receives them irregularly. The resulting heartbeat becomes irregular and rapid.

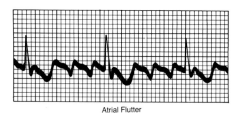

Atrial Flutter

Healthy individuals may occasionally experience brief episodes of atrial fibrillation, but a return to normal sinus rhythm usually follows without treatment. In such cases, called "lone atrial fibrillation," the patient feels a fluttering sensation in the chest, a feeling of fullness, and mild shortness of breath. No treatment is ordinarily required, but digitalis is sometimes used during an attack to prevent rapid heartbeats.

Atrial fibrillation more often occurs with such predisposing conditions as overactivity of the thyroid gland (hyperthyroidism) or severe lung disease. The most important therapy is correction of the underlying cause. In most cases the rapid contractions of the ventricles can be slowed with drugs. Sinus rhythm may be restored by means of an electrical shock administered to the heart, a technique called cardioversion, but in general sinus rhythm is restored through treatment of the underlying disease. A major complication of atrial fibrillation, particularly in long-standing cases and cases when rheumatic heart disease is present, is the risk of formation of blood clots in the left atrium. These clots may break off and travel to other parts of the body, resulting in potentially life-threatening stoppage of blood flow in the heart or brain. Patients with long-standing atrial fibrillation may benefit from anticoagulant (blood thinner) treatment.

Long-standing atrial fibrillation will usually not produce symptoms. Persons with narrowed coronary arteries may feel chest pain with the onset of fibrillation, especially if the ventricular rate is fast. In such cases, the heartbeat should be slowed at once with digitalis or electrical shock. In these circumstances an untreated rapid heart rate may produce heart failure, or even a heart attack.

Atrial tachycardia exists when the atrial rate is between approximately 160 and 220 beats a minute. If the rate is faster and the P waves appear somewhat differently, the condition is called atrial flutter. Although the exact mechanism causing these disturbances is not known, it appears that faster-than-normal beats originate in an area of the atrium outside the normal pacemaker-cell area. In both atrial tachycardia and atrial flutter, all the atrial impulses may not get through the AV node. This is somewhat similar to the situation in atrial fibrillation, where the AV node does not conduct all the impulses it receives. The ventricular rate, and thus the pulse rate, is kept slower than the atrial rate. This delay is actually built into the conduction system; the slower conduction of impulses at the AV node acts as a safeguard against excessive heart rates.

Atrial arrhythmias may occur in healthy persons and end spontaneously. Atrial tachycardia and atrial flutter seem to be caused by various diseases, including rheumatic heart disease, some congenital heart defects, hyperthyroidism, pneumonia, and blood clots in the lungs. Atrial tachycardia with a block in conduction may also be a result of excessive levels of digitalis in the blood.

A sense of fullness in the chest, lightheadedness, and chest flutters are characteristic symptoms of atrial tachycardia. Patients with different kinds of heart disease experience similar symptoms with atrial tachycardia and atrial fibrillation. Drug therapy is usually effective in treating tachycardias, including sudden onsets of the disturbance (paroxysmal tachycardia). The drugs used include digitalis, quinidine, procainamide, and propranolol. However, drug therapy is initiated only when the rhythm disturbances are frequent enough to cause considerable discomfort and annoyance. When the disturbance is related to an underlying disease, successful treatment of that disease usually restores normal heart rhythm.

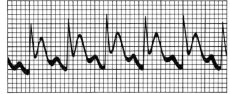

Paroxysmal Atrial Tachycardia

Junctional premature beats and junctional tachycardia are abnormal rhythms that result when specialized conduction tissue close to the AV node develops the ability to originate impulses. The symptoms and treatment of these conditions are much the same as for atrial premature beats and atrial tachycardia. Sometimes people are born with conduction pathways that bypass the AV node; these are called pre-excitation syndromes. People with this condition tend to develop recurrent tachycardias. Sometimes they develop atrial fibrillation which conducts to the ventricle at very fast rates. Medication must be carefully selected for this condition. Sometimes special studies by means of catheterization are necessary. Surgery to cut the bypass tract is not often required.

Occasionally an area of tissue in the ventricular muscle will develop pacemaker capability. The electrical activity then spreads throughout the ventricle and frequently back into the atrium. The kind of beat that originates in the ventricle usually occurs before the next regular beat initiated by the sinus node. These early beats are called premature ventricular beats. Some individuals with healthy hearts may occasionally experience premature ventricular beats, just as they may experience premature atrial beats, often in association with anxiety or excess use of coffee, tea, cigarettes, or alcohol.

VENTRICULAR RHYTHM DISTURBANCES

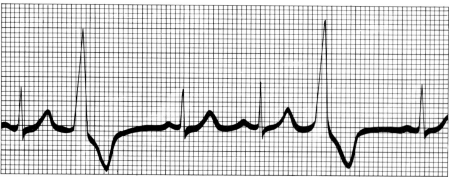
Premature Ventricular Contractions

Both atrial and ventricular premature beats may affect the sinus node pacemaker, with the result that the next normal beat (from the sinus node) is somewhat delayed. This delay allows more time for blood to fill the heart as it returns from the body and the lungs, and a stronger ventricular contraction results. The person then feels a stronger pulse beat, often described as an unusual awareness of the heart's beating, or a sensation of having skipped a heartbeat or of having gained an extra beat.

Although ventricular premature beats are sometimes experienced by persons in excellent health, they may be indicators of a heart abnormality and should be brought to the attention of a doctor. Even when a cause cannot be assigned to the symptoms, some doctors consider more than six premature beats a minute an indication that an attempt should be made to regulate the heart by such drugs as procainamide, quinidine, propranolol, or lidocaine. Ventricular premature beats may indicate heart muscle disease associated with virus infections, coronary atherosclerosis, heart valve disease, alcoholism, or other causes.

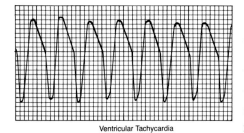
Ventricular Tachycardia

Ventricular tachycardia exists when more than two consecutive premature beats occur at a rate greater than 100 beats a minute. When this rhythm continues for any length of time, the volume of blood pumped by the heart decreases, resulting in shortness of breath, fainting, and possibly shock. This rhythm may also degenerate into the completely disorganized ventricular beating called ventricular fibrillation. If regular rhythm is not immediately restored, ventricular fibrillation results in sudden death.

CARDIOVERSION Normal heart rhythm may sometimes be restored through the shock of a direct electrical current, a technique called cardioversion. Electrical conversion causes an electrical discharge over the entire heart simultaneously, temporarily wiping out all electrical activity and allowing the sinus node to resume its normal function of initiating impulses. An analogy can be made with an orchestra that has begun to play completely out of tempo; the conductor stops all the players for a moment, then re-establishes the proper rhythm and tempo and allows the orchestra to continue.

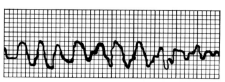
Ventricular Fibrillation

The electrical shock, delivered through the chest wall, is usually synchronized with the existing ventricular activity, so that the shock can be delivered at a predetermined period in the cardiac cycle. This synchronized cardioversion is used to stop atrial tachycardia, flutter, or fibrillation, and ventricular tachycardia. In ventricular fibrillation, when there is no clear cardiac cycle and no coordinated rhythm, synchronization is not possible, and electrical shock is an emergency measure.

In most cases of atrial fibrillation, cardioversion can restore normal rhythm. How long the normal rhythm remains constant after cardioversion depends on the underlying cause of the rhythm disturbance. Usually a drug (digitalis, quinidine, or propranolol), or a combination of drugs is given after cardioversion in an attempt to maintain normal rhythm. Anticoagulant drugs are often administered for several days before and after cardioversion because of the increased incidence of clot formation in cases of long-standing atrial fibrillation. The voltage required in cardioversion varies in different situations, but the procedure itself is safe and effective.

Digitalis, procainamide, lidocaine, quinidine, and propranolol are among the **DRUG TREATMENT** drugs most commonly used in treating arrhythmias. Each drug has particular properties and complications which determine its effectiveness in treating the various kinds of arrhythmias.

Digitalis, the oldest known and longest used of these drugs, is particularly effective in correcting atrial fibrillation, flutter, and tachycardia. Digitalis works by delaying transmission of the electrical impulse through the AV node, thus slowing the rate at which the ventricles beat. It also improves the strength of the beat of a failing heart, thereby possibly improving blood flow to the heart itself and relieving either atrial or ventricular arrhythmias. The disadvantage of digitalis in treating arrhythmias is that the drug itself, when taken in excess, can cause various kinds of arrhythmias. Toxic manifestations of digitalis include such rhythm disturbances as ventricular premature beats, heart block, and atrial tachycardia with a conduction block. (Other possible late signs of toxicity include nausea and visual disturbances. The toxic effects of digitalis are made more likely, or if they exist are worsened, if the patient has a potassium deficiency caused by diuretic drugs. This deficiency can be corrected by taking potassium in appropriate amounts, as prescribed by a doctor.

Lidocaine, a local anesthetic frequently used by dentists, has been found invaluable in the treatment of ventricular arrhythmias. The drug is most effective when given by injection in a vein; its action is immediate but of short duration. In spite of its limited duration, however, lidocaine can in most cases eliminate ventricular premature beats and ventricular tachycardia. Infrequent side effects, such as confusion, lightheadedness, and convulsions, wear off quickly because the drug's effects are so brief.

Procainamide is useful in the treatment of ventricular tachycardia and the prevention of ventricular premature beats. Because it can also be taken orally, it is more convenient than lidocaine for long-term use; however, with long use arthritis, skin rash, and other side effects are fairly common. The drug is used more frequently for ventricular than for atrial disturbances.

Quinidine is used to eliminate both atrial and ventricular rhythm disturbances. Mild diarrhea is a common side effect, but other, less common but more serious side effects—light sensitivity of the skin, fainting, bleeding, and convulsions—often require discontinuation of the drug.

Propranolol, a relatively recent drug, sometimes blocks some of the stimulating effects of the body's normal flow of adrenalin. It also decreases the force of the heartbeat and has an anti-arrhythmic effect similar to that of quinidine. Some doctors contend that propranolol is helpful in the treatment of atrial arrhythmias and, under special circumstances, of certain ventricular rhythm disturbances. However, except in a few specific instances, it is not the drug of choice. Because propranolol does not increase the strength of the heartbeat, it is not as a rule used in cases of severe heart failure. In some people the drug may aggravate the symptoms of asthma, and must be used with caution in diabetic patients on insulin as it may mask the signs and symptoms which warn of low blood sugar.

CONDUCTION ABNORMALITIES

Delayed conduction of electric impulses in the atria occurs at times, but this may not be a problem in itself. The same is true of delays within the ventricles, provided that the delay does not result in a complete failure of conduction. If, however, transmission in the AV node is delayed, a sinus or atrial beat may not be conducted to the ventricle. This condition is called second-degree AV block and results in slowing the ventricle's rate of beating. Occasionally every other beat is blocked—a condition called two-to-one AV block. Thus, if the sinus rate were 80 beats a minute, the ventricular rate would be only 40 a minute. When the ventricular rate is too slow, a decreased volume of blood is being pumped out of the heart. This may be caused by certain drugs or by disease in or around the AV node. The result is poor blood flow to the vital organs. The brain can be especially affected, with dizziness and even fainting resulting.

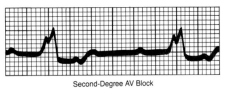
Second-Degree AV Block

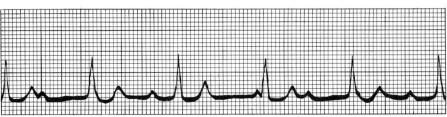
Complete AV Block

Atrioventricular conduction can become totally blocked as a result of a congenital condition, or disease either within or around the conduction system, or of the toxic effects of certain drugs. Complete AV block may also follow a heart attack which has damaged the conduction system. Symptoms vary, depending on the person's heart rate. When the block occurs above or in the AV node, tissues nearby may act as a pacemaker, in which case, the heart rate remains adequate, there are no symptoms, and treatment may not be necessary. This is often the case with congenital complete block. If, however, the block occurs below the AV node, the new pacemaker tissues are located below the area of the block and operate at a rate of 40 beats a minute or less. Further, blocks below the AV node often imply more widespread ventricular muscle involvement with the underlying disease. In this case the flow of blood through the cardiovascular system may be inadequate. Symptoms may be dizziness, shortness of breath, fatigue on exertion, fainting, and, possibly, heart failure. If this type of block develops suddenly, the patient may faint. If it develops gradually, the patient may experience dizziness or fainting during activity or upon standing up. The condition of chronic slow ventricular rate with inade-

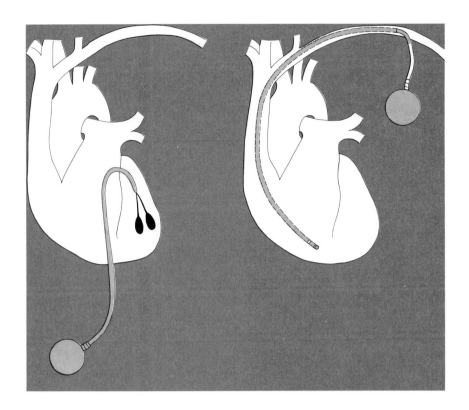

quate blood flow can now be treated quite satisfactorily with an artificial pacemaker.

ARTIFICIAL PACEMAKERS

An artificial pacemaker is an electrical source of energy produced by chemical means or, in the latest models, by a nuclear-powered generator. The two basic types of artificial pacemakers are the demand (synchronous) models and the fixed-rate (asynchronous) models. The demand pacemaker is designed to deliver periodic electrical impulses at a given rate whenever the patient's heart rate is slower than that set for the pacemaker; a special device shuts off the impulses when the patient's heart beats adequately. The fixed-rate pacemaker delivers constant electrical impulses, at a rate preset by a doctor. Pacemakers have also been designed to supply a rate which varies with the sinus node rate; this has proved to be a particularly effective way of increasing cardiac output during exercise.

The pacemaker delivers its electrical impulses by means of electrodes which are positioned either by insertion through a vein (transvenous) or by being sewn onto the heart (epicardial). The energy source on which the artificial pacemaker depends must be tested by periodic electrocardiograms and other electronic tests. In time, the source of energy weakens and the pacemaker must be replaced. Recent advances in technology have greatly increased the life span of artificial pacemakers.

Implanting the pacemaker is relatively simple. Two methods are used at the present time. In one, the surgeon makes an incision through the chest, and either one or a pair of electrodes is then sutured onto or screwed into the heart. From these electrodes, wire leads, placed just beneath the layer of flesh that covers the abdomen, are run down to a container usually implanted below

PRINCIPLES

1. *The normal heartbeat is caused by spontaneous discharge of a group of special cells in the heart called the sinus node, or pacemaker. Electrical impulses travel from these cells and spread along special pathways, finally reaching the heart's working muscle cells and causing them to contract and pump blood.*

2. *Arrhythmias are disturbances in the normal rhythm of the heartbeat. They may be of little consequence, but they may also signal a life-threatening condition.*

3. *An electrocardiogram, a visual record of the electrical activity of the heart, provides an extremely helpful report on a variety of cardiac disorders.*

4. *The heart's normal rate at rest is about 60 to about 100 beats a minute, with an average of about 70. A slow rate—under 60 beats a minute—is called bradycardia. It may be a sign of disease, but it may also be a sign of an efficiently functioning heart. A rapid heartbeat—more than 100 beats a minute—is called tachycardia. Under certain conditions, such as exercise or emotional excitement, this is a normal response, but sometimes it is a signal of an underlying disease.*

5. *Atrial premature beats are rhythm disturbances which may be caused by stimulants or by diseases of the heart or lungs. In the absence of other symptoms, the fluttering sensation of premature beats requires no treatment other than cessation of excess stimulants such as coffee, tea, or nicotine.*

6. *Premature ventricular beats may indicate some abnormality in the heart and may need to be eliminated or reduced in frequency, which is usually accomplished by drug treatment. They may sometimes occur as a response to stress and anxiety.*

7. *Ventricular rhythm sometimes degenerates into a completely disorganized effort, called fibrillation, which can have fatal consequences unless normal rhythm is immediately restored.*

8. *Permanent damage to the heart's natural pacemaker or to pathways of the conduction system may require implantation of an artificial pacemaker. Relatively uncomplicated procedures are used to connect the artificial source of electrical impulses with the heart, and patients are able to lead near-normal lives with little restriction of activity.*

the bottom left rib. The container, about the size of a package of cigarettes (to use an inappropriate comparison), holds both the timing mechanism and the long-life battery pack. Occasionally this type of pacemaker needs adjustment. In that case, a special instrument can be painlessly inserted through the flap of skin covering the pacemaker, and the controls can be manipulated without removing the battery pack. Batteries are easily replaced in a minor surgical procedure which does not require hospitalization. The open-chest procedure is also used to implant a pacemaker which coordinates the activation of the atrium and ventricle.

The second basic method of implantation does not involve exposing the heart. Using local anesthesia, the doctor exposes a large vein near the right shoulder. With a fluoroscope to guide him, he threads a pair of electrodes, encased in silicone tubes, through the vein and into the right ventricle. The electrodes are maneuvered into firm contact with the inner surface of the ventricle. The packet containing the timing mechanism and power supply is then mounted under the flesh below the right shoulder.

Complications from either method of pacemaker insertion seldom occur, and infections are no more frequent than with other kinds of operations. Such problems as dislodgement of electrodes are so rare that pacemaker implantation has become a trouble-free lifesaving procedure for thousands.

13

CONGESTIVE HEART FAILURE

Dean T. Mason, M.D.

Despite its threatening implications, the term "heart failure" does not necessarily imply imminent death from heart disease; it simply indicates that the pumping action of the heart is impaired (cardiac dysfunction). Depending on the extent of the impairment, which may range from mild to severe, the result is that the delivery of blood (cardiac output) becomes inadequate to satisfy the oxygen and nutritional needs of the body at rest and during normal physical activity. When there is a decrease in cardiac output, the volume of blood within the cardiovascular system becomes abnormally expanded. In cases of chronically reduced cardiac output, the increased volume in the vessels causes an excessive accumulation of fluids in the body. That excess fluid retention, combined with heart failure, is called congestive heart failure. It is not a specific disease but an abnormal condition resulting from any type of heart disease in which the function of either of the principal pumping chambers of the heart (the left and right ventricles) has been substantially impaired.

CAUSES   The specific kinds of impairment of heart functioning that lead to congestive heart failure can be classified into three general types:

1. Diminished force of contraction of the ventricles. Two kinds of heart disease —primary heart muscle diseases (cardiomyopathies) and coronary artery disease—result in impairment of the ability of the ventricles to contract properly.

2. Mechanical failure in filling the ventricles during the diastole phase of the cardiac cycle. Inadequate filling of the pumping chambers may be due either to narrowing of the mitral valve opening between the left atrium and left ventricle (rheumatic mitral stenosis) or to increased accumulation of fluid between the thin membrane surrounding the heart (pericardium) and the heart itself. The latter condition, called pericardial tamponade, causes pressure on the heart and prevents an easy flow of blood into its chambers.

3. Overloading of the ventricles during cardiac contraction (systole phase of the cycle). High blood pressure (hypertensive cardiovascular disease) leads to an excessive build up of pressure within the ventricles during the systole phase. Pressure also builds up when the aortic valve between the left ventricle and the aorta is partially obstructed and narrowed (aortic stenosis). The condition may also be the result of an excessive amount of blood within the ventricles at the beginning of systole, a situation which arises when the aortic valve fails to close completely (aortic valvular regurgitation) and there is backward flow of blood from the aorta into the left ventricle. A similar overload of blood volume may occur if there is a congenital heart defect (see Congenital Heart Defects, chapter 16) in which blood from the left side of the heart shunts to the right side (ventricular septal defect), resulting in extra recirculation of blood through the lungs.

COMPENSATORY   When the pumping action of the heart is impaired and begins to malfunction,
MECHANISMS   whether through primary disease of the heart muscle or through chronic overloading of blood volume and blood pressure, the body itself provides emergency relief in the form of compensatory mechanisms. These mechanisms are designed to help the ventricles carry on their function and maintain a normal

level of cardiac output. There are three basic cardiac compensatory mechanisms: dilation of the pumping chambers, increase of muscle mass (ventricular hypertrophy), and increased activity of the sympathetic nervous system. All three usually operate in concert to maintain normal output of the failing heart. Unfortunately, these adaptive processes are responsible for many of the symptoms that the patient with congestive heart failure experiences. And although the body attempts to compensate for the failing heart as long as possible, eventually the compensatory mechanisms themselves become insufficient.

DILATION OF THE PUMPING CHAMBERS Through dilation, or enlargement, the ventricle is capable of holding a greater than normal volume of blood at the completion of the relaxed or filling phase of the cardiac cycle (end-diastolic volume). The elevated volume of blood causes increased stretching of the heart muscle, which in turn leads to more forceful systolic contraction during the subsequent pumping phase of the cardiac cycle. The force of contraction is related to a fundamental property of muscle, including cardiac muscle, which is called the length-tension relationship, or Starling's principle (for the English physiologist, Ernest H. Starling, who first formulated it). According to this principle, an increase in the length (stretch) of a muscle during the relaxation phase leads to increased tension (stronger contraction) during the pumping phase. Through dilation the failing heart becomes capable of ejecting an increased amount of blood when it contracts, returning cardiac output toward a normal level in spite of the intrinsic malfunctioning. But while ventricular dilation provides an important process for maintaining the cardiac output of the failing heart, the mechanism results in excessive body fluid accumulation. Many of the physical symptoms characteristic of congestive heart failure will then appear.

VENTRICULAR HYPERTROPHY In this adaptive process the heart develops an increased muscle mass, thereby adding to the number of heart muscle units able to contract. The force of cardiac contraction is strengthened, and cardiac output is able to return toward normal. But as with ventricular dilation, the process of ventricular hypertrophy may be accompanied by serious side effects. For example, the cardiac muscle may develop to the point where coronary circulation is no longer adequate. The result is angina pectoris, the chest pain symptom of cardiac oxygen insufficiency (myocardial ischemia).

INCREASED ACTIVITY OF THE SYMPATHETIC NERVOUS SYSTEM The sympathetic nervous system is a component of the involuntary autonomic nervous system, which regulates tissues not under voluntary control, including the tissues of the heart. Increased activity of this system produces a greater force of contraction of the impaired ventricle and an increased heart rate. Like the two previously described, this adaptive mechanism frequently has serious side effects. There may be redistribution of peripheral blood flow, resulting in such symptoms as excessive sweating, cool skin, and retention of urine (oliguria). Other symptoms may be excessively rapid heart rate (tachycardia) and abnormal cardiac rhythm (tachyarrhythmias).

Compensated congestive heart failure is achieved when the body maintains cardiac output at a normal level through the combined involvement of the compensatory mechanisms. Decompensated congestive heart failure occurs when even the full range of adaptive mechanisms fails to preserve cardiac output at a normal level. That failure represents the final stage in the impairment of the heart's pumping function. In addition to the basic congestive signs that result from excessive fluid accumulation, patients with decompensated heart failure may experience low blood pressure (hypotension) and the symptoms associated with low cardiac output. These include marked tiredness, weakness, emaciation, mental confusion, and marked urine retention, and reflect the action of an adaptive mechanism in the peripheral arterial circulation which causes the blood flow to be preferentially distributed to the body organs with the greatest need for oxygen.

**FORMS OF
HEART FAILURE**

LOW-OUTPUT HEART FAILURE Reduced cardiac output is the most common form of heart failure. Patients with this form of cardiac dysfunction have a heart disease process which can be classified under one of the three types already described; impaired ventricular contraction, mechanical failures in ventricle filling, overloading of blood pressure or blood volume.

LEFT-SIDED HEART FAILURE This is the most common type of congestive failure and occurs when improper functioning of the left ventricle leads to fluid accumulation in the lungs and lung congestion. Heart disorders associated with left-sided heart failure include rheumatic disease of one or both left heart valves (aortic and mitral valves), coronary heart disease, and hypertensive heart disease.

RIGHT-SIDED HEART FAILURE Inadequate pumping by the right ventricle results in fluid accumulation and congestion of the liver and legs. Common causes are chronic lung disease with pulmonary hypertension (cor pulmonale) and diseases of the valves on the right side of the heart—congenital narrowing of the valve between the right ventricle and the pulmonary artery (stenosis of the pulmonary valve) and incomplete closing of the valve between the right atrium and the right ventricle (incompetence of the tricuspid valve).

BIVENTRICULAR HEART FAILURE This occurs when the pumping action of both ventricles is impaired. The failure can result from generalized heart muscle diseases such as inflammation of the muscular wall of the heart (infectious myocarditis) and other spontaneous diseases of the heart muscle (idiopathic cardiomyopathies), as well as in cases when long-standing primary left-sided heart failure has led eventually to secondary right-sided heart failure.

HIGH-OUTPUT HEART FAILURE This relatively rare condition develops because of an abnormal communication between the larger vessels in the peripheral arterial and venous systems (arteriovenous fistula), or because of increased activity of the thyroid gland (thyrotoxicosis). The term heart failure is nevertheless appropriate, for even though the total cardiac output is increased, the regional blood flow falls below the level to meet the oxygen needs of certain body organs. The condition is similar to that of a farm which has an adequate supply of water in its reservoir but whose irrigation system fails to deliver enough water to certain crops.

Heart failure may be acute or chronic, depending on the rapidity of its onset. In either case, the specific conditions that lead to heart failure and the consequences in terms of blood pressure and blood volume are essentially the same. Acute congestive heart failure, however, is precipitated by such catastrophic events as acute heart attack (myocardial infarction) and bacterial infection of heart valves(infectious endocarditis). The chronic form, by far the more common, usually develops over a period of several years and in association with rheumatic, congenital, coronary, and hypertensive heart disorders.

Cause of Fluid Retention

When impaired ventrical pumping results in a chronic lessening of cardiac output, certain abnormalities in blood pressure and blood flow and certain alterations in kidney function occur, causing an excessive accumulation of fluid in body tissues (edema formation). The expansion of blood volume and the elevation of pressures in the cardiovascular system lead to increased pressure within the vast network of capillaries in the lungs. In left-sided heart failure, higher pressure forces fluid into the lung tissues, resulting in pulmonary edema and congestion. In right-sided heart failure, the increased pressure within the capillary network of the peripheral circulation pushes fluid from the vascular space into the tissues of the body organs: the result is edema and congestion of the liver, legs, and feet.

The role of the kidneys in fluid retention is important. A low cardiac output means that the blood flow to the kidneys is reduced, and this in turn initiates a complex series of adjustments involving the kidneys and the adrenal glands. The result is that less salt and water are excreted. Along with diminished renal blood flow, there is a proportionally greater decrease in the amount of plasma filtrated from the renal blood vessel system into the small tubes of the kidneys (tubules). Consequently, greater quantities of salt and water are reabsorbed from the tubules and returned to the vascular system. Reduced renal blood flow also activates kidney secretion of the circulating hormone renin, which ultimately stimulates adrenal gland secretion of aldosterone. This circulating hormone acts on the kidney tubules to produce increased sodium and water reabsorption into the vasculature, and increased reabsorption (or decreased excretion, which is the same thing) means a greater volume of fluid in the body.

Clinical Symptoms

The most common symptom of congestive heart failure is shortness of breath (dyspnea), caused by the pulmonary congestion resulting from left-sided heart failure. If the impairment of left-ventricle pumping is minor, dyspnea occurs only with physical activity; more serious impairment produces dyspnea when the patient is at rest, or even, in particularly advanced cases, while the patient is lying down (orthopnea). In advanced cases, the breathlessness forces the patient to sleep with extra pillows elevating the head or sometimes to sit bolt upright in a chair while sleeping.

A particularly serious form of shortness of breath in marked congestive left-sided failure is paroxysmal nocturnal dyspnea, in which severe attacks of breathlessness occur at night and are so distressing that they wake the patient from sleep. Attacks are often accompanied by coughing and wheezing (cardiac asthma), which the patient tries to relieve by sitting up. Both orthopnea and paroxysmal nocturnal dyspnea are related to pulmonary congestion and edema, and both are aggravated by the sleeping position. When the body is prone, excessive blood volume is no longer concentrated in the lower extremities and there is an increased amount of blood in the vasculature of the lungs.

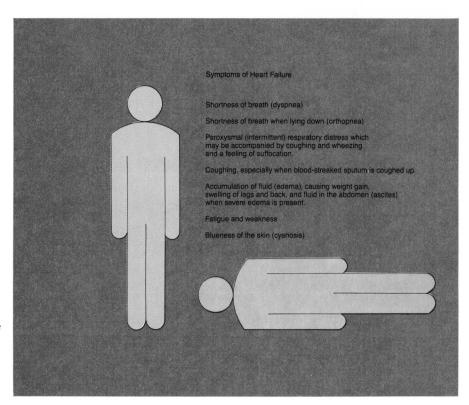

Symptoms of Heart Failure

Symptoms of Heart Failure

The most common symptoms in low-output heart failure are fatigue on exertion, weakness, and tiredness. In cases of severe heart failure, mental impairment and confusion may also appear, particularly in elderly persons with cerebral arteriosclerosis. A type of periodic breathing (Cheyne-Stokes respiration), characterized by alternating cycles of rapid breathing followed by stoppage of respiration (apnea), is observed in some patients with advanced heart failure and reduced cerebral blood flow. Other symptoms are coolness of the skin, excessive sweating, inability to tolerate heat, and reduced urine output. These result from a redistribution of regional blood flow in which the amount of blood delivered to the skin and kidneys is reduced.

Physical Signs When examining a patient with heart failure, a doctor can detect particular physical signs related to the side of the heart involved, the state of fluid congestion, and the extent to which cardiac output is limited. In left-sided heart failure with pulmonary congestion, a stethoscope placed at the bases of the lungs will enable the doctor to hear moist, noisy breath sounds (rales) when the patient breathes in. When the doctor taps the bases of the lungs, he may hear a percussion dullness, similar to the sounds made by tapping a barrel containing fluid. In either left- or right-sided congestive heart failure, fluid may collect within the pleural space between the chest wall and the lungs (pleural effusion). In right-sided congestive heart failure, the most common symptom is swelling of the lower extremities (edema). Gentle finger pressure produces pitting of the fluid-filled soft tissues, especially in the area of the ankles in patients who are able to walk. In bedridden patients, tissue edema may be either generalized (anasarca) or localized, with swelling of the lower back area. Distention of the jugular veins in the neck, caused by abnormally elevated pressure within the peripheral venous system, can be detected on physical examination. When the doctor presses on the liver for a time, blood is displaced upward toward the heart (positive hepatojugular reflux). The same elevated venous pressure may lead to an enlarged, tender liver (congestive hepatomegaly) and occasionally to enlargement of the spleen.

If the liver has been enlarged for a long time, the person's eyes and skin often have a yellow tint (jaundice). In some cases, fluid moves from the veins of the liver into the space between the abdominal wall and the intestine, producing swelling of the abdomen (ascites).

Reduced cardiac output often results in a diminished arterial pulse, most readily detected when the examining doctor feels the carotid arteries of the neck while listening to the heart with a stethoscope. The diminished pulse is often accompanied by a relatively fast heart rate and mildly elevated blood pressure during the relaxation phase (diastole) of the cardiac cycle (diastolic hypertension). Reduced blood flow to the skin may also be detected in facial pallor, sweating, and a blue tint to the lips and nail beds (cyanosis). When the pumping action of the left ventricle is severely impaired, there may be a cyclic alteration of blood pressure during the systolic phase, caused by successive strong and weak ventricular contractions. This phenomenon, called pulsus alternans, may be noted in the peripheral arterial pulse.

Physical examination of the heart itself, through palpation and listening with a stethoscope, may reveal cardiac enlargement (cardiomegaly) and characteristic extra heart sounds (gallops), which occur when the ventricles have become enlarged. Specific types of heart sounds, with characteristic locations and radiations of sound, are associated with particular kinds of heart valve diseases and other heart abnormalities.

Treatment

The best treatment of congestive heart failure is prevention. Obviously, cardiac function should never be allowed to become seriously impaired by congenital heart disease or acquired valvular disorders. Therefore, anyone with congenital heart disease should be given a definitive evaluation by cardiac catheterization and, if necessary, undergo surgery before severe symptoms develop. The same is true for patients with chronic rheumatic valvular diseases who experience cardiac symptoms during their ordinary daily activity. When heart valve malfunction is severe, the valve should be replaced before congestive heart failure develops; the depressed ventricular contraction associated with heart failure may remain even after the faulty functioning of a valve has been corrected by surgery.

Even when certain heart muscle diseases (idiopathic cardiomyopathies) are suspected, patients with chronic heart failure are given detailed right- and left-heart catheterization to establish the type of disease and to determine the extent to which the heart or heart muscle is impaired. In other cases of chronic heart failure, an unsuspected congenital or acquired heart disease may be detected by catheterization and corrected or alleviated by surgery.

In addition to making a systematic evaluation of the nature and degree of heart disease, the examining doctor looks for signs of conditions outside the heart that may be simulating or perpetuating its malfunctioning. A number of conditions can contribute to chronic heart failure. In many instances, however, no previously unrecognized diseases are revealed by the patient's history or in the results of physical examination, laboratory tests, and cardiac catheterization. In such cases, chronic heart failure is due to primary myocardial heart disease resulting in severely impaired ventricular contraction. Medical management of congestive heart failure that is the result of chronically reduced pumping action seeks to improve the four determinants of cardiac function, adjusting each so that the failing heart can deliver as nearly normal an output as possible. The determinants are: preload, or the volume of blood available just prior to the pumping stroke; contractibility, or the force of ventricular contraction regardless of the volume of blood in the ventricles; ventricular impedance, or the resistance offered to ventricular ejection during systole; and heart rate.

In advanced congestive heart failure, treatment is best begun in the hospital with bed rest and decreased physical activity. The treatment usually centers on improving impaired contractibility and on reducing salt and water retention by the body.

Since the basic problem in heart failure is the impairment of ventricular contractile force, the first principle in treatment is the use of agents that strengthen this force and increase cardiac performance. Drug therapy usually begins with the digitalis glycosides. These drugs directly stimulate the force of heart contraction, thus improving the contractile state. The cardiac output is increased and the ventricular end-diastolic pressure that produces symptoms of circulatory congestion is lowered. At the present time, the digitalis glycosides are the only such drugs that can be given orally over long periods of time to patients outside the hospital. Certain more powerful drugs, including isoproterenol and dopamine, can be given intravenously to hospitalized patients.

Recent experience indicates that drugs which alter cardiac loading are beneficial in chronic as well as acute cases of cardiac failure. These are peripheral vasodilator drugs which are effective because of certain physical properties of the cardiovascular system. The heart must pump against a certain amount of pressure, part of which is caused by the presence of blood already in the vessels. If these vessels can be dilated, or widened, resistance is lowered, making it easier for the heart to pump more blood (overload reduction). In congestive heart failure due to acute heart attack, reducing

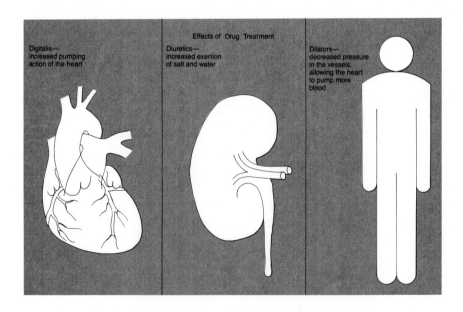

Effects of Drug Treatment

Digitalis—
increased pumping
action of the heart

Diuretics—
increased exertion
of salt and water

Dilators—
decreased pressure
in the vessels,
allowing the heart
to pump more
blood

ventricular overload with intravenously administered vasodilators such as nitroprusside or phentolamine has been shown to raise low cardiac output, decrease high left ventricular filling pressure, and diminish myocardial oxygen demands. Intravenous nitroprusside can also raise reduced cardiac output and lower markedly elevated ventricular filling pressures in cases of chronic heart failure. The same benefits that come from reducing the volume load on poorly functioning ventricles may be obtained by the regular use of long-acting nitrates taken orally.

There are also electrical methods that can be used to improve the pumping function of the heart. These include pacemaker catheters to step up markedly slow heart rates (sinus bradycardia) and when there is complete heart block. Ventricular filling can be improved, and thus cardiac output raised, when the "booster" pumping function of the atria is regained by direct electric current (electroconversion of atrial fibrillation). The atria are thus enlisted to fill the ventricles to their maximum capacity. Although it is difficult to maintain normal heart rhythm when the pressure or volume of the left atrium is increased, this procedure is sometimes worthwhile in cases of chronic heart failure.

When chronic ventricular malfunctioning is accompanied by abnormally slow heart rates, cardiac performance may be improved by increasing the frequency of contractions with electrical pacing catheters. Raising relatively slow heart rates to normal levels (and sometimes to the upper limits of normal resting rates), may enhance cardiac output by increasing the rate of cardiac contraction.

Careful selection of diuretic agents can reduce excessive salt and fluid accumulation. The recent development of such potent diuretic drugs as chlorothiazide, ethacrynic acid, furosemide, and spironolactone has greatly increased the possibility of relieving circulatory congestion. Modern diuretic therapy begins with oral thiazides, agents which prevent reabsorption of sodium in the renal tubules and thereby lead to the excretion of excess sodium and water. Since loss of potassium is a side effect of these diuretics, the patient may be given potassium supplements. If the thiazides alone prove inadequate, an orally administered aldosterone antagonist, either spironolactone or triamterene, is added. Aldosterone antagonists inhibit the exchange of potassium for sodium in the renal tubules, thereby aiding the excretion of sodium and water while retaining the potassium. The aldosterone inhibitors are less potent than thiazides, ethacrynic acid, or furosemide, but they do promote considerable loss of sodium when taken daily for several weeks. However, since aldosterone inhibitors retain potassium, the addition of oral potassium may be hazardous. If the combination of a thiazide with spironolactone or triamterene is unsuccessful, one of the more potent oral diuretics, ethacrynic acid or furosemide, may be substituted for the thiazide. These agents block the absorption of sodium in the renal tubules, resulting in the excretion of large amounts of excess sodium and water. In some cases of chronic congestive heart failure, the start of salt and water excretion seems to be aided by an initial use of intravenous ethacrynic acid or furosemide therapy.

When chronic congestive heart failure persists in spite of all medical measures and surgery is not feasible, a possible last alternative is heart transplant (cardiac homotransplantation). Such transplants, however, require careful selection of both patient and donor and involve a degree of surgical skill that is within the capability of only a very few specialists. The expenses involved, the high rate of failure, and the resistance offered by the patient's natural "rejection" system have restricted the application of this procedure.

Mechanical cardiac assist devices have not been useful in the management of chronic heart failure, although such devices have provided at least temporary benefit in the treatment of severe cardiac impairment due to acute myocardial infarction. The major hope for treatment of absolutely intractable heart failure perhaps lies in the development of a permanently implantable artificial heart.

RESEARCH ON DEVICES TO AID THE FAILING HEART

So much of the heart muscle may be damaged as a result of coronary occlusions that there is not enough left to pump the minimum amount of blood the body needs. Medical science has investigated the development of collateral circulation, which can revive dormant muscle tissue, and has studied the heart muscle's capacity to assume a greater work load under proper circumstances. Putting both concepts together, doctors have come to believe that some patients with heart failure can be saved if the heart can be given a temporary "boost" or some supplementary aid in circulation.

The experimental devices created so far are based on a simple principle; to allow the heart to recuperate from the damage it has sustained—that is, to reduce its work load—and at the same time to make sure that the body receives the oxygenated blood it requires. The supposition is that if the heart can rest, time will enable collateral circulation to develop and muscle tissue that remains alive but nonfunctioning to be revitalized.

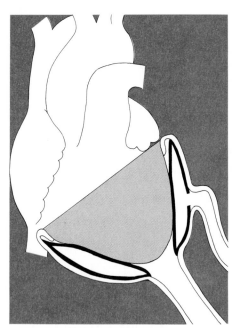

One mechanically simple device consists of a cup with a diaphragm inside it. This is placed around the outside of the left ventricle. A compressor, governed by a timing mechanism synchronized with the patient's heartbeat, intermittently pumps air between the rigid cup and the diaphragm. This forces the diaphragm to press against the ventricle, exerting an even pressure over the face of the chamber. The pressure helps to expel blood into the aorta with a minimal effort of the muscles of the ventricle. Since the diaphragm squeezes against the external wall of the heart, it has no contact with blood and thus blood damage is avoided, as is any increase in the potential for clotting. The obvious drawback is that, in order to use the device, the chest wall must be open and the heart exposed.

The cup and diaphragm devices assist the ventricle by adding compressed air power to the heart's own muscular contractions. In another mechanical assisting device, the ventricle contracts and relaxes on its own, but the resistance against which the heart must pump is lowered. A balloon is threaded through the femoral artery and into the aorta until it lies at the level where the left subclavian artery branches off the ascending aorta. A compressor then pumps air into the balloon, which is timed to inflate the relaxed phase (diastole) of the cardiac cycle and deflate in the contracting phase (systole). The inflation of the balloon forces the blood already in the aorta backward into the coronary circulatory out toward the peripheral system supplying blood to the heart. The deflation of the balloon during systole permits blood pumped from the ventricle to flow freely around the balloon toward the peripheral circulations supplying blood to the body's organs. This flow meets less resistance, since the inflation of the balloon during diastole has already

To assist a failing heart, a cup with a diaphragm inside it is placed around the inside of the left ventricle. A compressor timed to synchronize with the patient's heartbeat intermittently pumps air between the rigid cup and the diaphragm, helping to expel blood into the aorta with a minimal effort of the muscles of the ventricle.

removed some of the blood from the aorta. Clinical experiments with this device at Maimonides Hospital in Brooklyn, New York, proved encouraging; all but one of the critically ill patients on whom it was tried showed improvements. Seven recovered sufficiently to leave the hospital. It should be remembered that all such experiments are used on humans only after extended animal studies, and only as a last resort. In the study just mentioned, ten other potential candidates for the device were ruled out for various medical reasons, and all died within a short time.

The heart-lung machine is one of the most frequently used means of assisting a failing heart. Just as this machine may be used during "open heart" surgery to take over the work of the patient's own circulatory system, so it may take over the work of the natural organs for as long as ten hours as an emergency measure. After an extended period, however, the effects of total cardiopulmonary bypass diminish, and alterations of blood structure inevitably occur.

When the left ventricle does not empty during systole and thus does not deliver enough blood to the arteries, pressure remains high within the ventricle during diastole, when the chambers fill with blood. With the resulting high pressure, the right ventricle must pump harder to get blood through the pulmonary artery to the lungs, and lung congestion often results. While whatever has caused the left ventricle to fail may be resolved if time permits—an embolism that blocked a coronary artery may be removed, or collateral circulation may circumvent an area of an infarct and revive muscle tissue—delay can often be fatal. To win time, physicians, notably Dr. Michael De Bakey, experimented with a left ventricular bypass pump. The method employed a Dacron tube connected to the left atrium at the point where the pulmonary vein delivers freshly oxygenated blood. The blood was diverted from the heart chambers by means of a Dacron tube which carried the blood to the axillary artery, a continuation of the right subclavian artery. Thus the work load on the left side of the heart was lessened and a proper supply of oxygenated blood was still brought to all parts of the body.

The first patient Dr. De Bakey attempted the bypass upon was a dying forty-two-year-old man. The booster kept him alive for four days, but his heart was too badly damaged to recover and he had suffered extensive brain damage before the bypass could be operative. The second attempt was made on a thirty-seven-year-old Mexican woman, who stayed on the bypass pump for ten days. This woman's heart was able to regain its power, and she lived without cardiac problems for six years, until she was killed in an automobile accident.

The heart-lung machine and the bypass procedure have not only revived individual patients; their success has sparked the search for a mechanical replacement for the entire heart. Dr. Alexis Carrel, the French surgeon who won the Nobel prize in 1912, used his pioneering research in tissue transplantation and anastomoses (the technique of fastening together veins and arteries), proposed an artificial heart made out of glass. While more recent synthetic materials such as Dacron and Teflon make the notion of glass seem somewhat simplistic, Dr. Carrel's suggestion was perfectly reasonable: in his time, glass was the only available substance that would not produce a chemical reaction when in contact with tissue or blood.

Research workers today consider that a number of synthetic materials suitable for use on the heart have been developed. Silastic, for example, is a

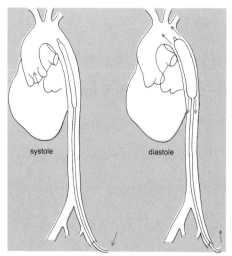

systole   diastole

A balloon threaded through the femoral artery and into the aorta is one of the devices used to assist a failing heart. Air is pumped into the balloon by a compressor in a rhythm timed to inflate in the relaxed phase (diastole) and deflate in the contracting phase (systole) of the cardiac cycle. The resistance against which the heart must pump is lowered by this means.

PRINCIPLES

1. *Congestive heart failure is a broad term used to describe conditions in which the heart's pumping capability is impaired. The term does not mean that death is imminent, and in fact the degree of heart failure may range from mild to severe. The condition may be associated with an accumulation of fluid within the body.*

2. *Congestive heart failure results from the inability of the heart's pumping chambers to contract forcefully enough. This may be due to weakness of the heart muscle, to failure of the ventricles to load blood fully, or to an overload of blood or pressure which excessively burdens the contracting power of the ventricles.*

3. *The body compensates for congestive heart failure in several ways. The pumping chambers of the heart may enlarge their capacity by stretching muscles, thus providing added force to the contraction. The ventricle itself may enlarge, adding to the over-all mass of muscle involved in the pumping stroke. The sympathetic nervous system may elevate the heart rate, thus improving the contraction power of the available heart muscle.*

4. *Congestive heart failure may involve either ventricle or both, with different causes and symptoms in left-sided and in right-sided heart failure.*

5. *When cardiac output drops, the imbalance of excessive pressure in the capillaries of the pulmonary circulation forces fluid into the lung tissue. This condition, called pulmonary edema, is due to left-sided heart failure. An imbalance of increased pressure that leads to fluid retention in other areas, such as the legs and feet, is a sign of right-sided heart failure. Diminished blood flow due to congestive heart failure causes the kidneys to reduce their salt and water excretion, leading to further edema.*

6. *Shortness of breath (dyspnea) is the most common symptom of congestive heart failure and is due to pulmonary edema consequent to left-sided heart failure. Dyspnea may be mild or it may be severe enough to wake the patient from sleep. Other common symptoms of congestive heart failure are tiredness on exertion and weakness. Examination of the chest by palpation and with the use of a stethoscope can detect many of the signs accompanying these symptoms.*

7. *Congestive heart failure is best treated by correction or amelioration of the conditions that lead to it. Defective heart valve or coronary artery disease should be treated by medication or surgery. Advanced chronic congestive heart failure is treated with restrictions of activity, with bed rest, and with drugs to improve heart pumping action and to eliminate fluid retention.*

synthetic that will not trigger the body's rejection response to a foreign substance. It is also smooth enough for blood to flow over it without damage and without stimulating clotting. It will not build up electrostatic charges from the friction of the blood moving over its surface (another possible cause of clotting). The material also appears to be strong enough to endure the hydraulic pressure necessary for heart pumping action and to last for years in spite of the wear and tear of constant expansion and contraction. Prototypes of artificial hearts made of Silastic have already been implanted in animals. The procedure that is usually adapted retains the original upper chambers but connects them to a pair of substitute ventricles, which are then anastomosed to the pulmonary artery and the aorta. During systole, gas or air pressure from an external source fills a section of each ventricle. This pressure forces blood to flow through the pulmonary and aortic valves in the same manner as it does in the natural heart. A timing mechanism then permits the pressure to drop and the artificial heart goes into the diastolic or relaxed phase.

A successful artificial heart must have the capacity to pump blood at varying rates according to the needs of the body. Since human responses to emotional stimuli vary from individual to individual, no artificial heart yet contemplated is capable of adjusting to emotional stress or mental stimulation or any of the other myriad commands of the central nervous system. But to be effective an artificial heart must adjust its output to meet physical stress. The means to build this flexibility into a mechanical heart are at hand, with miniature timing devices and computers capable of making such subtle changes. There is, moreover, proof that the working of the mechanical heart will not be seriously affected by its adjustment's being limited to merely physical stimuli. The experiments with heart transplants suggest this. In a typical heart transplant, the surgical procedure necessarily severs the links of the vagus and accelerator nervous systems to the transplanted heart; the borrowed hearts do not, therefore, respond to intellectual or emotional stimuli. Nevertheless, the hearts do adjust their output according to signals sent to them by changes in venous pressure. An artificial heart would do the same.

Although material for an artificial heart and an adequate sensing mechanism to regulate cardiac output are both theoretically possible, one vital element is still missing—an acceptable source of energy. Motors or pumps durable enough and small enough to fit into the human chest cavity already exist, but the means to power them does not. The problems are obvious; not only must the energy flow be constant, but the drive system must remain at a steady temperature and must not dissipate heat through the blood, since any significant change in temperature will produce dangerous alterations in blood chemistry. Perhaps the most promising approach to a safe, constant power supply may be in nuclear-powered devices.

14

PERIPHERAL ARTERIAL DISEASE

Victor G. deWolfe, M.D.

Peripheral arterial diseases are abnormal conditions affecting the blood vessels which carry blood away from the heart. The peripheral arteries discussed in this chapter are the aorta and the branches from it which supply the upper and lower extremities and the abdominal organs (except the kidneys). Peripheral arterial diseases are of four kinds: occlusive disease, in which the flow of blood through the artery is blocked; vasospastic disease, in which the small arteries go into spasm; functional disorders, in which the small arteries dilate; and aneurysm, a bulging or ballooning due to weakness in the artery wall. Arterial diseases affecting the brain and kidneys are also peripheral vascular disorders; these are discussed in other chapters (see Stroke, chapter 19, and Hypertension, chapter 10).

PERIPHERAL ARTERIES The aorta, the main artery receiving blood from the left ventricle, arises from the aortic valve at the top of the heart and to the right of the breastbone. It courses first toward the head and then curves down in an arch, descending to the left of the breastbone. The first branch of the aorta, the innominate artery, arises at the beginning of the aortic arch and then divides into the right subclavian artery, which supplies the right side of the chest, shoulder, and arm, and the right common carotid artery, which supplies the neck and head. Two other branches arise from the arch as it curves to the left; the left common carotid artery to the neck and head, and the left subclavian artery to the left side of the chest, shoulder, and arm.

As the aorta descends, small pairs of branches from it go to the ribs and the main vessel enters the abdomen through an opening in the diaphragm, at which point it becomes the abdominal aorta. A series of smaller arteries branch off to feed the major organs: gastric arteries supply the stomach; the hepatic artery supplies the liver, pancreas, and duodenum; the splenic artery supplies the spleen. Immediately below these, the superior mesenteric artery branches off, supplying the small intestine and the right side of the large intestine. The next branches are the paired right and left renal arteries to the kidneys. Below these and above the level of the navel, the inferior mesenteric artery branches to the left side of the large intestine and to the rectum. At the level of the navel, the abdominal aorta divides into the right and left iliac arteries, which pass through the pelvis to reach the groin, after which they become the common femoral arteries supplying the legs and feet.

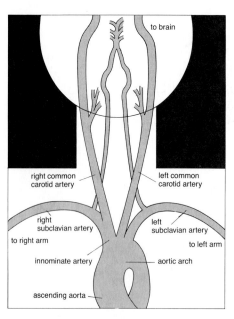

The blood supply to the lower extremities is provided by the common femoral arteries. These divide into the deep femoral arteries, which supply the thighs, and the superficial femoral arteries, the main source of blood to the lower part of the legs and the feet. At the top of the knees, the popliteal arteries arise from the superficial femoral arteries, then run behind the knees (popliteal spaces) and divide into the anterior tibial arteries, which supply the front of the legs, and the posterior tibial arteries, which supply the calves. From behind the inner ankle bones, the posterior tibial arteries enter the soles of the feet. The anterior tibial arteries, at the top of the ankles midway between the ankle bones, run into the top of the feet and become the dorsalis pedis arteries, where pulses can be easily felt. The dorsalis pedis and posterior tibial arteries join in the feet to form the plantar arches, from which arise small digital arteries that supply the toes.

The major vessels carrying blood to the upper extremities and the brain arise from the aortic arch.

The upper extremities receive their blood supply from the subclavian arteries. Emerging from the neck just above the collarbones, these descend into the armpits (axillary arteries) and continue down along the inside of the upper arms (brachial arteries) to the elbows. At the inside of the elbows (the antecubital space), the brachial arteries divide into the radial arteries (which go down toward the thumbs) and the ulnar arteries (which go down toward the small fingers). Where the radial artery comes close to the skin surface at the wrist, it provides a convenient place for taking the pulse. As the radial and ulnar arteries enter the hand, they connect to form the palmar arch. From the outer edge of this arch small digital arteries arise and travel to each side of the fingers.

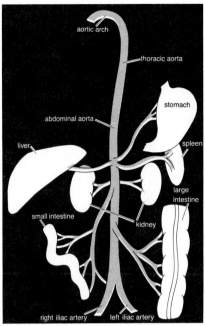

Descending Aorta

Smaller arteries branching from the aorta bring oxygenated blood to the abdominal organs and the legs and feet.

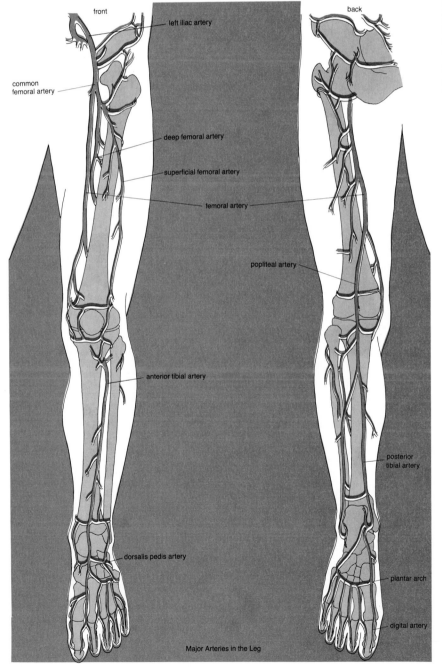

Major Arteries in the Leg

The arterial route through the legs begins at the branching of the abdominal aorta into the right and left iliac arteries, which subdivide until finally reaching the toes.

ARTERIOSCLEROSIS OBLITERANS (CHRONIC OCCLUSIVE ARTERIAL DISEASE)

The disease process that causes blockage of the arteries supplying the brain can lead to stroke. Similar blockage of the coronary arteries can result in myocardial infarction. When the arteries that supply the legs and feet are affected, the disease process is called arteriosclerosis obliterans. Its cause is atherosclerosis, a disease of unknown origin in which the inner layer of the artery wall becomes thick and irregular from the piling up of fatty deposits called atheromata. The disease develops slowly and insidiously over a period of years, progressively narrowing an artery until it eventually becomes blocked. To overcome the obstruction, the body develops a detour circulation, bypassing the blockage. Small arteries branching from the artery above the obstruction develop connections with small arteries below the obstruction, allowing the blood to continue to flow. This collateral circulation is adequate to keep the tissues alive, but it is not enough to prevent discomfort such as cramps or pain when the muscles are in use (intermittent claudication). If the disease progresses, the collateral arteries also become affected, and the severe decrease in the circulation causes pain even when the patient is at rest. Ultimately, the loss in blood supply to the tissues may be so severe that they will ulcerate or become gangrenous.

Although arteriosclerosis obliterans usually occurs in persons over fifty,

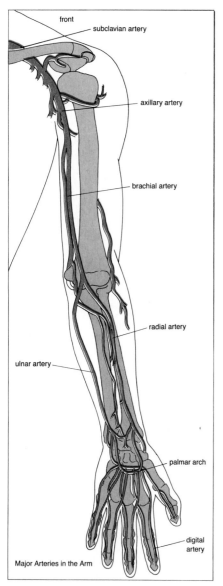

Arteries supplying the arm and hand branch off from the subclavian artery, descending into the armpit and down the inside of the upper arm, where they divide into the radial and ulnar arteries before connecting to form the palmar arch.

An obstructed artery supplying the legs and feet can be identified by feeling the pulse at four key points.

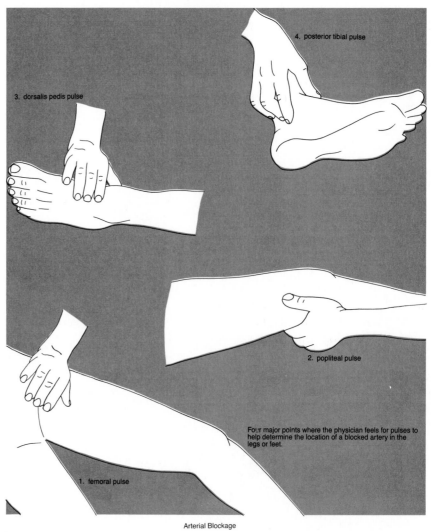

Arterial Blockage

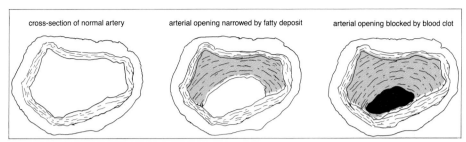

cross-section of normal artery   arterial opening narrowed by fatty deposit   arterial opening blocked by blood clot

Formation of atherosclerotic deposit in arterial wall

it also appears in younger persons as a result of diabetes mellitus, elevated cholesterol or other blood fats, hypertension, cigarette smoking, or a family history of premature atherosclerosis. Smoking is perhaps the most significant risk factor—studies show that 90 percent of persons with arteriosclerosis obliterans are smokers. About 20 percent of patients have overt diabetes and another 20 percent have abnormally high blood sugar levels. Men are more affected than women, in a ratio of four to one.

The earliest symptom of arteriosclerosis obliterans, called intermittent claudication, is discomfort on walking, caused by an inadequate supply of blood to an exercising muscle. Patients usually have sufficient collateral circulation to walk short distances comfortably, but longer walks—from as little as half a block up to a quarter of a mile—result in pain, aching, cramping, tightness, or severe fatigue, most often in the calf, but also in the foot, thigh, hip, or buttock. The location of the distress is related to the site of the blocked artery. When the lower abdominal aorta or the iliac arteries are affected, the hips, buttocks, thighs, and calves are involved. When the blockage is in the superficial femoral artery, the discomfort is felt in the calf; blockage in the arteries below the knee affects the foot as well as the calf. The pain disappears within a minute or two after the person stops walking and then recurs after walking the same distance.

Intermittent Claudication

When the disease has progressed to a point where collateral circulation no longer provides adequate blood to the tissues, pain is felt even when the patient is inactive. The characteristic severe and unrelenting pain in the foot usually occurs while resting in bed, because the horizontal position neutralizes the force of gravity, and not enough blood flows down into the foot. To obtain relief, most patients will hang the leg over the side of the bed or sleep in a chair with the leg dependent. Any further decrease in arterial circulation can result in the breakdown of tissue, usually on the toes, foot, or heel. These ischemic ulcers are small and shallow at first, but may increase in size with further breakdown of tissue. Gangrene, the final complication of lack of blood supply, usually requires amputation of a toe, the foot, or the leg.

Rest Pain

In the early stages of the disease, when the patient has only mild intermittent claudication, the foot receives an adequate supply of blood, and thus the skin temperature and color, as well as hair and nail growth are usually normal. The location of the affected artery can be determined, however, by examination of the various pulses. If the aorta is occluded, the pulses will be absent or severely diminished in the groin, over the femoral arteries, behind the knees

Physical Examination

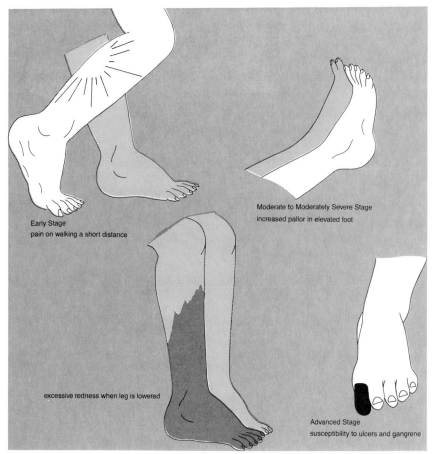

Early Stage
pain on walking a short distance

Moderate to Moderately Severe Stage
increased pallor in elevated foot

excessive redness when leg is lowered

Advanced Stage
susceptibility to ulcers and gangrene

Symptoms of Arteriosclerosis Obliterans

over the popliteal arteries, and in the feet. If one iliac artery is occluded, all the pulses in the affected leg will be absent. If the superficial femoral artery is occluded, the femoral pulse will be present and strong, but the pulses below the groin will be absent or weakened. If the lower popliteal artery or the arteries in the legs are occluded, the femoral and popliteal pulses will be present but the foot pulses will be absent.

In moderate to moderately severe cases, elevation of the limb results in changes in the color of the skin of the foot. Under these conditions, the insufficient flow and pressure in the collateral artery cannot overcome the force of gravity and supply blood to the limb. The blood continues to drain out through the veins, and the foot becomes pale. When the leg is lowered, however, it becomes excessively red, because the small arteries and capillaries dilate to compensate for the lack of blood flow while the leg was elevated. With further progression of the disease, the foot becomes cold to the touch, the skin rough and scaly, and hair and nail growth is poor. In the advanced stage, any injury to the foot, infections (including fungus infections, such as athlete's foot), or abnormal exposure to heat or cold can lead to ulcers and gangrene.

Diagnosis The diagnosis of arteriosclerosis obliterans is usually made quickly and accurately from a physical examination and a study of the patient's medical history. Instruments have been devised to give precise and objective measurements of decreased arterial circulation, and these may be used to confirm the diagnosis. They are useful in recording the progress of the disease. Angiography (the process of taking an X-ray picture after a blood vessel is injected with a contrast medium) is required to locate the precise site of arterial occlusion, especially if corrective vascular surgery is contemplated. A complete angiographic study in cases of arteriosclerosis obliterans consists of an aortogram (dye is injected into the aorta) and of femoral arteriograms (dye is injected into the femoral arteries). (When a vein is injected, the procedure is called venogram or phlebogram.) These procedures are performed either by inserting a needle directly into the aorta through the left side of the low back and into the femoral arteries through each groin or by inserting a catheter into one of the arteries in the groin or arm and threading it through the aorta and then into the extremity to be studied. When the needle or catheter is in place, the contrast medium is injected, and X-ray pictures are taken of the aorta, both iliac arteries, both superficial femoral arteries, and the arteries of the legs and feet. In addition to revealing the exact location of the blockage, the studies show the condition of the arteries above and below the occlusions and the extent of the collateral circulation. Such information is essential before reconstructive surgery is undertaken because it shows the surgeon whether it is possible to bypass the involved arteries or to remove short blockages by a procedure called endarterectomy.

Most cases of arteriosclerosis obliterans are treated medically. The goals **Treatment** are to maintain function of the affected limb, relieve pain, protect the limb from injury and infection that might lead to ulceration and gangrene, and to eliminate or lessen the impact of as many risk factors as possible. Unfortunately, there is no drug or medication that is of proven value in the treatment of arteriosclerosis obliterans. Although some drug manufacturers claim that their products (vasodilators) dilate the arteries in the extremities, the overwhelming experience of specialists in the field is that these are of no value to patients with any type of occlusive arterial disease, though they are occasionally helpful to patients with spasm of the small arteries.

It is absolutely essential for anyone with arteriosclerosis obliterans to stop smoking completely and permanently because smoking impedes the development of the collateral circulation and thus not only prevents improvement but may even worsen the condition. Meticulous care of the feet is also essential for all patients with reduced circulation. Each day the feet should be carefully washed with mild soap and water, rinsed, and then dried carefully with a soft towel, particularly between the toes. The toes should be dusted with an effective antiseptic foot powder. Stockings should be clean each day and shoes should be well-fitting and roomy but not so loose that they rub and cause friction. Any evidence of athlete's foot, corns, calluses, or other problems should be promptly attended to by a physician or podiatrist. Since any injury to the foot can initiate ulcerations and possibly culminate in gangrene, patients should never risk injury by walking barefoot or by exposing the feet to extremes of hot or cold.

Patients with arterial insufficiency are usually told to sleep with the head of the bed elevated 4 to 6 inches. Additional pillows only raise the trunk of the body; this does not lower the feet or enable them to benefit from the force of gravity. The entire bed should be elevated by placing blocks of wood, bricks, or books under the legs at the head of the bed. Then the feet are 4 to 6 inches below the level of the heart, a position which not only increases the blood flow to the feet but allows those suffering rest pain to sleep in a bed rather than a chair.

A structured walking plan is an indispensable part of the treatment program for patients with intermittent claudication. Walking to the point of pain or distress has been found to be the most important stimulus to the development of collateral circulation. In most cases, the patient is advised to walk for a half hour twice a day, resting when the pain and discomfort appear and then resuming the walk until the allotted period is completed. If age, arthritis, or other infirmity prevents such a schedule, the patient should walk as much as possible two or three times a day. There is conclusive proof that following this regimen will increase the daily walking distance significantly. Many patients have reached the point where they can walk for indefinite periods without pain or distress.

Ulcerations   Patients with severe arteriosclerosis obliterans are prone to ulcerations on the feet or legs resulting from injury. Local treatment of arterial (ischemic) ulcers is designed to maintain cleanliness and avoid infection—no salve or ointment has been found to induce healing of the ulcers. Healing occurs only if the circulation is improved by the development of collateral circulation or by surgery. Local treatment consists of daily cleansing in lukewarm water with mild soap or detergent; hot, cold, irritating, or sensitizing solutions must be avoided. The affected foot should be soaked for ten to twenty minutes once a day in a solution prescribed by a physician and then rinsed in clear water and carefully patted dry with a soft towel. The ulcer is then bandaged with a clean, nonbulky dressing that allows a shoe or slipper to be worn comfortably. Many physicians also prescribe a mild antibiotic ointment for application under the dressing to prevent infection. The antibiotic does not actually heal the ulcer itself.

SURGICAL TREATMENT
Revascularization   Surgical correction of arteries blocked by arteriosclerosis obliterans is called revascularization and can be accomplished either by construction of a bypass around a blocked artery (using a leg vein or a synthetic material such as Dacron), or by dissecting and separating short occlusions from the wall of an artery (endarterectomy). When either procedure is successful, blood flow is restored to the tissues below the previously obstructed artery.

Revascularization may be recommended for the patient with intermittent claudication due to disease of the superficial femoral artery whose circulation continues to deteriorate even after a scheduled walking program has been followed for a period of two to three months. Surgery in this case bypasses the occlusions of the artery by means of a vein from the patient's leg. Unfortunately, from 40 to 60 percent of the grafts become blocked over a five-year period. When the graft fails, the symptoms may be severe and the affected leg may ultimately have to be amputated because the collateral circulation becomes quiescent when the bypass graft functions successfully. Therefore, when the graft fails, there is no circulation to replace it; reoperating then becomes an emergency measure and often again results in failure. The high incidence of graft failure and the loss of collateral circulation are the

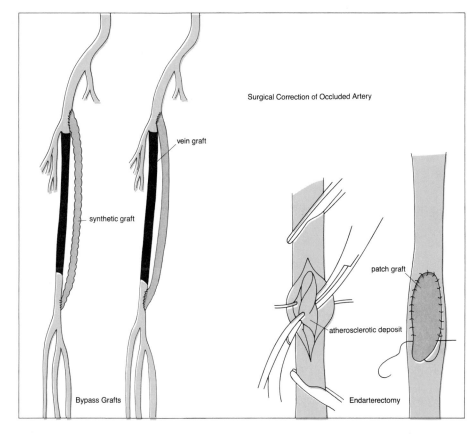

Surgical Correction of Occluded Artery

vein graft

synthetic graft

patch graft

atherosclerotic deposit

Bypass Grafts

Endarterectomy

A bypass graft attached above and below a blocked segment of an artery allows blood to reach tissues formerly deprived of adequate oxygen.
Short atherosclerotic deposits can be surgically removed and a patch graft attached to replace the damaged arterial wall.

reasons that grafting in superficial femoral disease is seldom done by choice. Revascularization should be done if possible when the patient suffers severe rest pain, ulcerations, or minor gangrene. In such cases medical treatment is usually not successful, and the operation is no longer a matter of choice, but an essential procedure to save the limb.

Revascularization is most successful in patients with moderate intermittent claudication due to blockage of the lower aorta or the iliac arteries. Operations on arteries this high in the body are successful in nine of ten cases, with a long-term period of functioning predicted for the graft. In these operations, synthetic grafts of Dacron or Teflon are used because the aorta, which supplies blood to the graft, is large and delivers blood at a high rate and under high pressure, and leg veins are not large enough in diameter to replace occluded sections of the aorta.

In all forms of revascularization, the patient must be well enough to tolerate the stress of major surgery. Because patients with arteriosclerosis obliterans frequently have atherosclerosis in other parts of the body as well, they must be carefully screened before an operation. Any pre-existing heart disease or diabetes must be under good control, the kidneys must function well, and circulation to the brain as well as lung function must be adequate to withstand anesthesia and the stresses of the postoperative period. Arteriosclerosis obliterans affecting the lower extremities is rarely life-threatening. Death rate in patients with this disease is usually caused by other manifestations of atherosclerosis, such as heart disease or stroke, particularly if these follow major amputation or a revascularization procedure.

Lumbar Sympathectomy   Patients with severe rest pain, ulcerations, or small areas of gangrene, who cannot undergo reconstructive surgery, will sometimes benefit from an operation called lumbar sympathectomy (surgical removal of the sympathetic nerves). The sympathetic nerves affect the blood vessels and the sweat glands of the extremities, causing the small arteries to constrict. When these nerves are removed by surgery, the small arteries dilate, thereby increasing the blood supply to the skin and the tissues under the skin. With blood supply to the foot improved, the ulcer will often heal. This "last resort" operation is done to save a threatened extremity and is successful in about half the cases. The high rate of failure results from the inactivity of the sympathetic nerves in the elderly and in patients with diabetes. Fortunately, a lumbar sympathectomy is a relatively minor procedure, is well tolerated by most patients, and is well worth trying to save a leg or foot.

Amputation   When arteriosclerosis obliterans reaches the stage where there is extensive death of tissue, the toes and feet may be affected by large areas of gangrene. At this point amputation becomes necessary. It is only occasionally possible to amputate across the foot just behind the base of the toes, because the circulation at that level is usually not adequate to heal the incision. However, this is done whenever possible and is often tried first. If it is not successful, the surgeon will amputate just below the knee. This level is preferred because rehabilitation is more likely if the patient has a functioning knee joint. Only if the gangrene extends to the level of the knee is it necessary to amputate above the joint, and this happens infrequently.

With careful postoperative care, most below-knee amputations heal and vigorous physical therapy then enables the patient to learn to walk with crutches and eventually with a below-knee artificial limb. Many months of supervised physical therapy and rehabilitation are necessary, requiring patience and perseverance on the part of the patient and encouragement and reinforcement from family, therapist, and physician. Only in the very elderly and severely debilitated is rehabilitation unlikely after below-knee amputation.

Diabetes Mellitus   Patients with diabetes mellitus tend to develop arteriosclerosis obliterans at an earlier age than do nondiabetics for reasons not well understood. Characteristically, the arteries below the knee and the small arteries of the foot are involved. The disease tends to be widespread and is usually associated with poor collateral circulation. Revascularization (bypass grafting or endarterectomy) is therefore not feasible. Moreover, most diabetic patients are not good candidates for lumbar sympathectomy, because the disease destroys the function of the sympathetic nerves. For these reasons, arterial insufficiency in diabetics, which manifests itself as severe intermittent claudication, rest pain, and ulceration, is best treated by medical procedures and by careful foot hygiene, avoidance of injury, and treatment of ulcers to postpone or avoid amputation.

Another complication of diabetes mellitus is diabetic neuritis (or neuropathy), in which nerves supplying the lower extremities cease to function. When this occurs, there is a significant lessening or a total loss of sensations of pain, vibration, and temperature. Occasionally, in the late stages of diabetic neuritis, the patient loses position sense, develops weakness of muscles, and finds walking difficult. Diabetic neuritis is believed to be caused by a deficiency in circulation to the tiny arteries that supply the nerves, the vasa nervorum. With the loss of sensation, the diabetic person does not feel the pain that normally accompanies injury, exposure to extreme heat or cold, or a corn or callus. Many continue to have adequate circulation of the main arteries, and their feet are warm and have good pulses. However, the diseased nerves cause deformities of the bones of the feet, resulting in abnormal weight bearing and the formation of corns and calluses. The patient without pain sensation can be unaware that corns or calluses have split open and become infected. Such untreated infections may spread to the bone, which can become infected and gradually destroyed (osteomyelitis).

Prevention, therefore, is the most important part of the treatment in diabetic neuritis. The feet must be kept scrupulously clean, injuries to the feet and legs must be avoided, and corns and calluses must be promptly treated by a podiatrist. Special footwear and appliances may be needed to protect deformed or pressure areas from injury. Once an ulcer forms, it can penetrate deep into the tissues and require drainage and trimming. Oral antibiotics are frequently prescribed for prolonged periods of time, especially if osteomyelitis has set in. If the ulcer, infection, and osteomyelitis are persistent and if the bone deformities are severe, amputation may be necessary. Because such patients usually have adequate circulation through the large blood vessels, removal of one or more toes or amputation across the middle of the foot is often successful.

Thromboangiitis obliterans, more commonly called Buerger's disease after **Buerger's Disease** the American physician who first described it in 1908, is an inflammatory disease affecting the arteries, veins, and nerves. Although the exact cause is unknown, it has been well established that the disease occurs only in cigarette smokers, is immediately arrested when the patient stops smoking, and progresses relentlessly if the patient continues to smoke. (There have been occasional reports of the disease's occurring in non-smokers, but most authorities believe that these were errors in diagnosis.) The exact nature of the relationship between Buerger's disease and cigarette smoking is not known, but a sensitivity or allergy to tobacco is suspected. This allergy produces the characteristic inflammatory reaction in the arteries, veins, and nerves. Pathological changes brought on by the disease result in a thickening of the walls of the arteries and veins due to infiltration of inflammatory cells (white cells). Eventually the arteries and veins become occluded. Similarly, inflammatory cells surround the nerves, often causing severe pain.

The disease usually begins in the small arteries of the toes and foot and if not arrested, will progress upward to the knee and thigh. At this point, amputation of one or more toes, the foot, or the lower leg is often required. In approximately half the cases, inflammation and blood clotting affect a superficial vein, usually of the foot or leg (superficial thrombophlebitis), which becomes raised and red and tender. In about two of five cases, the arteries of the upper extremities are involved.

Buerger's disease occurs almost exclusively in men below the age of forty-five and is rare among women. It seems to be less prevalent than it was about three decades ago, probably because of more precise diagnosis. Previously, cases of arteriosclerosis affecting the small arteries were attributed to Buerger's disease.

Symptoms   Since Buerger's disease initially involves the small arteries, the first symptom is usually coldness, or blueness of a finger or a toe. Ulcerations at the tips of the fingers and toes eventually develop, with accompanying pain that is often severe enough to prevent sleep. The pain is most intense when the patient is lying down, but is somewhat relieved by sleeping upright in a chair or by hanging the foot over the side of a bed to bring more blood to the foot. Pain in the foot or calf on walking is common, because the exercising muscle does not receive enough blood. The distance that can be walked without experiencing discomfort is often limited to two blocks or less. About half of those with Buerger's disease also complain of raised, tender, red superficial veins on the foot or leg, a condition which persists for several weeks, subsides, and then reappears in another area. As the disease progresses, larger arteries in the lower leg or thigh become involved and the toes or foot may become gangrenous. Amputation may then become necessary.

Diagnosis and Treatment   The characteristic case of Buerger's disease involves a young, male cigarette smoker in whom the small arteries and veins of the legs and arms are affected. Physical examination reveals painful ulcers on the toes or fingers, absence of one or more pulses of the feet or wrist, and often palpable red, hard, and tender veins (phlebitis) on the top of the foot or on the lower leg. The feet have a bluish tint and are cold and sweaty as a result of overactive sympathetic nerves. When the leg is elevated, the affected foot becomes extremely pale, because there is not enough pressure or flow to bring blood to it. When the leg is lowered, it becomes deep red or bluish-red as the capillaries dilate to compensate for the deprivation of blood to the tissues when the leg was raised.

The single most important therapeutic measure in Buerger's disease is the immediate and permanent cessation of smoking. If the patient stops smoking soon after symptoms appear, the disease will be arrested and improvement will follow as collateral circulation develops. If the patient stops smoking at a later stage in the disease and the subsequent improvement is insufficient or the ulcerations do not heal, a lumbar sympathectomy operation often provides dramatic improvement. Severing the nerves that normally cause the small arteries to constrict and the sweat glands to excrete allows the small vessels to dilate and bring more blood to the foot. The foot then becomes warm and dry, pain disappears, and the ulcers heal. The local treatment of ulcerations is similar to that described for arteriosclerosis obliterans.

ACUTE THROMBOSIS AND EMBOLISM   A serious and often catastrophic condition occurs when an artery becomes suddenly blocked by a clot (thrombosis) which forms in an atherosclerotic area. The same effects occur when a clot that arises in the heart is carried by the bloodstream to a peripheral artery (arterial embolism). The sudden blocking of an artery does not allow time for collateral circulation to develop, and there is a rapid onset of severe pain, numbness, coldness, and often paralysis of muscles in the extremity involved. At first the limb has a deathly pale color, feels cold to the touch, and has no discernible pulse below the blocked artery. If the condition does not improve, or worsens, within two hours, immediate surgery is necessary to remove the embolus or to bypass the

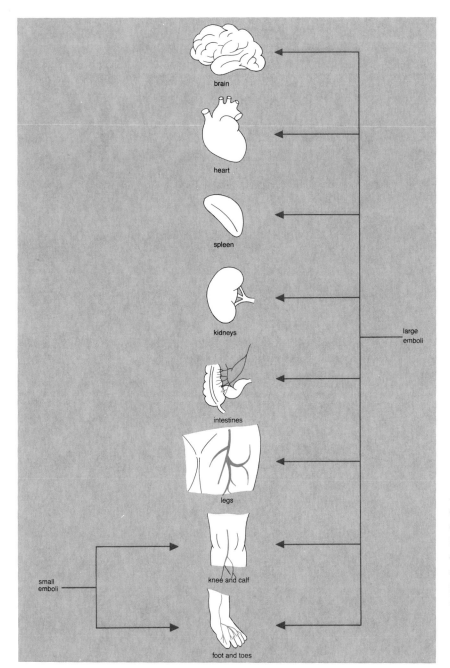

brain

heart

spleen

kidneys

large
emboli

intestines

legs

knee and calf

small
emboli

foot and toes

Large embolisms or clots that originate in the heart may be carried to any part of the body. Small embolisms, which arise from an occluded artery, or from the abdominal aorta, usually affect the peripheral arteries of the lower leg, foot or toes.

thrombosis. If treatment is delayed, the limb becomes a mottled blue and white color and then turns a deep blue. If the limb becomes gangrenous, amputation is necessary. If gangrene does not develop, surgical removal of the embolus or bypass of the thrombosis is possible even as long as three or four days after the onset of the acute blockage.

In some cases of arterial blockage the symptoms remain mild and surgery is not indicated. Such patients may suffer intermittent claudication or they may have no symptoms as collateral circulation develops.

There are two types of arterial embolism; those that arise from the heart, which are quite large and may travel to any part of the body, and those that arise from the lining of an atherosclerotic artery or from an aneurysm of the abdominal aorta or of any of its branches supplying the lower extremities. The small, multiple emboli released from an artery usually lodge in the small arteries of the toes, the foot, or occasionally the lower leg.

The larger emboli which arise from the heart form in the left atrium or its appendage in patients with rheumatic heart disease, stenosis (narrowing) of the mitral valve, and irregular heart rhythm (atrial fibrillation). They may also form on damaged muscle in the lining of the heart following a heart attack. These large emboli can be carried to any part of the body (brain, kidneys, intestines, for example), but when they are carried to the upper or lower extremities, the artery involved is related to the size of the embolus. The location of the embolism can be determined by palpating the pulses. The obstruction is usually detected just below the last pulse that can be felt, and only occasionally is it necessary to use angiography to locate the embolus.

Small emboli usually lodge in the tiny arteries of the toes or the soles of the feet, producing small, round, blue or reddish areas, or occasionally bluish mottled areas. Both feet will be involved if the emboli arise in the aorta; if they arise in an iliac, superficial femoral, or popliteal artery (or in aneurysms of these arteries), only one leg or foot will be involved. The pulses in the involved foot can still be felt, however, because these tiny masses cannot pass through closed arteries.

Emboli tend to recur, and therefore the source must be found and removed if possible. In patients who have rheumatic heart disease, the narrowed mitral valve is corrected or replaced. Clots can be removed from the atrium or the atrial appendage (the appendage, not necessary for heart function, is usually removed). Thrombosis and embolism usually do not recur after such procedures. When the embolus arises from the lining of the heart after a heart attack, direct removal of the clot is not possible. In that event, oral anticoagulants, prescribed for an indefinite period, are usually effective in preventing recurrence.

Small emboli that arise from atherosclerotic deposits or from an aneurysm require surgical removal of the affected areas of the artery and replacement with a suitable graft. A Dacron graft is used in the aorta or the iliac arteries and a vein graft in the superficial femoral or popliteal arteries. When the sources of the emboli are removed, the small discolored areas or small ulcerations of the toes and soles will disappear. Patients who have experienced one minor episode of small emboli, without recurrence, are sometimes treated with aspirin or dipyridamole (Persantin). These medications may prevent recurrence because they inhibit blood-platelet clumping, a part of the clotting process. However, medical authorities are not certain whether these agents are effective in themselves or whether their apparent effectiveness is simply coincidence—that is, there would have been no recurrence, regardless of the use of medications.

ARTERIAL INJURY Injuries to arteries are considered a surgical emergency, requiring the immediate attention of a vascular surgeon or a general surgeon who has had experience in vascular surgery. Arterial injuries are generally of three types: penetrating injuries, such as those caused by a knife or bullet; blunt injuries, such as those which occur when an extremity is crushed or injured by fall or accident; and compression injury, caused by fractured bones or dislocated joints pressing upon or lacerating an artery. Such injuries may cause an artery to be severed and bleed or to become blocked by a thrombus. In such cases, careful examination of the injured extremity will reveal an absence of the pulses below the injury, and the injured part is usually cold and pale. If an artery is severed, a pulsating mass is felt in the area of the injury. When the injury is in the chest or abdominal area, the victim may suffer shock and severe loss of blood.

In all cases where surgery is necessary, examination by arteriography prior to surgery can determine the exact location of the vascular injury. Prompt surgical treatment can prevent death from internal bleeding or amputation of a limb as a result of the trauma.

Occasionally an artery becomes blocked following the insertion of a catheter into the brachial or femoral arteries for the purpose of performing an arteriogram or when the femoral artery is used for cardiac bypass during heart operations. Under these circumstances, the blockage is readily recognized and easily corrected by opening the artery and removing the thrombus.

An arteriovenous fistula is an abnormal, direct flow of blood between an artery and a vein. One type is congenital, a developmental abnormality resulting in multiple connections between arteries and veins. However, an arteriovenous fistula can also occur as a result of a penetrating injury which seals the artery to the vein and results in a short-circuit of the blood flow from the artery directly into the vein. When an arteriovenous fistula occurs in the extremities, the superficial (surface) veins become dilated and pulsate in the same manner as an artery. Because of the great increase in pressure in the veins, the extremity becomes swollen and venous ulcers often appear (see Peripheral Venous Disease, chapter 15). With arterial blood being shunted into the veins, there is evidence of arterial insufficiency, with decreased pulses in the extremity below the fistula. A hand placed over the fistula can feel a vibration, or "thrill," and a stethoscope can detect a continuous noise, called a bruit.

ARTERIOVENOUS FISTULA

If the quantity of blood flowing through the fistula is great, it may put an abnormal strain on the heart. The heart becomes enlarged and, over a period of time, may not be able to handle the burden. Heart failure may result. In congenital arteriovenous fistula, or in the fistula resulting from an injury that occurs in childhood during the period of bone growth, the long bones in the involved extremity grow faster than the normal limb. An involved leg thus becomes longer and greater in girth. The reason for this abnormal growth is not fully understood.

Surgery is the best treatment for a large arteriovenous fistula which causes arterial or venous insufficiency or cardiac enlargement. The procedure involves tying off the vein (other veins compensate for this loss) and then restoring blood flow within the artery. Whenever possible, the surgeon simply sews the hole closed. When that is impossible, the surgeon removes a small segment of the damaged artery and either connects the ends together or replaces the segment with a vein or a Dacron graft. Surgical treatment of congenital arteriovenous fistulas is often much more complicated and is sometimes unsatisfactory because there are numerous communications between the arteries and veins. In many cases, multiple communications are found in a finger or toe and these can be easily monitored without special treatment. But if the communications are large or tend to become larger with time, several operations may be required to remove all the communications.

ANEURYSMS   Aneurysms (from the Greek word for opening) are of three types: true, false, and dissecting. A true aneurysm, the most common, is a localized, abnormal dilatation or ballooning of an artery. A false aneurysm is caused by blood leaking from a rupture in an artery and being contained by surrounding tissue. A dissecting aneurysm occurs when a tear in the inner lining of the artery wall allows blood to enter the middle layer, creating a new channel within the wall. An aneurysm that ruptures is a catastrophic event accompanied by sudden, potentially fatal loss of blood.

True Aneurysm   A true aneurysm is the result of a weakening of the wall of an artery. Because of pressure and the pulsating nature of blood flow, the artery tends to become progressively larger, and frequently ruptures. The majority of true aneurysms are the result of arteriosclerosis (they may, but rarely, be caused by syphilis or other infections). The aneurysm either dilates throughout its entire circumference or balloons out like a large bubble at only one place on the artery wall. The opening between the main arterial channel and the sac may be quite small.

Although a true aneurysm may develop in any artery, the abdominal aorta below the origin of the renal arteries is the most common site. The iliac arteries are also frequently involved. The patient may be totally unaware of an aneurysm in the abdominal aorta until it is discovered on physical examination as a pulsating mass. The growing aneurysm produces pulsating sensations in the abdomen or, if the aneurysm presses on neighboring organs, back pain or abdominal pain radiating into the groin or testicle on the left side. The aneurysm may also be filled with clots which can break off and travel to the legs, causing mottled discoloration of the skin of the leg and foot or small blue spots or ulcers on the toes and soles. If the aneurysm leaks, there is severe, unrelenting abdominal or back pain. A ruptured abdominal aneurysm produces sudden, severe back or abdominal pain, tenderness over the abdomen, and rapid shock. Immediate surgery has been lifesaving in half the cases of ruptured aneurysm.

When an aneurysm occurs in the thoracic aorta, frequently there are no symptoms and the problem is not discovered until a routine chest X ray is taken. As the aneurysm enlarges, it presses on other organs, resulting in pain in the upper back, difficulty in swallowing, coughing, and hoarseness. An aneurysm in the femoral artery in the groin or in the popliteal artery behind the knee is easily felt as a pulsating mass. It usually causes no symptoms until it ruptures, is involved in a thrombosis, or throws off small emboli into the legs or feet.

Treatment of the true aneurysm is surgical resection and replacement with a graft. Poor-risk patients with small thoracic or abdominal aneurysms should be monitored by periodic X rays or imaging with ultrasound. If the aneurysm progressively increases in size, it should be removed despite the risk, because the chance of survival following rupture of an aortic aneurysm is small. Femoral and popliteal aneurysms should be removed whenever possible to avoid the complications that can necessitate amputation.

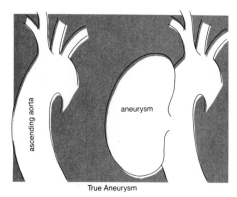

True Aneurysm

Weakened arterial wall balloons out in a bubble-like protrusion which may rupture under the pressure of blood flow.

A false aneurysm results from the rupture of a true aneurysm, from a hole in an artery caused by a penetrating wound, or from a leak through the suture line between a graft and the host artery. The latter situation is common when a Dacron graft is sewed onto the femoral artery in the groin. The blood that leaks from an artery into an enclosed space will form a pulsating mass which can be felt on examination. True and false aneurysms are distinguishable by arteriography, or they become apparent at the time of surgery.

False Aneurysm

An aneurysm that dissects into the wall of an artery creates a false channel along the course of the artery and may block branches of it, causing a variety of complications. If the dissection occurs at the origin of the aorta and proceeds along the aortic arch, circulation to the arms and head (via the subclavian and carotid arteries) may be blocked, resulting in arterial insufficiency in the arms, a severe stroke, or even death. If the circulation to the intestines or the kidneys is compromised, gangrene of the bowel or failure of the kidneys may result. A channel that runs along the back of the aorta will not interfere with blood flow to the intestines or the kidneys, but it may cut off the circulation to one or both legs.

Dissecting Aneurysm

The symptoms of dissecting aneurysm of the thoracic aorta are sudden and severe, usually involving severe pain in the chest, which radiates through to the back and often into the neck and down the arms. As the dissection proceeds into the abdomen, severe pain in the abdomen or back or both may result, along with coldness and numbness in the lower extremities. Pain is usually so severe that the patient sweats profusely and frequently goes into shock. A routine X ray may suggest the presence of the aneurysm, but an exact diagnosis is made by aortography, which shows the tear in the lining of the artery, the false channel, and the extent of the aneurysm.

Patients with dissecting aneurysms may die before any treatment is possible. The prognosis is particularly poor when the ascending aorta and the aortic arch are involved, because the dissection may involve the aortic valve (resulting in heart failure) or may rupture into the pericardial sac surrounding the heart (resulting in pressure on the heart and death). If at all possible, surgical correction should be attempted in such cases. Surgery usually involves replacing the aortic valve with an artificial valve and replacing the aneurysm with a graft. If the aortic arch and the vessels supplying the arms and brain are involved, most patients do not survive surgery.

The type of dissection with the most favorable prognosis is that which starts just beyond the origin of the left subclavian artery and involves the descending aorta. Treatment with medication to lower blood pressure and reduce the contractile force of the blood flow may result in thrombosis of the false channel. The patient has a chance of recovery with this treatment, but the weakened aortic wall tends to enlarge with time, causing the development of a true aneurysm. Periodic chest X rays are therefore desirable. If the aneurysm becomes larger, surgical correction can be performed with a fair chance of success.

One of the ways the body controls its internal temperature is by constriction and dilation of the small arteries. Exercise in hot weather will bring on considerable perspiration and a flush to the face and other parts of the body as

CONSTRICTION OF BLOOD VESSELS

PRINCIPLES

1. *Peripheral arterial diseases are those affecting the blood vessels which carry blood from the heart. They are of four kinds: occlusive, in which blood flow is blocked; vasospastic, in which small arteries constrict or go into spasm; functional, in which small arteries dilate; and a ballooning or bulging of the wall of the artery due to weakness (aneurysm).*

Raynaud's Phenomenon

2. *Arteriosclerosis obliterans is a chronic, progressive arterial disease in which the build-up of plaques in their walls interferes with blood flow. The disease affects the legs and feet by reducing circulation. Diabetics are particularly susceptible. The symptoms are discomfort on walking (intermittent claudication), affecting most often the calf, but also the foot, thigh, hips, or even the buttocks. At first, new connections in the circulatory system develop to bypass the affected arteries (collateral circulation), but when this becomes insufficient to nourish tissues, the victim will feel pain even at rest, and may develop ulcers and gangrene. Bypass surgery is reserved for severe cases.*

3. *Buerger's disease is an inflammatory condition that affects small arteries, veins, and nerves. Although the precise cause is not known, Buerger's disease has been definitely associated with cigarette smoking. Cessation of smoking often halts the development of the disease and allows the development of collateral circulation.*

4. *A thrombus, or clot, sometimes occurs suddenly in arteries and blocks them. When such clots are formed in the heart and carried to a peripheral artery, they are known as emboli. Sudden blockage of an*

the arteries in the skin dilate and more blood is brought to the surface, allowing the body to lose heat. This mechanism helps to keep one cool during hot weather. In cold weather, the arteries constrict, shunting blood away from the cold surface into the deeper arteries, allowing the body to conserve heat. The finely tuned mechanism which causes the arteries to dilate and constrict can, at times, function abnormally, producing a series of disorders called vasospastic diseases.

Certain mild vasospastic disorders are simply exaggerated responses of normal body functions to the environment. The condition, called vasomotor instability, usually occurs in women (men are sometimes affected) who complain of cold hands and feet. Their circulation is normal, but nervous tension causes their small arteries to constrict, and the hands and feet become cold. This is not a disease and requires no treatment other than a physician's reassurance and his advice to wear warm clothing, especially gloves and socks, in cold weather.

Raynaud's phenomenon is a condition in which the smallest arteries supplying the fingers or toes constrict (go into spasm) on exposure to cold or as the result of emotional upset. Because the small veins are usually open, the blood drains out of the capillaries and the fingers or toes become pale, cold, and numb. If there is a spasm in the small veins and the blood becomes trapped in the capillaries, the fingers or toes become blue as the blood loses its oxygen. The condition clears when the spasm is released by rubbing the part affected or by returning to a warm environment. The fingers or toes then become redder than normal as capillaries dilate to the maximum extent to compensate for the prior deprivation of oxygen. The condition is episodic and involves one or more fingers or toes, but usually not the thumb. It never progresses beyond the bases of the fingers or toes into the hands or feet.

Raynaud's phenomenon can be primary or secondary. The primary type, usually in young women, affects either the hands or the feet or both. Pulses in the wrists or feet are strong and ulcerations rarely occur. If such sores do develop, they are minor and never necessitate amputation. Although the condition continues for many years, there is no evidence to suggest that primary Raynaud's phenomenon is associated with any underlying disease. The treatment is to reassure the patient that the condition is not serious, and is merely a nuisance, and to advise avoidance of a cold environment and to dress the entire body warmly when it is necessary to go into the cold.

When primary Raynaud's is especially annoying and limits activities, or when small sores or cracks appear on the ends of fingers or toes, a medication called reserpine can be injected directly into an artery at periodic intervals. Reserpine can be taken by mouth for indefinite periods, but the patient must be followed closely because it sometimes causes depression. Sympathectomy is reserved for the more severe cases.

Secondary Raynaud's phenomenon is a complication of some underlying disease, such as scleroderma (hardening of the skin), or other diseases of connective tissue (collagen diseases), such as rheumatoid arthritis or systemic lupus erythematosus. Occasionally Raynaud's phenomenon may be secondary to Buerger's disease. The secondary type usually occurs in persons over the age of forty and more frequently in men than in women. It may be associated with painful ulcers and small areas of gangrene. Often one or more pulses in the wrists or in the feet are absent and an arteriogram will show blockage of the small arteries in the fingers or toes. Because of the underlying disease, the skin on the fingers may be tight, the joints may show evidence of arthritis, or aches and pains, fever, anemia, and other manifestations may occur.

Treatment of secondary Raynaud's phenomenon is directed to the underlying disease. The patient is also instructed in the care of ulcerations and in ways to protect the extremities and the entire body from cold. Reserpine is sometimes prescribed, but it is not as effective in secondary Raynaud's phenomenon as it is in primary. Medications used to dilate the arteries are usually ineffective, and sympathectomy is not considered helpful. Finally, there is no evidence to suggest that smoking causes or affects the course of either the primary or secondary type.

This may occur following injury or operations, or as a result of using pneumatic or vibratory tools, grasping and squeezing machine tools, typing or playing the piano. Treatment consists of changing jobs, using an electric typewriter, modifying piano technique or avoid playing for a period of time, and, of course, protecting the hands and body from exposure to cold.

Post-traumatic Raynaud's Phenomenon

Acrocyanosis is a condition in which young women experience persistent coldness and blueness of the hands and feet. It is presumably due to spasm of the smallest arteries and veins, which cause the blood to pool in the capillaries and become dark. The circulation appears to be normal, since the arterial pulses are present. The condition is painless and is primarily a cosmetic nuisance. Although the symptoms are worse on exposure to cold, the blue color is persistent even in a warm environment. Since the condition is never associated with ulcerations or gangrene, treatment is ordinarily not necessary. Some medications may be used to dilate the arteries, and sympathectomy may be helpful but is rarely necessary.

Acrocyanosis

Livedo reticularis is a mottled appearance of the skin of the arms and legs and occasionally of the trunk, affecting both sexes but mostly young women. The condition is due to constriction of the small arteries which supply the capillaries of the skin. Because these capillaries are distributed in the skin like a network, the bluish-red discoloration looks like a net with clear spaces between the mesh. The mottled appearance is made worse by exposure to cold and often by emotional upset. The condition is not serious or a danger to health, and no treatment is required. The discoloration can be eliminated temporarily by vigorous massage, and it sometimes disappears altogether when the arms or legs are elevated.

If the mottled areas of the skin are painful and tender to the touch, and if they persist for long periods, the condition is usually secondary to some other disease which causes a blockage of the capillaries, such as small emboli or cryoglobulinemia, a disease which causes the blood to become jelly-like in consistency. In such cases the primary disease must be treated. Only rarely does severe and persistent primary livedo reticularis cause small skin ulcerations of the toes, feet, or ankles.

Livedo Reticularis

artery by a thrombus or embolism does not permit development of collateral circulation, and immediate treatment is necessary. Angiography can locate a thrombus or embolism, and various surgical techniques can remove them or provide alternate routes for circulation.

5. *Injuries to arteries are medical emergencies requiring immediate treatment. They may result from penetrating wounds, blunt injuries, or compression. Surgery is usually the only possible treatment.*

6. *An arteriovenous fistula is an abnormal direct communication between an artery and a vein, caused either by congenital defect or by a penetrating wound. The increased pressure in a vein from a fistula may produce swelling, varicose veins, and sores. Below the*

fistula there may be marked decrease in arterial circulation with coldness, numbness, paleness, or pain. Congenital forms of the condition sometimes produce abnormal bone growth in children. Surgery is the preferred treatment in serious cases.

7. *True aneurysms are due to the ballooning out of the walls of an artery. Rupture can bring death from sudden loss of blood. They are due to a weakness in the artery wall, most commonly caused by arteriosclerosis and occasionally as a result of syphilis or some other infection. The most common site is the abdominal aorta, with the*

Cold Injuries

connecting iliac arteries frequently involved. Dissecting aneurysms are due to a splitting of the artery wall with the production of a false channel. This causes blockage of arteries to vital organs and death may occur if surgical repair is not possible.

8. *In Raynaud's phenomenon, the smallest arteries supplying fingers or toes go into spasm or constrict as a result of exposure to cold or perhaps from emotional upset. Digits wlll feel cold or turn white or blue from lack of oxygenated blood. Primary Raynaud's is not a serious threat to health and does not progressively worsen. Secondary Raynaud's develops as a complication of some other disease and can produce painful sores and even gangrene.*

9. *Acrocyanosis and livedo reticularis are two conditions in which some of the smallest arteries go into spasm. The former causes a dark blue color of hands and feet; the latter, with mottling of the skin, appears on legs and arms and occasionally on the trunk. Neither condition is a serious threat to health.*

10. *Cold injuries include frostbite, chilblains (pernio), and trenchfoot. Frostbite is a condition in which blood and tissue are frozen from prolonged exposure to cold, with symptoms of coldness, numbness, and even paralysis of affected parts. Treatment is by rapid thawing in warm water (105°-110°F) until affected parts are soft and red and feeling returns. Chilblains (pernio) are small surface sores on the lower legs and the feet which erupt on individuals susceptible to the cold. The ulcers usually heal by themselves. Trenchfoot or immersion foot results from prolonged exposure of the feet to a cold, wet environment in which the foot is unable to move or to dry out. The condition results in pale, cold, swollen, and painful feet with ulcerations. Recovery is rapid when the person is removed to a warm, dry environment.*

FROSTBITE This is a condition in which circulation is arrested because prolonged exposure to cold results in freezing of the tissues, including the blood within the vessels. In the acute phase of frostbite, the affected part of the body becomes cold and numb but is usually without pain. On examination, the part is cold, pale, hard to the touch, and often paralyzed. The severity of frostbite cannot be determined until the part is thawed, when the amount of tissue damage is classified into degrees, a classification similar to that used for burns. In first-degree frostbite, the part, on thawing, becomes red or reddish-blue and may burn or itch. It is an inflammatory reaction without serious freezing of the tissues. Second-degree frostbite is associated with pain, swelling, and the formation of blisters. Third-degree frostbite results in the death of the skin and the tissues beneath it and is caused by prolonged lack of blood supply. With adequate medical treatment recovery without loss of the finger or toe is possible. Fourth-degree frostbite is characterized by gangrene and ofen requires amputation of the part involved.

The treatment of acute frostbite is rapid thawing: the part is immersed in warm water (between 105° F and 110° F) until all the tissues become soft and red and sensation returns, usually within a half-hour to an hour. Contrary to folklore, the part should never be rubbed with snow or placed in cold or very hot water. If warm water is not available, the frostbitten part should be placed next to normal warm skin or wrapped in blankets until warm water can be obtained. First-degree frostbite requires no treatment except thawing, but the other degrees of frostbite must be treated by a physician. Sometimes hospitalization is advisable to avoid infection of the tissues, and in severe cases sympathectomy is occasionally helpful.

CHILBLAINS (PERNIO) Some individuals with unusual susceptibility to cold develop small, superficial ulcers of the lower legs and feet called chilblains. The ulcers usually heal in a matter of weeks, but new ones appear from time to time. Protection from cold is the most effective treatment, and only rarely is it necessary for a person to move to a warmer climate.

TRENCH FOOT This condition (and a similar one called immersion foot) results from prolonged exposure to a cold, damp environment, during which a person is inactive and the feet are immobile, usually in a dependent position. The blood flow becomes sluggish as a result of spasm of the small arteries, the feet become pale or blue, cold, painful, and swollen. At times, the poor blood exchange produces ulcers. The condition was first recognized during the First World War in combatants who had been confined to cold, wet trenches or spent long periods in water or wet lifeboats.

When the patient is moved to a warm, dry environment, the foot becomes red, more painful, and swollen. Recovery, particularly of ulcerated tissue, may take weeks or months. After recovery, the patient may develop Raynaud's phenomenon on exposure to cold. The best treatment is prevention by avoiding long exposure of the feet to cold and wetness whenever possible and by wearing warm clothing if exposure is necessary.

15

PERIPHERAL VENOUS DISEASE

Stanford Wessler, M.D.

Peripheral venous disease is the medical term for any interference with the passage of deoxygenated blood back to the heart and lungs. In the human body's closed circulatory system, the veins function by returning blood to the heart from the capillary network in all the organs. The arteries arise from the left side of the heart and deliver oxygenated, enriched blood to the capillaries. The venous system, progressing from the minute capillaries, forms into larger and larger vessels that finally terminate in the two largest veins, the inferior vena cava and the superior vena cava. The inferior vena cava empties blood into the right atrium from the legs, abdomen, and lower chest; the superior vena cava, which also flows into the right atrium, carries blood from the head, neck, arms, and upper part of the chest.

Leaving the left side of the heart by way of the aorta, oxygenated blood is transported through branching arteries that progressively decrease in diameter until they form a network of threadlike vessels (capillaries). Here, carbon dioxide and other waste products are exchanged for oxygen and nutrients by the cells of all organs of the body except the lungs. At the venous side of the capillaries, the blood begins its journey back to the heart through a system of veins that progressively increase in diameter, converging from the lower part of the body in the inferior vena cava and from the upper part in the superior vena cava. Oxygen-depleted blood from these two large veins is deposited in the right side of the heart and then transported to the lungs, where carbon dioxide and oxygen are exchanged. The replenished blood is returned to the left atrium, to begin anew its circulation in the body.

The venous system labors under one natural handicap—the upright stance that mankind has adopted in the course of evolution. The vessels that carry blood from the parts of the body below the heart must work in opposition to the force of gravity; only the veins in the head, neck, and shoulders enjoy the downhill assistance of gravity. The blood in the veins is not entirely at the mercy of gravity, however. Medium-sized veins, particularly in the arms and legs, are equipped with valves which prevent the blood from flowing backward: that is, away from the heart and toward the extremities. The direction of venous flow is also aided by muscle contractions, especially in the legs and feet.

The role of the one-way valves in the larger veins is particularly important because of the nature of the veins themselves. The walls of the veins, unlike those of the arteries, are not strongly muscular, nor do the veins have the built-in elastic tension of the arteries. Because veins lack these properties, and because they are not rigid, neither muscular contraction nor the pumping action of the heart itself would be sufficient to maintain the flow of venous blood to the heart without the safeguard of the valves.

The two types of peripheral venous diseases discussed here—varicose veins and phlebitis—most commonly manifest themselves in the legs. To understand how each condition develops and how it can be treated, something about the venous system in the legs should be known. There are three separate but interconnecting venous systems in the legs: the superficial veins, those just under the skin; the deep veins, within the muscles; and the connecting veins which form bridges between the superficial and the deep systems. In addition, between contiguous veins within each system there is a network of vessels. This intricate network of leg veins makes it possible for surgeons to replace a blocked artery by removing a leg vein to serve as a bypass without reducing the flow through the venous system (see chapter 20, Cardiovascular Surgery). Another advantage of the network is that if a vein becomes blocked, the other open veins can readily return blood to the heart.

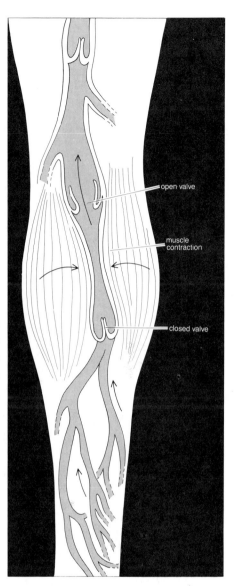

open valve

muscle contraction

closed valve

One-way valves in the large veins guarantee that blood returning to the heart will not be pulled downward by the force of gravity. The valves, combined with pressure from contracting muscles, compensate for the relative lack of elasticity and muscular strength in the walls of the veins and the dissipated force of heart contractions.

VARICOSE VEINS   In a common, almost always benign condition affecting adults of both sexes, one or more superficial veins, usually in the legs, may become dilated. What actually causes varicose veins remains uncertain, although heredity seems to be a possible predisposing factor. Weaknesses in the walls of veins have been shown to be congenital in origin, and the condition appears earlier in persons one or both of whose parents had the problem. Varicose veins may also develop because the valves fail to function properly in preventing backward flow. The leakage of blood backward adds to the resistance in the venous system, causing the blood to stagnate and form pools in the veins, which become dilated with the added fluid.

Varicose veins are so common that a considerable folklore about them has grown up. For instance, there is a widespread belief that varicose veins are an occupational disease among people who spend a great deal of time on their feet. Statistical comparisons between persons who stand while working as opposed to those with sedentary jobs do not support this notion. Naturally, prolonged standing is likely to aggravate a pre-existing weakness in the veins or an inherited susceptibility to varicose veins. Moreover, con-

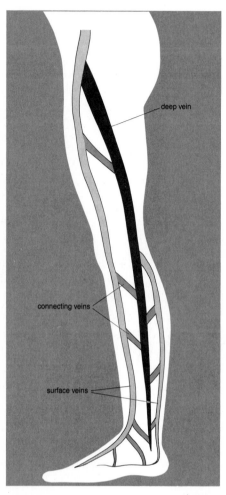

deep vein

connecting veins

surface veins

Blood returns from the legs through three separate but interconnecting venous systems: superficial veins that lie just beneath the skin, deep veins within the muscles, and connecting veins linking the surface and deep veins.

tinuous constriction or compression of the legs with tight garters, girdles or clothing may contribute to the development of varicosities. Folklore also associates varicose veins with pregnancy, on the assumption that the added weight of the unborn baby causes the mother's veins to become dilated. Actually, the dilation of the veins often shows up as early as the second or third month of pregnancy, well before there is any significant increase in weight. Although some factor other than weight appears to be involved, medical science so far cannot determine it. Similar uncertainty surrounds another apparent association between weight gain and varicose veins. Obesity, or extreme overweight, seems to be related to varicosity, but the way in which excess weight may contribute to the development of the condition is not known.

Most varicose veins cause no noticeable symptoms beyond the cosmetic unattractiveness which often accompanies them. The vast majority of people with varicose veins experience no discomfort, although painful symptoms do appear in some individuals. These may include a heavy or tired sensation in the leg or soreness along the veins. If the deep veins are obstructed with clots, some blood accumulates in the lower leg and ankle, creating chronic swelling, or edema. The poor blood flow in the extremity may then result in pigmentation, itching skin, or scaly eczema over all or a part of the foot or leg. If the damaged skin is not treated, it may finally ulcerate, resulting in sores that can become infected and last for long periods of time.

In addition to the obvious manifestations of varicosity in the superficial veins, many individuals have what are called "spider bursts," or "sky burst" varicosities on the leg—collections of small veins directly under the skin that dilate in a cluster and give the skin a blotchy discoloration. They may occur in one or more areas, but they bear no relationship to varicose veins as such and present no risk to normal health. They are at most a cosmetic problem and require no treatment at all. Attempts to obliterate the clusters by injection almost invariably fail, and the procedure itself may produce discomfort.

Treatment   Only under special circumstances do varicose veins require specific treatment either by injection or surgical removal of the varicosities. Unfortunately the varicosity often returns after surgery. If, however, inflammation or weal pain recurs in a small segment of a superficial varicosity, this section can be easily and safely removed, usually in the surgeon's office without the need for hospitalization. For patients with physical distress or discomfort, elastic stockings or bandages are sometimes prescribed. It is important that the supporting stockings be carefully fitted to the patient's feet and legs, for they must give the greatest pressure at the foot level, with gradually diminishing pressure up the leg. Patients who have debilitating diseases and pregnant women who have varicose veins are in particular need of such external supports. If discomfort or pain continues even after properly fitted elastic stockings are worn, it is likely that the symptoms derive from a cause other than the varicose veins.

Phlebitis is a term used to describe the presence of a clot, or thrombus, in a vein that partly or completely stops the flow of blood. A thrombus is a solid mass that forms from the different components of the blood: plasma proteins, red blood cells, platelets, and white blood cells. In today's medical usage the terms phlebitis, venous thrombosis, thrombophlebitis, and phlebothrombosis are used synonymously to refer to a clot within a vein. A number of other terms are used in referring to phlebitis that appears in specific veins or in a vein under specific conditions. Mondor's disease refers to thrombosis of the superficial veins over the mammary glands of the adjacent chest wall. Budd-Chiari syndrome refers to thrombosis of the hepatic veins, the veins that return blood from the liver to the heart. Phlebitis migrans is a condition of recurrent venous thrombosis in the superficial veins and occasionally in the deep veins of the extremities and in veins draining other areas. Effort

PHLEBITIS

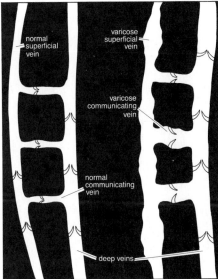

The swelling and expansion of one or more superficial veins, particularly in the legs, may result from congenital weakness of the walls of the veins or from defective (incompetent) valves which permit blood to leak backward in the vessels. The blood becomes stagnant and pools in the veins, which then swell with the excess fluid.

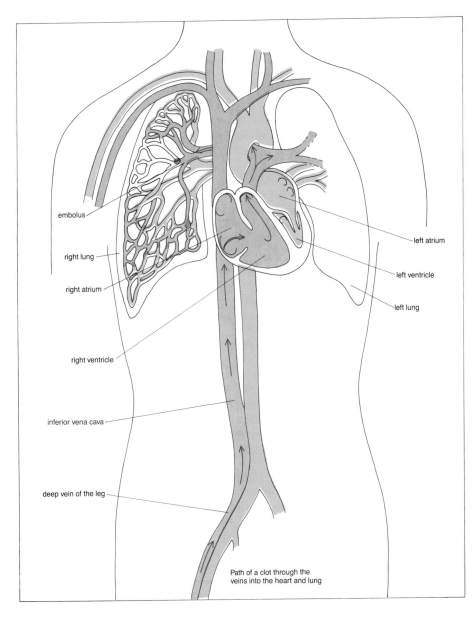

Path of a clot through the veins into the heart and lung

A small portion of a blood clot which partially or completely obstructs blood flow in a leg vein may break free and be carried to the heart and on into the lung, where it may lodge in one of the smaller arteries.

or strain phlebitis occurs in the axillary and subclavian veins of the arm following injury or some sudden or unusual effort, such as when the arm is forcibly pulled away from the body. Chemical phlebitis is venous thrombosis occurring at a site where needles or catheters have entered the vein for diagnostic studies or for intravenous infusions. Finally, phlegmasia alba dolens (white or milk leg) and phlegmasia cerulea dolens (blue leg) are terms applied to extensive thrombosis of the legs associated with massive swelling of the limbs.

Phlebitis, together with a potential complication, pulmonary embolus (a clot that has moved from the leg to the lung), are responsible for the hospitalization of some 300,000 patients in the United States annually. More than 50,000 of these die. The cost of hospitalization is in excess of $750 million a year, not including the out-patient costs of treating patients with venous thromboembolism and the loss in wages sustained during the recovery period, which may range from days to months. Venous thromboembolism may occur in an apparently healthy person, but it is more likely to strike the elderly, those who are immobilized for a long period (for example, stroke and arthritis victims and patients in plaster casts), and in persons who have recently undergone surgery, childbirth, heart failure, or shock. Thromboembolism may also occur after certain infections and malignant tumors have developed, or with the use of oral contraceptives. Venous thromboembolism is, in fact, one of the most common causes of death in patients hospitalized for major orthopedic procedures, such as hip and knee reconstruction and repair of long bone fractures. It is the most frequent nonobstetrical cause of after childbirth death and a major cause or contributing factor for death among chronic cardiac and pulmonary disease patients.

Causes and Symptoms

Doctors do not fully understand why clots develop in the veins, although certain predisposing conditions seem clear. Among these are direct injury to the lining of the vein by trauma, bacteria, or chemicals, and changes in the blood itself that create a condition known as hypercoagulability. Slowing of blood flow in the veins (stasis), which occurs when a person is bedridden, in a plaster cast, or immobilized for long periods in an occupation that requires prolonged sitting or standing, can accelerate the growth of an already formed clot. It seems likely, however, that several factors are simultaneously involved, with one predominating.

The symptoms of venous thrombosis vary, depending on the location of the clot. In the deep veins, venous thrombosis may occur at one or several sites. Sometimes the clot causes no discomfort, and the person is unaware of its presence. In other cases, there may be one or more symptoms, including spontaneous pain, tenderness on applying pressure over the vein, swelling of the limb (with subsequent pigmentation or ulceration of the skin), increased warmth of the extremity, fever, and bluish discoloration of the skin. When the clot is in a superficial vein, it appears as a linear, thickened, cordlike structure under the skin. There may or may not be pain, tenderness, redness, and warmth over the area. Recurrent clots in superficial veins may occur in different areas, a condition called migratory thrombophlebitis.

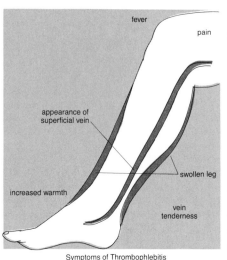
Symptoms of Thrombophlebitis

Diagnosis and Treatment

Deep venous thrombosis can often be inferred from examination of the patient. A limb may be swollen or have a bluish tint (cyanosis), or extreme pain may be felt when pressure is applied. The affected limb may also be warmer to the touch than the limb on the opposite side. A definite diagnosis, however, often requires use of phlebography—an X ray of the limb following injection of a radio-opaque dye into the veins. Examination is also conducted through noninvasive instruments that are able to detect an obstruction to the flow of blood in the veins. Diagnosis of superficial phlebitis, on the other hand, can almost always be made through clinical examination.

A clot in a deep vein of the leg is serious because of the potential complications. If extensive clots travel to the lungs, they can result in death. Extensive clotting can remain in the veins and produce disabling pain, swelling, discoloration, and eventually ulceration. Phlebitis of superficial veins, even when recurrent, is less serious; it never leads to death from clots going to the lungs or even to massive leg swelling or ulceration.

When an individual recognizes the symptoms of phlebitis, they should be reported to a doctor. Signs of possible phlebitis are pain or tenderness in the calf or thigh, a red streak on the leg, or swelling of the ankle. If the deep venous system is involved, hospitalization and further tests and treatment may be required. The mainstay of treatment is the use of anticoagulants to stop the clotting from progressing further up the legs. Physicians now rely on two types of anticoagulants—heparin, given by injection either into the vein or under the skin, or an oral medication, such as warfarin, taken in tablet form. Drug dosage must be monitored by blood tests to guarantee that the precise amount needed to stop excessive clotting without causing bleeding is being taken by the patient. Treatment usually requires a hospital stay of one to two weeks.

Anticoagulant medication is continued for two to six months after the patient leaves the hospital. If there has been swelling, fitted elastic stockings are worn to reduce the swelling by external pressure. The patient is advised to avoid prolonged periods of standing or sitting, and physical activity is encouraged. No special diets are required during the recovery period, but cigarette smoking should be avoided because it may favor further clotting. A patient who is on anticoagulants should take no other medications without the specific approval of a doctor. This restriction includes common aspirin along with dozens of other drugs which can increase the risk of bleeding and can affect the efficacy and safety of oral anticoagulants. In rare cases where anticoagulants are either ineffective or are prohibited because of some problem associated with bleeding or a tendency to hemorrhage, phlebitic veins can be tied off (usually in the abdomen) to prevent clots from reaching the lungs.

When surgery of any kind is planned for a patient who has previously suffered from phlebitis, anticoagulants may be prescribed before, during, and after the operation to prevent postoperative formation of clots in the veins of the legs. This is a relatively new form of preventive medicine in which treatment is instituted before rather than after the occurrence of phlebitis.

Patients who are on anticoagulants after hospitalization should be aware of certain warning signs. The doctor should be informed at once if the urine becomes red, brown, or "smoky" in color, if there are red or black bowel movements, if menstrual flow is prolonged or profuse, if the gums bleed, or if there is abdominal pain or severe and prolonged headache. Because any ill-

Precautions

PRINCIPLES

1. *Veins are the collecting vessels that carry blood back to the heart after it has passed through the capillary network. Some veins, particularly those in the arms and the legs, have one-way valves that help prevent a backward flow of blood.*

2. *The legs have three sets of interconnecting venous systems: the superficial veins, located just beneath the skin; the deep veins, embedded in the musculature; and the connecting veins, which bridge the superficial and deep systems.*

3. *Varicose veins are swollen or twisted veins, usually in the legs. Varicose veins in the superficial venous system are frequently the result of obstructions in the deeper veins.*

4. *Elastic support stockings or bandages, as well as elevation of the legs, can help relieve swelling or painful symptoms should they occur. While surgery can remove varicosities without impairing the circulatory system, the dilated veins often recur in time.*

5. *Phlebitis is a clot within a vein partially or completely stopping the flow of blood. There are a number of types of phlebitis, classified according to the cause or the location of the vein in which a clot has formed.*

6. *Although sometimes there are no obvious symptoms, phlebitis is often characterized by pain or tenderness over the afflicted vein, swelling of the leg, bluish discoloration of the skin, and warmth in the area. Phlebitis in a superficial vein may be troublesome but not serious; in a deep vein phlebitis can result in a clot detaching itself from the vein and floating to the lung, not infrequently with fatal consequences.*

7. *Treatment of phlebitis in the deep veins usually involves anticoagulant drugs to stop further clotting. Swelling can be contained and pigmentation and ulceration prevented by the use of specially fitted elastic stockings and by avoiding sitting or standing for prolonged periods.*

ness may produce bleeding among patients on anticoagulants, the doctor must be kept informed of all signs of illness, especially such symptoms as diarrhea, weakness, faintness, or dizziness. Pregnancy, spontaneous bruises, and other injuries should also be reported, even when there is no visible sign of hemorrhage. Patients who take anticoagulants should avoid occupations and sports that carry the risk of injury or accident. Every patient should carry an emergency medical identification card or wear a metal disk around the wrist or neck, giving the specific name of the anticoagulant, the doctor's name, the patient's name, and their telephone numbers and addresses. Identification cards can be obtained from a doctor or from a local chapter of the American Heart Association.

Phlebitis sometimes occurs as a complication of some underlying disease or after a serious surgical procedure and is more likely to be found in persons with sedentary occupations or habits, as well as in obese (extremely overweight) persons. Certain preventive measures would probably be beneficial, especially avoidance of prolonged periods of immobilization, whether at a job, while riding in an automobile or airplane, and during periods of relaxation.

16

CONGENITAL HEART DEFECTS

Mary Allen Engle, M.D.

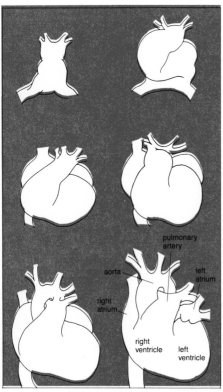

Development of Fetal Heart

Development of the fetal heart, from a single tube to the four-chambered fully developed organ with its dividing walls and four regulating valves.

In a marvel of orchestrated timing, the human heart begins as a simple tube that loops and bends and starts to beat as walls divide what will become the right and left sides, and valves form to direct the forward flow of blood from the upper to the lower chambers and then to the two major arteries. One of these great arteries is the pulmonary artery, which transmits blood from the lower right chamber, the right ventricle, to the lungs. The other is the aorta, the vessel that carries blood from the left ventricle to the various parts of the body. The pulmonary artery divides, one branch going to the right lung and the other to the left, and these branches in turn divide into smaller and smaller vessels that become capillaries, the minute channels by which carbon dioxide and oxygen are exchanged in the air sacs of the developing lungs. Two coronary arteries arise from the aorta, one to the right ventricle and one to the left ventricle, to supply oxygen and nutrients to the beating heart. The aorta then gives off branches to the arms and head as it arcs first upward and then downward to supply blood to the organs of the body and the legs. At the same time, venous connections are made to bring unoxygenated blood to the upper chambers, the atria. The superior vena cava returns blood from the upper part of the body, and the inferior vena cava returns blood from the lower part to the right atrium. Four pulmonary veins carry oxygenated blood from the right and left lungs into the left atrium. Blood from the coronary arteries collects in a channel that empties into the right atrium as the coronary sinus.

The stage is thus set for the heart to receive oxygen-poor blood from the tissues and to pump it to the lungs to pick up oxygen and give off carbon dioxide. The blood entering the lungs from the right side of heart is a dark bluish-red, which becomes bright red as it is saturated with oxygen. This oxygenated blood enters the receiving chamber on the left side of the heart and is then pumped to the body, delivering oxygen to all the tissues. This development is accomplished in the first eight weeks of the fetus's life. In the months that follow, the heart beats and grows and then undergoes other changes when the baby is born.

The fetus does not need to breathe; the mother does that, sending blood to the placenta, a vascular organ in the uterus which supplies oxygen to the fetus by way of the umbilical cord. The blood entering the right side of the fetal heart does not need to flow through the lungs until the moment of birth. To bypass the lungs, two channels are open, and these normally close in days and weeks after birth. One of these openings is in the wall that divides the right and left atria. This is the patent foramen ovale, a slitlike opening which has a flap that permits blood to pass from right to left but guards against flow in the opposite direction. The other passageway is a tube that connects the pulmonary artery near the point of its branching with the aorta just below the origin of the artery to the left arm, the left subclavian artery. This tube contains nerve endings and muscle which make it constrict or dilate and allow it to close off after birth. In the fetal state, when the tube is open, it is called patent ductus arteriosus; when it seals off, it is called ligamentum arteriosum. When it is open, the tube transmits the oxygen-poor blood that enters the right ventricle and the main pulmonary artery to the descending aorta at a high pressure equal to that in the aorta, which is connected to the placenta.

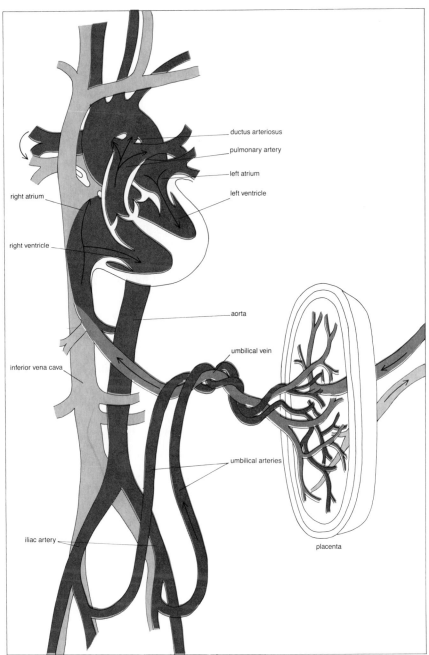

ductus arteriosus

pulmonary artery

left atrium

left ventricle

right atrium

right ventricle

aorta

umbilical vein

inferior vena cava

umbilical arteries

iliac artery

placenta

Circulation in the Unborn Child

When the baby is born, two important changes occur: the umbilical cord is clamped, and the lungs expand as the infant begins to breathe. From that moment on, the left ventricle builds up sufficient pressure to supply all the tissues with oxygen. It becomes stronger and more muscular than the right ventricle, which pumps blood to the lungs into a network of blood vessels which offers little resistance to the flow of blood. Because the right ventricle no longer has to pump blood at as high a pressure as it did in fetal life, the pressure drops over the next few days and weeks to about one-quarter of that in the left ventricle, and the muscular wall becomes thinner. This relationship between pressure and wall thickness of the two ventricles is normally maintained for the rest of life.

During the baby's first few heartbeats, the two fetal passages, which now have no function, begin to close. In the normal situation, the ductus closes completely, but the foramen ovale does not seal closed in one out of five normal persons. It remains a potential opening through which oxygen-poor blood can enter the left atrium and mix with the oxygen-rich blood transmitted by the pulmonary veins from the lungs.

ABNORMALITIES IN DEVELOPMENT

In any process as complex as the development of the human heart, critical alignment of structures or formation of tissues may not occur at the appropriate time. In fact, one baby in about a hundred is born with a congenital abnormality of the cardiovascular system. The causes are not well understood, and in only about 3 percent can the cause be ascribed. One cause is rubella, or German measles. If the mother contracts this viral illness in the first two months of pregnancy, its effects on the development of the fetus can be damaging to the heart—for example causing the ductus to stay open; to the eyes, causing cataracts; and to the brain, producing mental retardation. Fortunately, immunization against rubella can prevent this cause of congenital heart defects.

An abnormality of the chromosomes (on which the genes are carried) is associated with certain congenital heart lesions. In the most common of these, Down's syndrome or mongolism, there is often a malformation of the walls and the valves between the atria and the ventricles, in addition to mental retardation and unusual physical appearance, especially a mongoloid slant to the eyes. Mothers in the older childbearing years are more likely than young mothers to give birth to infants who have this chromosomal disorder. In the early childbearing years, the incidence is about 1 in 2,000 live births; for mothers over forty, it rises to 1 in 50 live births.

In some rare instances, congenital heart disease is related to an inherited genetic disorder. An example is the Marfan syndrome, which results in cardiovascular abnormalities in heart valves or the aorta and an exceptionally tall, thin physique. Another rare occurrence is the clustering of heart defects in otherwise normal families.

Most cardiovascular malformations result either in an obstruction of the flow of blood or in a rerouting of the flow, but unusual disorders can also occur; for example in congenital complete heart block, the electrical impulse responsible for the heartbeat may be blocked in its passage from the normal pacemaker in the right atrium down the pathway to the ventricles. These various disorders may appear in mild, moderate, or severe forms, with the severe form least common. Two major categories of malformations are based on the presence of a shunt—an abnormal entry of blood from one side of the heart to the other. In a right-to-left shunt, some poorly oxygenated (venous) blood appears in the aorta and therefore throughout the systemic circulation. The venous blood imparts a bluish tint to the skin, lips, and nailbeds. A person with that condition has cyanotic heart disease, and infants who have it are called "blue babies." In a left-to-right shunt, arterial blood spills abnormally into the right side of the heart. Since this is oxygenated blood, no cyanosis is present, and the person's color is normal. Another common malformation impairs the flow of blood, usually by obstructing it; here again cyanosis does not occur.

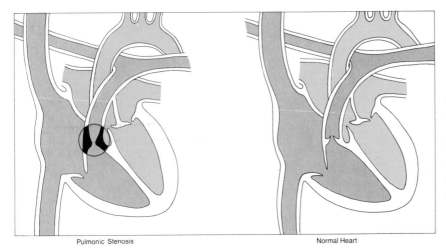

Pulmonic Stenosis   Normal Heart

When the pulmonary valve is narrowed (stenotic), the passage of blood is impeded and the right ventricle becomes enlarged because of the increased work load required to pump blood through the artery and into the lungs.

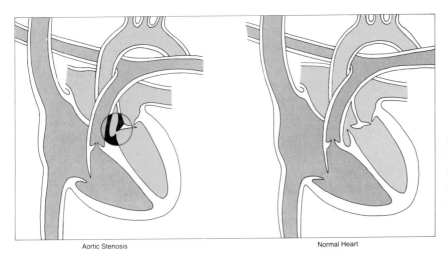

Aortic Stenosis   Normal Heart

The narrowing of the aortic valve forces the left ventricle to pump at a higher pressure as the heart struggles to maintain normal blood pressure beyond the point of constriction.

The most common malformations which impair blood flow by obstruction are pulmonary stenosis, aortic stenosis, and coarctation of the aorta. Any one of the four heart valves—aortic, mitral, tricuspid, and pulmonary—may be narrowed (stenotic), or without an opening (atretic), although aortic and pulmonary stenosis are more common. Congenital stenosis usually is localized to the valve itself, but it may also lie just below (subvalvular) or just above it (supravalvular). Blockage at all three locations is rare. In most cases of stenosis, the edges of the valve leaflets fuse and cannot open fully. Sometimes a valve has only two cusps instead of the normal three (see Heart Valve Disease, chapter 18). The narrowing that occurs in stenosis blocks the passage of blood and causes the ventricle to pump at a higher pressure in order to achieve a near-normal pressure beyond the point of blockage. In pulmonary stenosis, the work load falls on the right ventricle, resulting in enlargement of the muscle (hypertrophy). The enlarged muscle fiber can achieve a pressure as high as ten times normal (250 millimeters of mercury or more) to drive blood through the narrowed passageway. In aortic stenosis and in coarctation of the aorta, the left ventricle bears the burden of pressure overload.

In coarctation of the aorta, movement of oxygenated blood from the left ventricle through a narrow segment of the aorta and the lower part of the

Impaired Blood Flow

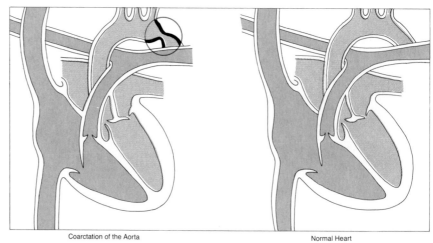

Coarctation of the Aorta   Normal Heart

When the aorta is narrowed or pinched (coarcted), oxygenated blood cannot move freely from the left ventricle. The resulting build up of pressure can cause heart failure in infants.

body is impeded. Pressure builds up, particularly in the head and arms. In the infant, the result may be heart failure; in an adult, headache, nosebleed, and poor circulation in the legs.

Left-to-Right Shunts The three most common forms of left-to-right shunt abnormalities are a defect in the wall separating the two atria (atrial septal defect), a defect in the wall (septum) between the ventricles (ventricular septal defect), and

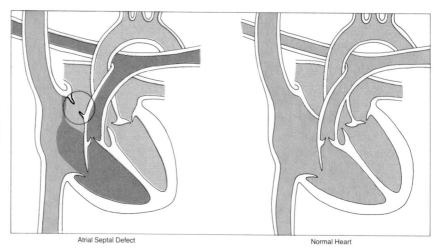

Atrial Septal Defect   Normal Heart

The opening in the wall separating the left and right atria results in a greater than normal volume of blood in the right side of the heart, with resulting enlargement of the right chambers and the pulmonary artery.

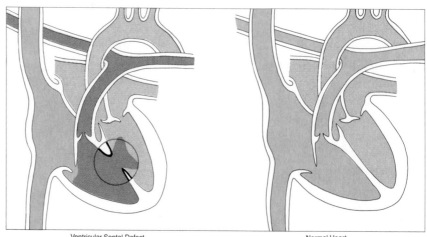

Ventricular Septal Defect   Normal Heart

An opening between the two lower chambers results in the movement of blood from the left to the right ventricle and then out through the pulmonary artery. A large volume of blood passing through the defect will raise the pressure in the right ventricle and the pulmonary artery.

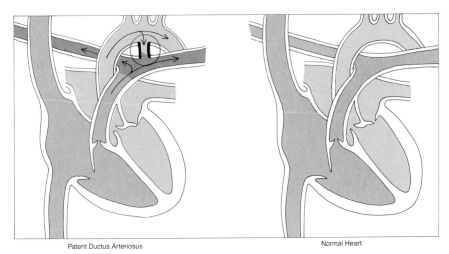

Patent Ductus Arteriosus   Normal Heart

When the fetal opening between the aorta and the pulmonary artery fails to close after birth, blood flows into the pulmonary artery, flooding the lungs and forcing the heart to pump more strenuously.

patent ductus arteriosus. The last condition results when the duct between the aorta and the pulmonary artery fails to close after birth.

An atrial septal defect results in a greater-than-normal volume of blood in the right side of the heart, which leads to enlargement of the right atrium, the right ventricle, and the pulmonary artery. When the defect is in the wall between the ventricles, some oxygenated blood is pumped from the left to the right ventricle and out to the pulmonary artery. If the defect is small and the volume of blood flowing through it is small, the heart and the lungs are not burdened. If the defect is large, however, the volume of shunted blood may increase the pulmonary blood flow to two or three times normal, raising the pressure in the right ventricle and the pulmonary artery. The result is pulmonary hypertension due to excess blood volume (hyperkinetic pulmonary hypertension); the right ventricle has both a volume and a pressure load; and the left ventricle has a volume overload. Both ventricles increase in size and their walls thicken.

When the fetal passageway between the aorta and the pulmonary artery fails to close within a few weeks after birth, the effect on the infant's heart and lungs resembles that of a ventricular septal defect. There is a difference, however. In a ventricular septal defect, blood flows through the opening when the ventricle contracts, but with an open ductus, blood flows through the opening during both the contraction (systolic) and the relaxation (diastolic) phases of the cardiac cycle. During both systole and diastole, the pressure in the aorta is normally greater than the pressure in the pulmonary artery. Arterial blood therefore continuously flows into the venous blood through the open ductus.

Right-to-Left Shunts

The three most common malfunctions with a right-to-left shunt at birth are tetralogy of Fallot, complete transposition of the great arteries, and underdevelopment of the left side of the heart. All three result in cyanosis.

Tetralogy of Fallot (named after the French physician Etienne Fallot who first described the condition in 1888) is a congenital malformation with four distinct aspects. One of the two most important of these is the presence of a large hole in the wall between the right and left ventricles—a ventricular septal defect—which allows the pressure in the two ventricles to become equal and at the same time permits unoxygenated blood to move from the right to the left ventricle and from there into the aorta. Since it has not

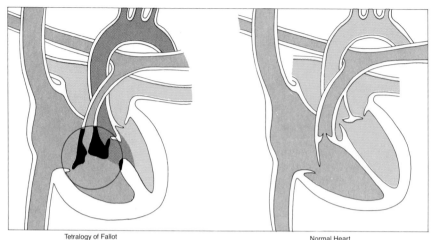

Tetralogy of Fallot   Normal Heart

The two major aspects include the presence of a large hole between the left and right ventricles, and a narrowing of the pulmonary artery or valve. As a result of these defects the right ventricle becomes enlarged and the aorta receives blood from both left and right ventricles.

passed through the lungs, this part of the blood remains unoxygenated. The second major aspect is a narrowing, pulmonary stenosis, which blocks the movement of blood from the right ventricle through the pulmonary artery into the lungs. The obstruction is usually subvalvular, but it may also be valvular or supravalvular. In the most extreme form, there may be no opening at all, a condition called pulmonary atresia. The other two effects are consequences of the two major ones; the right ventricle becomes excessively muscular or enlarged, and the aorta receives blood from both ventricles by overriding the septal defect. This combination of abnormalities obstructs the normal flow of venous blood to the lungs and diverts some of it through the hole in the ventricular septum and into the aorta. Venous blood is thus shunted into the arterial system; a veno-arterial or right-to-left shunt occurs. At the same time, the pulmonary blood flow is lessened as part of it bypasses the lungs and returns directly to the body.

In complete transposition of the great arteries, the aorta and the pulmonary artery arise from the wrong sides of the heart: the aorta from the right ventricle and the pulmonary artery from the left ventricle. The aorta thus receives venous blood returning from the body instead of oxygenated blood from the lungs via the left ventricle. The pulmonary artery, receiving oxygenated blood from the left ventricle, transmits it back to the lungs in a

The aorta arises from the right ventricle (instead of the left) and the pulmonary artery from the left ventricle (instead of the right). On occasion, an opening in the wall between the ventricles or the atria permit some mixing of oxygenated with venous blood. The foramen ovale and the ductus arteriosus may also remain open, permitting the same mixing of blood and sustaining the infant's life for a period.

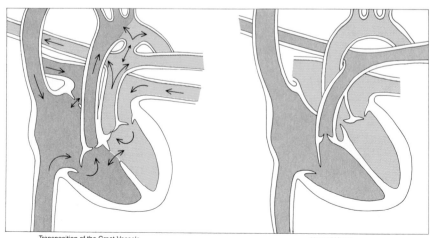

Transposition of the Great Vessels   Normal Heart

needless recycling. Unless there is some mixing of the oxygenated blood with the venous blood, the defect usually proves fatal within a few hours or at most, days. However, in most cases, the heart is otherwise normal, and the temporary persistence of the fetal channels, the patent foramen ovale and the patent ductus arteriosus, permits some mixing to take place for a short time. On occasion, a defect in the ventricular septum or the atrial septum permits mixing of oxygenated with venous blood, sustaining the infant for some time. In contrast to the situation in tetralogy of Fallot, where blood flow to the lungs is decreased because of pulmonary stenosis, transposition of the great arteries increases blood flow to the lungs. Blood is trapped in a recycling circuit, with the patent foramen ovale creating a one-way passage from right to left atrium and preventing passage in the opposite direction. Both conditions result in increased muscle size of the right ventricle, which is obliged to pump blood at a systemic pressure into the aorta.

The third cyanotic condition is one in which there is an underdevelopment (hypoplasia) or even absence (aplasia or atresia) of one or more structures on the left side of the heart; this is called the hypoplastic left heart syndrome. The left ventricle may be rudimentary in size; either the mitral or the aortic valves, or both, may be narrowed or underdeveloped; the aortic arch may be inadequately formed; and sometimes the descending aorta is constricted (coarctation of the aorta). The fetus is not handicapped by this abnormal development, but at birth the situation changes. When the infant begins to breathe on its own and the pulmonary blood vessels are opened to the flow of blood, the underdeveloped left side of the heart is unable to receive the oxygenated blood returning from the lungs or to pump it to the body. Survival in this situation for a brief time is possible if there is a defect in the septum between the atria to reroute blood from the left atrium to the right atrium and right ventricle and then into the pulmonary artery. This results in complete mixing of arterial and venous blood in the right heart chambers, but these are overloaded in the process. The aorta receives its blood through the fetal patent ductus, which permits some blood in the pulmonary artery to flow down the descending aorta and a smaller portion to flow back up around the malformed aortic arch. Often the ascending aorta is so small or so narrowed that it is difficult for blood to enter the coronary arteries. These abnormalities create one of the few conditions in which medical or surgical intervention is of little aid.

The nine malformations discussed comprise about 90 percent of all congenital heart defects. In most cases, a malformation occurs singly, but sometimes there is more than one defect. Certain combinations tend to occur together. One is ventricular septal defect with coarctation of the aorta and patent ductus arteriosus. Another is atrial septal defect with severe pulmonary stenosis or with a severe abnormality of the tricuspid valve, which results in cyanosis.

In addition to the malformations in the septa and the valves of the heart and the defects in the great arteries, the position of the heart is sometimes different from the normal. Normally, the heart lies in the left side of the chest (levocardia). Sometimes the heart is located in the right side of the chest (dextrocardia), either because it has been displaced or because it has rotated (dextrorotated heart) or is a mirror-image dextrocardia. If the heart is in the middle of the chest, the condition is called mesocardia. These variations in the position of the heart can occur with or without any of the previously mentioned congenital malformations. Moreover, other internal organs are sometimes transposed, and if all organs are the mirror-image of normal, the condition is called situs inversus.

EFFECTS OF CONGENITAL ABNORMALITIES   The effect of a congenital heart abnormality may be felt in infancy or it may be delayed until school age and even early adulthood. Certain mild lesions, such as a small ventricular septal defect and mild pulmonary valve stenosis, place no excessive burden on the heart and lungs, and the patient can live a normal, healthy life span. Other abnormalities, such as atrial septal defect, are of little consequence in childhood but cause disability or premature death in early adult life. Still others result in retardation of growth and fatigue or breathlessness upon exertion from early childhood on; two such conditions are moderate-sized ventricular septal defect and patent ductus.

The consequences of more serious congenital abnormalities are likely to be seen in the first weeks or months of infancy, when there is the greatest risk of death from heart defects. The critical symptoms of a severe heart defect in the newborn infant are rapid breathing (tachypnea), extreme difficulty in breathing (dyspnea), and persistent, pronounced cyanosis. After the first week, these symptoms may be augmented by others, including slow gain in weight and fatigue during feedings, which is often mistaken for a feeding problem. Death occurring during this period is usually from severe oxygen lack (hypoxia) or congestive heart failure.

A large left-to-right shunt eventually alters the structures of the pulmonary arterial bed. At first, the vessels begin to resemble arteries in the systemic circulation, and then, as additional changes occur, the opening in the vessels (lumen) is obliterated. These changes accompany pulmonary hypertension with elevated pulmonary vascular resistance. This pathological state tends to develop in children who have a large ventricular septal defect or a patent ductus and an initial excessive flow into the pulmonary arteries with normal or somewhat elevated resistance. However, the conditions may take some time to develop, often not appearing until early adult life when there is an atrial septal defect. With that malformation, large volumes of blood are pumped at normal right ventricular pressure for a long time before pulmonary hypertension begins and progresses. A left-to-right shunt diminishes as resistance to pulmonary flow rises. When the pulmonary resistance exceeds the resistance to blood flow into the systemic vascular bed, a right-to-left shunt appears. The cyanosis which appears at this late stage—cyanose tardive, according to Dr. Maude Abbott—is symptomatic of the Eisenmenger syndrome (ventricular septal defect plus pulmonary vascular obstruction). That term has come to be applied to any kind of arteriovenous shunt in which pulmonary vascular resistance is high and the shunt reverses to right to left.

Other effects of congenital heart defects associated with right-to-left shunt and cyanosis are clubbing of the fingers and toes, in which the tips become bulbous and the nails curved. There is also an increase in red blood cells (polycythemia), in which the body tries to increase the amount of oxygen carried to the tissues.

Not all congenital heart defects produce such obvious symptoms, however. Infants and children who are not cyanotic may in fact show no symp-

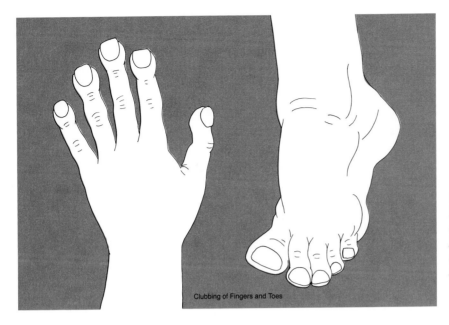

Clubbing of Fingers and Toes

The tips of the fingers and toes become bulbous and the nails curved as a result of a congenital heart defect which allows poorly oxygenated blood to circulate in the aorta or arteries.

toms, even when the heart defect is severe. In making a diagnosis, a doctor must look beyond the obvious symptoms, or even their absence, to determine the real status of a defect. Often, the child's family does not realize how debilitating the defect is until surgery has corrected the problem. After surgery, many children have a remarkable spurt of growth and an unanticipated increase in vitality.

Diagnosis of heart defects is essential for early treatment and even surgical intervention to save the life of an infant, but it is complicated by several factors. Heart disease manifests itself somewhat differently in an infant than it does in a child or in an adult; physical examination of an infant or a very young child is a difficult process at best (it includes inspection, palpation, and auscultation as well as blood pressure readings), and other problems can give rise to many of the "symptoms" of a heart defect (cyanosis, for example, can be caused by disease of the respiratory system as well as by a heart malformation).

Usually it is the presence of a heart murmur that first alerts a doctor to the possibility of a congenital heart defect. The murmur is characteristic of the heart defect and must be distinguished from the soft, innocent murmur that most children normally have. Not all children with a heart defect have a murmur, however. For example, cyanotic patients with pulmonary atresia have no murmur, and generally healthy-looking patients with coarctation of the aorta may have no murmur. In the former, the cyanosis is the clue to a congenital heart problem. In those with coarctation of the aorta, a discrepancy in the strength of the pulse and blood pressure in the upper and lower extremities is the clue. In the rare cases of complete heart block the slow pulse rate supports a positive diagnosis. For the baby who has extreme difficulty in breathing, the grandmother's well-known clinical acumen is the tipoff to diagnosis. If the doctor suspects pneumonia and takes X rays of the chest, the picture of an enlarged heart and congested lungs enables him to recognize congenital heart disease.

DIAGNOSIS OF CONGENITAL HEART DEFECTS

Every diagnosis begins with the simplest procedure: history-taking followed by direct observation of the patient. Color, as has been noted, is an essential clue. Others are respiratory rate and effort. Pulses in all the extremities and blood pressure measurement for both arm and leg must be checked. The contour of the chest often reveals the presence of possible defects. A bulge in the chest to the left of the breastbone (sternum) indicates right ventricular enlargement, while a bulge or lift at the apex (the conical-shaped tip) of the heart suggests left ventricular enlargement. A purring sensation (thrill) beneath the palpating hand accompanies most loud murmurs.

Examination with a stethoscope helps determine the timing, point of maximal intensity and radiation of cardiac murmurs, along the course of aortic blood flow up the arteries of the neck or along the direction of pulmonary blood flow over the lungs. The timing and intensity of heart sounds to the left of the sternum and between the second and third ribs may reveal valve defects, for there the aortic and pulmonary valves can be clearly heard. The physician will also palpate the liver, since enlargement of this organ is a sign of right-sided cardiac failure. Consequences of birth defects such as congestive heart failure and bacterial endocarditis (inflammation of the inner layer, or endocardium, of the heart) may cause enlargement of the spleen (splenomegaly), which is easily detected by palpatation.

The physician will also look for fluid accumulation (edema), a symptom of congestive heart failure. Edema in an infant is usually generalized and may appear as swelling of the eyelids in one who sleeps on his abdomen. In the walking child, pitting edema (when pressure applied to a swelling leaves an indentation or pit in the skin) appears on the back of the foot, the ankles, and the shinbone. Edema in the lungs creates abnormal chest sounds (rales) in a child or an adult, although rales are unusual in infants and appear only after pulmonary edema is far advanced.

Information gathered from these examinations may be sufficient to confirm a diagnosis of congenital heart defect, but the physician usually takes an electrocardiogram and a series of chest X rays involving frontal, side, and oblique (partially rotated) views. The electrocardiogram provides data on heart rate, rhythm, conduction, enlargement of cardiac chambers, and heart strain. Together with X rays, these findings help to substantiate a diagnosis and assess the severity of the defect. The chest X rays permit an analysis of over-all heart size, individual chamber enlargement, location and size of aorta and pulmonary artery, and the relative amount of pulmonary blood flow.

A newer diagnostic tool, echocardiography, can provide additional information on cardiac chamber size, muscle-wall thickness and functioning capability, valves and structural relationships of valves, aorta, chamber walls, and septa. The echocardiograph, as the name suggests, is a device that echoes very high frequency sound waves off cardiac structures. These echoes, not audible to human ears, are then visualized on a screen and recorded for analysis. Echocardiography is a noninvasive tool—that is, it does not involve penetration of the body or any cardiac chamber—and can be performed with no discomfort or danger to the patient.

In cases where further diagnostic confirmation is necessary or surgery is likely, an invasive study called cardiac catheterization with angiocardiography is performed. For this procedure the patient is hospitalized. A catheter is inserted through the skin, then advanced into the right and left sides of the heart, where pressure and oxygen saturation are measured. An opaque fluid is injected into the desired areas and the course of the contrast agent is filmed. Analysis of the films defines precisely the location and extent of the malfunction.

Standardized tests of exercise tolerance on a treadmill or bicycle, or continuous tape recording of the electrocardiogram for several hours or a day may be used in diagnosis.

Treatment of patients with heart defects must be based on accurate diagnosis and a decision as to whether medical management or surgical intervention is the preferred course of action. In either case, the physician offers guidance to the parents, selects the kind of intervention and the time, prepares the patient for diagnostic studies, and instructs the parents on the future needs, liabilities, and potentials of the child. **MEDICAL MANAGEMENT**

Among the immediate problems that the physician faces is the danger of cardiac failure, which is most likely to occur in the first three or four months of life. The infant usually has difficulty feeding, is easily fatigued, grows slowly or else shows rapid weight gain from edema, has rapid and labored breathing patterns, and may wheeze and cough. The chief causes of heart failure in the first weeks of life are severe obstructions to aortic blood flow (due to coarctation of the aorta, often in association with ventricular septal defect, or underdeveloped left heart) and obstructions to pulmonary blood flow (due to pulmonary stenosis). Symptoms of heart failure may, however, not appear for several weeks or even months after birth, particularly when there is a large left-to-right shunt. Only when the pulmonary vascular bed has opened sufficiently to accommodate excessive blood flow do the heart failure symptoms appear—the result, most commonly, of a ventricular septal defect or patent ductus arteriosus. Heart failure rarely results from an atrial septal defect, but it may occur if there is total pulmonary venous return or atrioventricular canal. In childhood and adolescence, heart failure is unusual except as a sequel to surgery, e.g. correction of tetralogy of Fallot, or as a result of complications of bacterial endocarditis. In adulthood, heart failure can occur as a result of a congenital defect which had been reasonably well tolerated for a long time.

Treatment of heart failure begins with the administration of digitalis, which must continue as long as the cause of the failure is not corrected (for example, by surgery to close a patent ductus). Other measures include the use of diuretics to eliminate edema and the restriction of salt intake to prevent the retention of fluid. Morphine helps to relieve pulmonary edema, and oxygen is useful until the lungs become less congested. A semi-upright position helps the patient to breathe more comfortably. An infant who is quickly fatigued or who vomits after feeding may respond to smaller, more frequent feedings.

The critically ill infant must be referred to a pediatric cardiology center for immediate diagnosis and treatment. These centers provide emergency relief of cardiac faliure and the acidosis that results from the inability of the lungs to remove carbon dioxide. If the condition is amenable to surgery, the center is equipped to perform it in an emergency. The development of miniaturized diagnostic tools and the advances in cardiac surgery have made it possible to save the lives of victims of cardiac defects in infancy, the period when they are at greatest risk.

Bacterial endocarditis is a particular danger to any patient with a serious congenital heart defect. (An exception is atrial septal defect, where the complication is very rare.) The patient with a heart defect who has an otherwise unexplained fever must be suspected of having this infection, which inflames the inner lining of the heart (endocardium) and affects previously damaged or defective heart valves and major arteries. Patients are exposed to the greatest risk of infection when undergoing surgery of the mouth or throat, the gastrointestinal tract, or genital and urinary organs. Invasive examination with surgical instruments, even without surgery, may also provide entry for bacteria. Under any of these circumstances, bacteria that normally inhabit organs of the body are released into the bloodstream. If the bacteria lodge on a defective valve or in a cardiovascular abnormality, infection may result.

Diagnosis of endocarditis is made when bacteria are found in the blood. Two very common types are streptococcus viridans in the mouth and streptococcus fecalis in the gastrointestinal tract. Once the organism is identified and its sensitivity to antibiotics tested, medication is begun. Penicillin is given intravenously for a minimum period of four weeks, although fever usually abates promptly with the beginning of treatment. Recovery is usually complete if complications do not develop before antibiotics are administered. Severe complications include infected blood clots (septic emboli) that may travel to the brain; erosion of a valve, making it incompetent (unable to close completely); and heart failure.

To guard against the possibility of endocarditis infection, physicians usually prescribe therapeutic doses of antibiotics before surgery or invasive examinations and for several days after these procedures. A patient about to have dental extraction will, for example, be treated with penicillin before and after the surgery. Such prophylactic measures must be considered a lifelong part of the medical management of all patients with congenital heart defects.

Brain abscess is an uncommon medical emergency among patients with congenital heart defects, but the mortality rate (about 50 percent) and the chance of residual damage to the central nervous system are high. Patients with cyanotic heart disease are especially susceptible to brain abscess after the age of five, probably because blood entering the systemic and cerebral circulations has not undergone normal filtering in the lungs. The infection in the brain substance results in persistent, localized headache. The physician may find evidence of elevated pressure inside the cranium when examining the eyes. Electroencephalograms may reveal abnormalities that help to locate the lesion, although precise confirmation is possible only with a computerized brain scan. Since the infection that produces brain abscesses is usually due to several bacteria (as opposed to a single cause in endocarditis), treatment includes use of broad-spectrum antibiotics for a prolonged period, together with neurosurgery to drain the abscess.

Stroke from blood clot or hemorrhage may affect patients with cyanotic heart disease, particularly infants who are anemic or patients who show an unusually large increase of red blood cells. In the latter instance, the patient may have problems related to blood clotting because normal clotting factors are disrupted.

Infants with tetralogy of Fallot may be subject to attacks in which the skin becomes deeply cyanotic. These attacks often occur early in the morning and seem to take place with little or no provocation. The infant becomes anxious, cries uncontrollably, breathes with difficulty, and may lose consciousness. The cause of such life-threatening episodes is spasm of the enlarged muscle in the right ventricle. The spasm pinches off the beginning of the pulmonary artery, preventing blood from reaching the lungs. Holding the infant in a knee-chest position against the shoulder will often help the attack to pass. An injection of morphine sulfate brings relief, as do oral doses of propranolol. Although medication will temporarily lessen the frequency and severity of the attacks, corrective surgery offers the best long-term solution.

HOSPITALIZATION FOR EMERGENCY CARE OR SURGERY

The critically ill infant, the child who requires cardiac surgery, and the patient recovering from medical emergency or from surgery are usually cared for in special units staffed by trained medical personnel. Electrocardiograms and arterial pressures are continuously monitored, central venous pressure is recorded, and arterial and venous pH and blood gases, as well as electrolytes and blood counts, are sampled frequently. Fluid intake by mouth or intravenously is measured. Respirators and respiratory physiotherapy are available if needed.

When a newborn infant is to be admitted for such care, the physician acquaints the parents with the condition of the infant and explains the operation of the emergency care unit. The cardiologist will explain the nature of the diagnostic tests and the treatment he institutes and interpret the results. When treatment is completed, the parents will be told what follow-up procedures must be undertaken to guarantee success of the treatment.

Preparing a toddler or young child for emergency care is likely to be more complicated and requires reassurance and support to allay anxiety. An older child, who may in fact be well acquainted with the hospital and its routine from previous visits, is usually told in advance about the testing he will undergo and any discomfort he is likely to feel—the finger prick for a blood test, for example, or the numbing sensation when the skin is prepared for a catheter insert. Nurses who are experienced with young patients spend time with each child, explaining various procedures by using toy models or diagrams. Such sessions often benefit anxious parents as much as they do the young patients themselves.

Special sensitivity is needed in dealing with an adolescent or young adult who is being hospitalized for treatment of a congenital heart defect.

TRANSITION FROM CHILDHOOD TO ADULTHOOD

PRINCIPLES

Unfortunately, most individuals born with cardiac defects are likely to need supervision and medical attention throughout their lives. (An exception is the patient who has had a successful patent ductus operation after which the murmur disappears and electrocardiogram and X ray are normal.)

The chances of living a normal, active life are greatly enhanced if the patient's heart defect can be corrected in infancy or early childhood and if a mild condition that does not require surgery is understood by the patient, and the adults caring for him, to be benign. Many patients do not require restrictions in activity, but in those with enlargement of the heart, mild or moderate aortic stenosis, or complete heart block, certain kinds of

1. *Congenital defects in the cardiovascular system occur in approximately 1 out of every 100 births, although the cause can be determined in only about 3 percent of the cases. German measles (rubella) early in pregnancy may*

damage the fetal heart as well as other organs.

2. *Impaired blood flow is a common form of defect. Causes may be narrowing of a heart valve (stenosis) or constriction of the aorta (coarctation).*

3. *Another common defect is a left-to-right shunt, in which some oxygenated blood moves from the left to the right side of the heart instead of emptying entirely into the arterial system. The cause may be a hole in the wall (septum) between the atria (atrial septal defect) or a hole in the wall between the two ventricles (ventricular septal defect), or a patent ductus arteriosus (the continuation, after birth, of the tube between the aorta and the pulmonary artery).*

4. *A right-to-left shunt results from the complex of defects known as the tetralogy of Fallot. In this condition, there is usually a large ventricular septal defect and a stenosis of the*

COMMUNITY RESOURCES

pulmonary valve. Right-to-left shunts also result from transposition of the large arteries, when the aorta and the pulmonary ateries rise from reverse positions in the heart, and from an underdeveloped left ventricle.

5. *Some congenital defects are so mild that they pose no serious threat to growth or health. Defects can usually be detected at birth or within a few weeks after birth. Symptoms include cyanosis (the bluish tint that results from lack of oxygenated blood), rapid breathing, fatigue, and in babies difficulty in eating.*

6. *Some congenital defects repair themselves, some require medication and medical management, and others need surgical correction. Ventricular septal defects may close of themselves, but in other instances surgery is necessary. Stenosis of the valves, patent ductus, and coarctation of the aorta as well as septal defects, transposition of the great arteries and other less common defects, are effectively handled with surgery.*

strenuous physical activity should be discouraged. (Guidelines for activity, frequency of checkups, vocational choices, and insurability are available in a publication of the Study Group on Congenital Heart Disease, Intersociety Commission on Heart Disease Resources, Table II.) It is essential that the child's condition be known to the school nurse or supervisor, and if some activities are to be curtailed, all who take part in the child's development should try to create a balance between overexertion and a potentially dangerous habit of invalidism.

Other problems arise with maturity, among them the question of marriage and the desirability of pregnancy. Most adults with congenital heart defect can marry and even rear a family. Two individuals with congenital defects should receive genetic counseling before marrying, since there is an increased danger that their offspring will inherit the defect. Pregnancy requires special consideration, since the critical periods of increased burden on the circulatory system (the seventh and eighth months, labor, and the immediate postpartum period) are particularly dangerous. Heart failure is always a danger in these circumstances, and a pregnant woman must receive constant reevaluation of her condition. Since the degree of danger varies with the nature of the heart defect, it is particularly important for the physician to have the patient's medical history. Fortunately, many of the emergencies that may arise late in pregnancy and during and after delivery can be dealt with if the medical staff is alerted to the existing heart condition.

There are a number of organizations and institutions that can help the family with an infant, a child, or with an adult who has a congenital heart defect. Expert consultation and care are available at cardiac diagnostic and treatment centers. Community hospitals offer many facilities to cope with ordinary tests and minor emergencies. Cardiac clinics in conjuction with medical schools or health departments are available for ambulatory patients. Federal, state, and local funds, obtainable through programs for physically handicapped children, help defray the costs of hospitalization for diagnostic studies and for surgery. Visiting nurse services help the family that must care for a convalescing patient at home. Vocational training and counseling services provide assistance to the individual who is incapacitated as a result of heart defect. Information on all these services can be obtained from the appropriate federal or state sources. The American Heart Association also provides information on a variety of aids to individuals and their families.

17

RHEUMATIC FEVER

Lewis M. Wannamaker, M.D.

Many people think of heart disease as some kind of mechanical breakdown—an assumption perhaps made because heart disease is not contagious and infection of the heart by bacteria or viruses is uncommon. And yet the heart is composed of living tissue, and like all other organs of the body it can be threatened by agents of infection.

There is one kind of common infection that can result in serious damage to the heart, particularly in children. The disease—not an infection but rather a delayed reaction to infection—is known as rheumatic fever. Its name is derived from its two most frequent symptoms: rheumatism and fever. The disease may manifest itself in other parts of the body as well, especially in the heart muscle and heart valves. In fact, some patients have the characteristic cardiac findings without ever having been aware of the two most common symptoms.

The trigger that sets off events leading to rheumatic fever is a streptococcal infection of the upper respiratory tract—the back of the throat, the tonsils, or related areas. Not all streptococcal infections lead to rheumatic fever: of the several kinds of streptococcus, only one group, the group A hemolytic streptococcus, is responsible for rheumatic fever. How this comes about is not yet known, but one possible explanation is that the streptococci produce a number of toxins, some of which are known to damage heart and other tissue cells. These toxins may be responsible for the initial damage. The infected person also produces many antibodies to various components of group A streptococci, and these in turn may also react with heart muscle, valves, and other tissue. Some patients escape involvement of the heart during an attack of rheumatic fever, while others have mild to severe damage to the heart muscle and connective tissues and particularly to the heart valves. Moreover, certain conditions seem to predispose a person to rheumatic fever itself.

FREQUENCY AND
PREDISPOSING FACTORS

It has long been recognized that rheumatic fever tends to run in families, but whether as a result of genetic factors or of environmental conditions is still uncertain. The disease is most prevalent among children and adolescents between the ages of six and fifteen and is rare in infants and older adults. However, adults who have had rheumatic fever as children or as adolescents and have residual heart disease are particularly susceptible to recurrences. Studies of incidence seem to indicate that brothers and sisters who develop rheumatic fever tend to have the same form of the disease even when it occurs a number of years apart.

Rheumatic fever and rheumatic heart disease occur about equally in males and females, but certain manifestations are more common in one sex than the other. Females are more often affected by narrowing of the mitral valve of the heart (mitral stenosis). Scarring of the aortic valve, which prevents it from closing properly and leads to leakage (aortic regurgitation), is more often seen in males. (For a more complete discussion, see Heart Valve Disease, chapter 18.) Chorea, or St. Vitus' dance, a disorder of the central nervous system, affects about one out of ten children with rheumatic fever and is much more frequently found in prepubertal girls. This manifestation may not appear until months after the acute stage of rheumatic fever.

In the United States, the percentage of known cases of rheumatic fever is higher among blacks than among whites. Studies indicate that the percentage is also higher among certain ethnic groups, but these differences are more likely to be due to living conditions such as overcrowding, which may favor the spread of streptococcal infections, than to genetic or racial characteristics.

Each year an estimated 100,000 new cases of rheumatic fever and rheumatic heart disease develop in the United States. The actual incidence may be appreciably higher, but the figure is not available because many cases are not reported or the symptoms are so mild that medical attention is not sought. About half the persons found to have rheumatic heart damage in their adult years have no history of rheumatic fever. Obviously, the illness had not been detected in its initial stage.

In the United States about 14,000 deaths per year are reported for rheumatic fever or rheumatic heart disease (almost 1 percent of all deaths). Death is rare in the first attack; most occur in adults with chronic heart disease, but the initial attack usually dates back to childhood.

Although rheumatic fever has traditionally been considered an ailment found only in temperate climates, it appears throughout the world. In tropical climates, the acute form with fever and pains in the joints may be less often recognized, but rheumatic heart disease seems to be as common as in temperate climates. In most sections of the United States, rheumatic fever is primarily a winter and spring illness, although in the south, it may be more frequent in the fall.

In recent decades in the United States and in Western Europe the incidence of rheumatic fever, especially recurrent attacks, seems to have declined, and the form of the disease has become less severe. This can be attributed in part to improved socioeconomic conditions. In addition, ever since medical research disclosed that rheumatic fever and rheumatic heart disease are related to streptococcal infections, there have been new, practical approaches to control of the disease, particularly in the prevention of recurrent attacks, which carry the risk of further heart damage. However, the problem has not disappeared in the United States. Studies conducted in Baltimore, Maryland, show that about 24 out of 100,000 children and adolescents (five to nineteen years old) develop acute rheumatic fever each year. Moreover, rheumatic heart disease is still one of the most common heart abnormalities detected in American schoolchildren; it is found in about one in 1000 or 2000.

Unfortunately, the improved picture does not hold true for many of the poorer countries of the world or for the large areas of substandard living conditions in the United States. In these places, rheumatic fever and rheumatic heart disease are still widespread and often serious health problems.

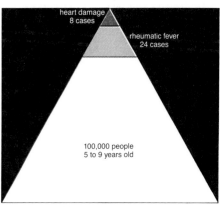

Incidence of Rheumatic Fever

Incidence of rheumatic fever. A study in Baltimore showed that out of every 100,000 children and adolescents 5 to 19 years old, an average of 24 each year develop acute rheumatic fever, and that in an average of 8 out of these cases there is damage to the heart.

Since rheumatic fever can involve different organs of the body, the clinical picture varies from patient to patient. Moreover, its onset may be acute or it may progress slowly. In many children the disease starts rather abruptly with fever, ranging as high as 104 degrees by the second day. The fever may continue for weeks but it usually lasts only from ten to fourteen days. If the findings are not obscured by aspirin or other anti-inflammatory treatment, the patient may experience the typical pattern of arthritic pain and tender-

SYMPTOMS AND SIGNS OF RHEUMATIC FEVER

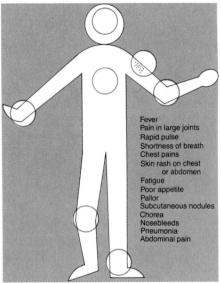

Fever
Pain in large joints
Rapid pulse
Shortness of breath
Chest pains
Skin rash on chest
              or abdomen
Fatigue
Poor appetite
Pallor
Subcutaneous nodules
Chorea
Nosebleeds
Pneumonia
Abdominal pain

Possible Signs of Rheumatic Fever
and Rheumatic Heart Disease

ness moving from one joint to another (migrating polyarthritis). Pain is most commonly felt in the larger joints, particularly in the knees, ankles, elbows, and wrists. Discomfort or pain in the extremities must be evaluated carefully, since it may be due to many causes other than rheumatic fever and may be confused with benign "growing pains." In acute attacks of rheumatic fever, the joints are usually exquisitely tender and may show swelling, redness, and heat. In contrast to many other kinds of arthritis, permanent joint damage is almost unheard of in rheumatic fever. If heart disease develops, as it does in about one fourth to one half of the first attacks of the illness in which arthritis is manifested, it usually occurs within a week or two.

The disease is more difficult to recognize when there are no joint pains or other obvious or localized complaints. There may also be no symptoms that point directly to the heart, even though the heart is affected. Parents may notice that a child tires easily, eats poorly, or is very pale. There may be shortness of breath or chest pains, which are related to heart involvement. On examination, a doctor may hear an abnormal heart murmur, the most common indicator of heart involvement, or he may discover that the heart is enlarged. Less frequently, fluid collects in the sac surrounding the heart (pericardium) or the heart is in failure (see Congestive Heart Failure, chapter 13). Since so-called innocent murmurs can often be found in normal children and appear with fever from almost any cause, they do not necessarily indicate inflammation of the heart (carditis) or of the heart valves (valvulitis) unless they have some special characteristic of abnormal murmurs. The rapid pulse rate which often accompanies rheumatic fever may also be due to excitement, uneasiness, or fever from another cause.

Other characteristic but uncommon manifestations of rheumatic fever occur in or beneath the skin. A lacy or wavy form of skin rash, called erythema marginatum, is most often seen over the chest or abdomen or on the inner surface of the arms or thighs. The rash is transient, sometimes lasting only a few hours, does not itch, and may come and go spontaneously or with the application of heat. Subcutaneous nodules—hard, painless, long-lasting swellings beneath the skin—are most commonly felt over the outer surface of the joints, especially the knuckles and the elbows, and also on the scalp and along the spine. These nodules usually appear in combination with carditis, but since they do not appear in the early stages of rheumatic fever they are generally not helpful in making an initial diagnosis.

A bizarre manifestation of rheumatic fever is Sydenham's chorea or St. Vitus' dance (the fourth-century Christian martyr was invoked against the disease). The child with full-blown chorea has rapid, uncontrolled movements involving at times most of the muscles. Chorea may not appear for as long as six months after the streptococcal infection, and it often develops so slowly that it may pass unnoticed for some time. Parents or teachers may begin to notice clumsiness, facial grimacing, a change in personality, or a tendency to fits of crying. Emotional factors play an important role in chorea, and rapid and unexplainable swings in emotion may be the first hint that it is developing. Chorea commonly occurs without other signs of rheumatic fever (pure chorea), or it may appear after other signs have disappeared. Fortunately, chorea is of limited duration and ultimately subsides without leaving any permanent damage to the nervous system. Parents should be assured that the uncontrolled body movements are not indications of any harm to the child's intellectual capabilities.

The manifestations of rheumatic fever may also include nosebleeds (epitaxis), an unusual form of pneumonia called rheumatic pneumonia, or abdominal pains which may be mistaken for acute appendicitis.

There is no specific laboratory test for rheumatic fever. However, laboratory tests can be helpful in confirming the presence of inflammation and the likely occurrence of a recent streptococcal infection and may provide supportive evidence of cardiac abnormalities. Examination of heart tissue at surgery or after death may provide definitive pathologic evidence of rheumatic heart disease.

LABORATORY AND PATHOLOGICAL FINDINGS

Rheumatic fever is an acute inflammatory disease. The presence of inflammation can be confirmed by laboratory tests, including one that measures how fast the red blood cells settle out on standing (erythrocyte sedimentation rate or ESR) and one that detects the presence of an abnormal protein in blood serum (C-reactive protein). Although none of these tests is specific for rheumatic fever, since the abnormalities are common to a variety of inflammatory diseases, the tests are useful for indicating that an inflammatory disease process actually exists and for following the course of rheumatic fever. These tests of inflammation register normal in patients who have passed the acute stages of the disease as well as in most patients with "pure" chorea and those with chronic rheumatic heart disease. Abnormalities may also be suppressed if the patient is taking aspirin or steroid hormones.

Throat cultures and streptococcal antibody tests help to indicate the possibility of a recent streptococcal infection that could have triggered acute rheumatic fever. The antistreptolysin O (ASO) test, the most frequently used of the many streptococcal antibody tests available, measures the ability of antibodies in the patient's blood serum to inhibit the rupture of red blood cells (lysis) by a streptococcal product, streptolysin O. An elevated ASO measurement (titer) is good evidence of recent streptococcal infection, occurring in about 80 percent of those convalescing from streptococcal sore throat, regardless of whether they develop rheumatic fever. Other tests that examine blood serum (serological tests) which may be useful include the anti-DNase B, the anti-hyaluronidase, the anti-streptokinase, and the anti-NADase tests. (Opinions vary about the validity of the new streptozyme test which is still under study.) Patients with normal titers for several of these tests are unlikely to be suffering from acute rheumatic fever.

Chest X rays of patients with active or chronic rheumatic heart disease may show enlargement of the heart shadow (cardiomegaly). The electrocardiogram may also show abnormalities.

Microscopic examination of heart tissue reveals a distinctive lesion, the Aschoff body, not found in any other disease process. These lesions consist of large cells with many nuclei in a rosette formation around pink granular material surrounding blood vessels.

The heart valves, particularly those of the left side of the heart—the mitral and aortic valves—may also be affected. About 60 percent of patients with mitral stenosis (narrowing of the valve between the left atrium and the left ventricle) have a history of acute rheumatic fever. Valves may show leakage of blood back into the chamber from which it came (regurgitation), or they may slowly become scarred and narrowed by calcium deposits, which results in restricted flow of blood.

TREATMENT Rheumatic fever is not a contagious disease, and patients need not be isolated. But it is very important that they be protected against its precursor, streptococcal infection, which may result in a repeat attack and further injury to the heart, and also against bacterial infection of damaged heart valves, which may occur after dental or surgical procedures (see following two sections). Bed rest is usually required during the acute stage, but prolonged bed rest is rarely necessary except for those in heart failure. Special diets are generally not needed, but restricting the amount of salt may be necessary for heart-failure cases.

Aspirin, or steroid hormones such as prednisone or cortisone, may be prescribed to suppress the acute inflammation of rheumatic fever, particularly when joint pains are severe. Doctors often delay using these drugs until the diagnosis is certain, however. Steroids are frequently prescribed for patients with carditis, but while they are usually effective in suppressing acute inflammation, their effect on the development or persistence of heart disease is uncertain. If the suppressive drugs are discontinued before the disease has run its course, the patient may suffer a "rebound." To avoid such occurrences, suppressive medications are generally withdrawn gradually.

Patients with chorea need a quiet environment and possibly a sedative, such as phenobarbital, or a tranquilizer, such as chlorpromazine. If the disorder is severe, the patient will need to be protected against injury resulting from uncontrollable movements. If heart failure is present, the doctor may prescribe digitalis or a related drug to stimulate the heart, or diuretics to increase urine output. Patients who do not benefit from digitalis, salt restriction, and diuretics or other medications may require surgical repair to relieve the obstruction of blood flow caused by scarred valves or leakage of damaged valves. In some cases, replacement by an artificial valve may be indicated. (Replacement of valves is discussed in Cardiovascular Surgery, chapter 20.)

PREVENTION OF REPEAT ATTACKS Patients who have recovered from rheumatic fever and those who have residual heart disease risk a recurrent attack and further heart damage if they acquire another streptococcal infection. Since these infections may not always be symptomatic, it is best not to wait until an infection is recognized. These high-risk individuals must have continuous protection against the development of a new streptococcal infection; this is accomplished by monthly injections of long-acting penicillin (benzathine penicillin G) or by daily oral sulfonamide or penicillin.

The likelihood of a recurrent episode of rheumatic fever is greatest during childhood, in adolescence, and in adults exposed to children or to crowded living conditions. The risk is also high in the years immediately after an attack, especially during the first five years. Patients with rheumatic heart disease are more likely to develop a recurrence than those who escape that complication. Continuous protection with penicillin or sulfonamides is therefore recommended for a long period of time, perhaps throughout life, although some doctors consider the risk low enough in older adults to discontinue these drugs.

Patients with rheumatic heart disease are prone to develop infection of the heart valves or the lining of the heart (endocarditis). Bacteria entering the bloodstream during dental and surgical procedures may locate and multiply on damaged heart valves. Therefore, rheumatic heart disease patients should be protected against endocarditis by administration of appropriate antibiotics at the time of the procedure.

PREVENTION OF INFECTION OF DAMAGED HEART VALVES

The group A hemolytic streptococcal infections of the respiratory tract that lead to rheumatic fever are known as streptococcal pharyngitis, streptococcal tonsillitis, streptococcal sore throat (strep throat). Streptococcal infections of the middle ear (otitis media) and of the lymph nodes or glands of the neck (cervical adenitis) may also result in rheumatic fever. Streptococcus also causes impetigo, a skin infection, but this does not lead to rheumatic fever.

STREPTOCOCCAL INFECTION THE PRECURSOR OF RHEUMATIC FEVER

The clinical picture in streptococcal sore throat varies, but in the typical case the illness starts suddenly, with the patient complaining of soreness on swallowing. Body temperature is usually above 100 degrees, and this symptom may be accompanied by headache, nausea, and vomiting at onset, as well as by abdominal pain, especially in children. On examination, the throat looks red and inflamed, and by the second day of illness patches of pus (exudate) may appear. The glands (lymph nodes) in front of the neck or under the angle of the jaw may be tender and swollen. Young children may show raw areas (excoriation) around one or both nostrils. The infection may, in some cases, spread to the middle ear or to the sinuses, causing pain in these areas. Occasionally a skin rash, red and about the size of "goose pimples," develops on the upper chest and back. The rash blanches on pressure and eventually peels. Streptococcal infections showing this rash are known as scarlet fever. Symptoms that are uncommon in streptococcal infection include simple runny nose (except in infants), hoarseness, coughing, and inflamed eyes (conjunctivitis). Almost half of all patients with streptococcal infections have minimal symptoms or none, and yet these infections, difficult to detect and to distinguish from carrier states (see section on streptococcal carriers below), may also result in rheumatic fever.

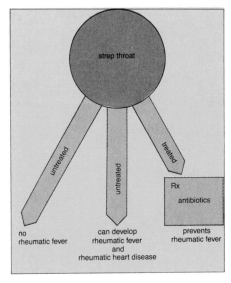

Most sore throats are not caused by streptococci but by viral infections which, unlike bacterial infections, do not benefit from treatment with antibiotic drugs. A throat culture is therefore an important help in confirming the possibility of a streptococcal infection. (Cultures are taken with a cotton swab firmly rubbed against the back of the throat and over the tonsil area.) A throat culture will usually reveal large numbers of the infecting bacteria. These hemolytic streptococci are recognized by their ability to break down (hemolyze) red blood cells when they are grown on a media containing blood (sheep blood is generally used). Other streptococci, found normally in all human throats, produce green or partial hemolysis on blood. Hemolytic streptococci can be divided into a number of groups, which are identified by the letters of the alphabet. Group A streptococci cause most of the streptococcal infections of the throat and upper respiratory tract; they are also the only bacteria that can trigger the development of rheumatic fever. There are more than sixty different types of group A streptococci, and infection with one does not result in immunity to the rest, which is the reason most people suffer a number of streptococcal infections during a lifetime. Many of the types of group A streptococci that commonly cause sore throat have the potential of causing rheumatic fever. It has been hypothesized that certain strains or types of streptococci are "rheumatogenic," but there is no clear method of identifying such strains.

Streptococcal sore throats occur most commonly in schoolage children, on an average of one every three to five years. Adults may also be infected, particularly those exposed to children or living under crowded conditions. Like most respiratory infections, streptococcal sore throats are less frequent in the summer months. This age and seasonal pattern is in general reflected in that of rheumatic fever.

Close contact with an infected, or recently infected, person is usually required to contract the infection. Although group A streptococci can be found in the environment of an infected person, contact with such contaminated objects as bed clothing does not result in spread of respiratory infection. Untreated patients are generally contagious for one to two weeks, although those with chronic streptococcal sinusitis or draining ears infected with streptococci may be contagious for longer periods. Infecting streptococci in the throat are suppressed after one or two days of penicillin treatment and are usually eradicated if treatment is continued for ten days. Patients are, therefore, no longer contagious after a 24- to 48-hour program of treatment with penicillin.

Streptococcal sore throats can also be acquired by individuals and even by large numbers of people if they eat food contaminated with group A streptococci (food-borne epidemics). Contamination usually takes place when the food has been prepared by someone with current or recent streptococcal infection. Storage of the food at room temperature or in large quantities in a refrigerator may permit the growth of streptococci. Egg salad or other salads such as tuna salad containing eggs are a common source of food-borne streptococcal infection. Milk-borne infections, usually acquired by drinking unpasteurized milk from infected cows, are now rare.

Streptococcal throat infection usually lasts only a few days, even without antibiotic treatment. Antibiotics may prevent the spread of infection to such nearby sites as the ears or the sinuses (conditions called suppurative complications since they are associated with discharge of pus). Adequate antibiotic treatment, however, is most important because it may prevent the development of rheumatic fever (see section on prevention of first attacks of rheumatic fever). Under epidemic conditions, rheumatic fever can develop in about 3 percent of patients with untreated streptococcal sore throat. In nonepidemic situations, the frequency of rheumatic fever after such infection appears to be less. Exact figures are, however, difficult to determine and may depend on the way streptococcal infection is defined or on the virulence of the infecting streptococci.

Rheumatic fever does not usually develop until after the patient appears to have recovered from the streptococcal sore throat. The hiatus between

PRINCIPLES

1. Rheumatic fever, a complication that sometimes follows streptococcal infections of the upper respiratory tract, most frequently strikes children of school age. A particular kind of streptococcus, group A streptococcus, has been identified as the agent responsible for the illness.

sore throat and signs of rheumatic fever, called the latent period, averages about eighteen days but may be several months in patients with chorea.

Another complication of group A streptococcal infection is a kind of kidney disease called acute nephritis (acute form of Bright's disease). In contrast to rheumatic fever, this complication may develop after impetigo as well as after throat infections. The latent period after sore throat is about ten days, and penicillin treatment is often ineffective in preventing this complication.

2. Rheumatic fever affects various parts of the body, with clinical findings including fever, joint pains, inflammation of the heart, skin rash, and a disorder of the nervous system, which may appear singly or in various combinations. Sometimes the initial attack is so mild it goes unnoticed.

Streptococcal Carriers

Individuals who carry group A streptococci in the throat or other areas but are not themselves currently infected are known as streptococcal carriers. Group A streptococci may remain in the throat for many weeks or for months. Chronic throat carriers have usually passed the time period in which they are likely to develop complications or to spread the infection, so they are generally harmless to themselves or others. They may, however, become a source of confusion to a physician who is trying to determine whether an individual is presently infected with group A streptococci. The carrier state may be difficult to eradicate with penicillin, and in fact many physicians do not advise such treatment for chronic throat carriers. Group A streptococci may also be carried at such other body sites as in the nose or in the area around the anus (opening of the rectum). Nasal and anal carriers may spread infection more readily than throat carriers.

3. There is no specific laboratory test for rheumatic fever. Laboratory tests can provide evidence of a recent streptococcal infection (the set-up that fits with the possible development of this complication) and can confirm the presence of some kind of inflammatory process.

4. Although streptococcal infections are contagious, rheumatic fever itself is not. The usual treatment includes bed rest and drugs to reduce fever

Prevention of First Attack of Rheumatic Fever

Adequate antibiotic treatment can reduce by as much as 90 percent the risk of first attacks of rheumatic fever in patients with recognized streptococcal infection. Prevention of repeat attacks by this approach is less dependable (see section on prevention of repeat attacks). Effective treatment must get rid of all the group A streptococci, which can usually be achieved by a single injection of long-acting penicillin (penzathine penicillin G) or by oral penicillin taken regularly for ten days. Oral treatment is less painful than injections and less likely to result in penicillin reactions but may be less effective, largely because the patient fails to take the penicillin for the full period. Improvement usually comes within the first few days, and the patient who begins to look and feel healthy again may forget about the necessity of continuing to take the medication regularly.

Erythromycin may be used if a patient is allergic to penicillin. Some of the newer antibiotics may also be effective. Although some group A streptococci are resistant to certain antibiotics (the tetracycline antibiotics, for example), no laboratory tests have shown them resistant to penicillin. But in spite of penicillin's effectiveness, it may be difficult or impossible to kill all of the group A streptococci in some infected patients and particularly in some carriers.

Since sore throats are not clear indicators of streptococcal infection, many doctors prefer to wait for the results of the throat culture before starting antibiotic treatment, knowing that a delay of from twenty-four to forty-eight hours does not reduce the effectiveness of penicillin in preventing rheumatic fever. Some doctors, however, may start treatment before the culture result is available, particularly if the clinical impression of infection is strong and if the patient is extremely uncomfortable.

and to suppress other symptoms during the acute stage. If there is cardiac involvement, a doctor may also prescribe drugs to assist the heart.

5. Most attacks of rheumatic fever subside in a few weeks and with the exception of heart damage do not result in chronic conditions. About one fourth to one half of the rheumatic-fever patients with arthritis also have inflammation of the heart, manifested most often by abnormal heart murmurs.

6. Patients with severe inflammation of the heart may be left with permanent heart damage. Rheumatic heart disease may also occur in persons whose symptoms are so mild that no medical assistance is sought.

7. Because victims of rheumatic fever and rheumatic heart disease who contract a new streptococcal infection are at high risk of developing a repeat attack, continuous protection with penicillin or sulfonamides for a long period of time, perhaps for life, is needed.

8. *Patients with rheumatic heart disease are also susceptible to bacterial infection of damaged heart valves and therefore are often advised to have additional prophylactic antibiotics when undergoing surgery or even with mild dental procedures.*

RESEARCH GOALS

9. *The risk of first attacks of rheumatic fever is much lower than the risk of recurrent or repeat attacks. First attacks can be prevented by recognition and appropriate treatment of streptococcal infections of the upper respiratory tract, which most commonly appear as a sore throat. Accurate diagnosis is greatly improved by the use of throat cultures along with clinical findings. Patients with mild or minimal symptoms of streptococcal infection are difficult to detect and to differentiate from streptococcal carriers. To reduce the risk of rheumatic fever, treatment with penicillin or another appropriate antibiotic must be continued for ten days, even though symptoms usually disappear after the first few days.*

10. *In recent decades, improved socioeconomic conditions and medical and surgical treatments, especially the prevention of recurrent attacks of rheumatic fever, have reduced the severity of rheumatic fever and rheumatic heart disease in the United States. In many less developed countries and among the poor of the United States, these continue to be common and often serious health problems. Further research is needed to discover the causes of rheumatic fever and improved methods for its prevention, since rheumatic heart disease is still the leading cause of death from heart disease in school age children and adolescents and a major cause of death in adults.*

Throat cultures as part of school health programs are taken in some areas, although the need for and the effectiveness of these in preventing rheumatic fever is uncertain. This is especially true in areas where rheumatic fever has not been demonstrated to be common. Differentiating between the carrier state and acute infection is a difficult problem in such programs, particularly if cultures are taken routinely or with minimal clinical indications of streptococcal infection. Such programs should not be started without careful evaluation of local conditions and the introduction of strict control over the procedures used in taking, handling, and interpreting cultures.

Although the impact of rheumatic fever is now being reduced, it continues to be the leading cause of death from heart disease in the 5- to 24-year-old group. An effort to improve approaches to the control and treatment of the disease must provide more accurate and easier ways of diagnosing streptococcal infections, of distinguishing acute infection from the carrier state, and of recognizing an infection which does not show symptoms. Further research is needed on a safe and effective vaccine for streptococcal infections, but this is complicated by the number of different types of group A streptococci. There is also the danger that a vaccine may result in reactions or even in the development of rheumatic fever.

New research is required to determine how rheumatic fever develops and why it appears in some and not others. Such knowledge would allow doctors to concentrate preventive measures on susceptible individuals before the occurrence of the first attack. Practicing physicians and their patients would be helped by development of new and better methods of diagnosis and prevention of rheumatic fever. Continuing research is also needed to find curative rather than suppressive drugs for treating rheumatic fever and to improve surgical approaches to remedying the heart damage of rheumatic fever.

18

HEART VALVE DISEASE

Robert O. Brandenburg, M.D.,
Dwight C. McGoon, M.D.

The passage of blood through the four chambers of the heart and on into the principal vessels that lead to the rest of the body requires delicate controls to maintain an efficient system constantly at work. Like all mechanisms involved with the flow of liquids or gases, the circulatory system relies on a pump to propel the flow and a series of valves to regulate it. The pumping action is achieved by the contraction and relaxation of the heart, assisted by a valve system throughout the arteries and veins. The heart itself has four valves: the tricuspid, the pulmonary, the mitral, and the aortic. Each valve consists of thin, fibrous, elastic sheets of tissue attached to the walls of the heart as if on hinges. When closed, the tissue leaflets that make up the valve meet in the center and seal the valve opening. The opening and closing of the valves takes place in response to changes in pressure within the chambers of the heart.

Schematic showing location of the four heart valves. The tricuspid, pulmonary, and aortic valves have three leaflets; the mitral valve has two.

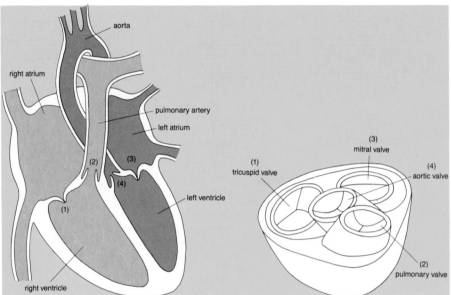

Location of Heart Valves

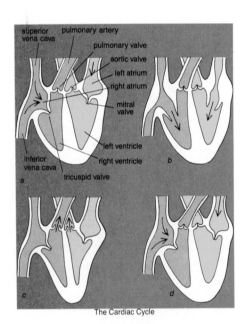

The Cardiac Cycle

a. All four heart valves are closed as atria fill with blood.
b. Pressure in atria opens tricuspid and mitral valves, allowing blood to pass into ventricles.
c. Pressure in ventricles closes tricuspid and mitral valves and opens pulmonary and aortic valves. Blood flows into aorta and pulmonary artery.
d. All valves close, atria fill with blood, the cycle begins again.

Blood returning to the right atrium (the upper right chamber of the heart) by way of the venous system must pass through two sets of valves before it is recirculated throughout the body. As it moves from the right atrium to the right ventricle, it passes through the tricuspid valve, so named because it is composed of three leaflets. The next valve, located at the outlet of the right ventricle, is called the pulmonary. It separates that ventricle from the pulmonary artery leading to the lungs. The oxygenated blood returning to the left side of the heart from the lungs must pass through two other valves before being propelled to the tissues of the body. The valve separating the left atrium from the left ventricle resembles a bishop's hat—a miter—and is called the mitral valve. The valve located at the outlet of the left ventricle, separating it from the aorta, is the aortic valve. The aorta, the largest artery in the body, is the major vessel transporting oxygenated blood from the heart to all the organs.

When the blood enters the right atrium, it fills that chamber until pressure there is greater than in the lower chamber, the right ventricle. The difference in pressure occurs between heartbeats, when the ventricle, having expelled its load of blood into the pulmonary artery, is empty. The pressure in the blood-filled atrium forces the tricuspid valve open, allowing the oxygen-depleted blood from the veins to flow into the lower ventricle. When the ventricle is filled it contracts or beats, raising the pressure in the ventricle, which in turn causes the pulmonary valve to open and the tricuspid to close. Blood is pumped into the lungs, where the waste gas (carbon dioxide) is released and where the red blood cells pick up oxygen. The oxygen-rich blood now enters the upper left chamber of the heart, the left atrium. Between heartbeats, the pressure of blood in the left atrium causes the mitral valve to open, and blood flows down into the left ventricle. When the heart contracts, the rise in pressure in the ventricle closes the mitral valve and at the same time opens the aortic valve. Blood is thus sent to all the organs of the body via the arterial system.

There are many ways in which valves can be injured, a common one being the result of rheumatic fever. Although this disease may affect the body joints and heart muscle, it is especially likely to cause permanent valve damage. Other common threats are bacterial infections, congenital defects, and a variety of conditions that weaken the supporting structures of the valves. **CAUSES OF MALFUNCTIONING**

A defective valve is one that fails either to close or to open fully. An improperly closing valve allows blood to leak back into the chamber from which it has just flowed, a condition called regurgitation, or insufficiency, or leakage. With the next heartbeat, the regurgitated blood must again flow through the valve, together with the normally flowing blood. This abnormally large volume of blood passing through the heart puts an increased demand on the heart muscle. The inability of a valve to open fully is called stenosis. Since heart disease symptoms usually do not develop until the valve opening becomes quite markedly narrow, doctors, using modern diagnostic tools, may discover stenosis of a valve many years before a patient complains of discomfort. Valves may be affected either by insufficiency or by stenosis, but in many instances, particularly following rheumatic fever, both problems develop in the same valve.

Symptoms from valve disease vary so greatly from individual to individual that some may experience no difficulty at all for years and others feel only mild discomfort for equally long periods. Valve problems gradually tend to worsen, however, and eventually cause serious disabling symptoms. These depend in part on the severity of the valve lesion and in part on the valve involved. Since blood pressures are higher on the left side of the heart, abnormalities of the mitral and aortic valves usually cause symptoms earlier than does valve disease on the right side (tricuspid and pulmonary valves). Patients with regurgitation of either of these valves notice that their heart becomes overactive during periods of increased work or play or with emotional distress. The extra stress is placing further demands on a heart already doing extra work because of the leakage. The left ventricle gradually increases in size, and its muscular wall thickens in order to cope with these demands. While the heart can often continue to function in this way for long periods, particularly if the valve defect has come on gradually, eventu-

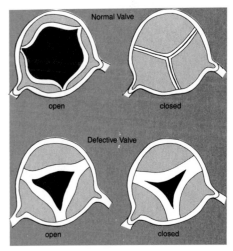

Aortic Stenosis

Narrowing of the valve prevents it from closing completely and blood leaks back into the left ventricle.

ally it begins to lose its ability to pump adequately. In spite of the enlargement of the chamber and the increased thickness of the wall, the ventricle cannot empty completely with each contraction. Pressure builds up in the ventricle, resulting in a slowing of the natural flow of blood from lungs to ventricle to arteries. Pressure transmits backward from the ventricle to the atrium and from there to the blood vessels of the lungs. The normally elastic lungs become stiffened as a result of being distended with blood, and the patient experiences shortness of breath.

An overtaxed, enlarged heart may also have difficulty in maintaining an adequate forward output of blood. When the body's muscles fail to receive their normal supply of oxygenated blood, fatigue develops during periods of increased activity. The kidneys, too, react to the reduced flow of blood by retaining salt and water, which in turn causes body tissues to retain fluid (edema), particularly in such dependent parts as the ankles.

When the problem is stenosis (inadequate opening) of the mitral valve, the ventricle is not overworked, but the blood vessels of the lungs are under high pressure. The lungs react by narrowing the small arteries, which in turn elevates blood pressure in the arteries of the lungs. As a result, the right side of the heart is burdened with the task of pumping blood against the resistance of the lungs. The right side of the heart is eventually unable to meet the abnormal demands placed on it, pressure in the veins leading into it rises, and fluid is retained in body tissues—the liver, the legs, the ankles, and occasionally even within the abdomen (this swelling is called ascites). As with leakage, the patient with stenosis experiences shortness of breath.

In stenosis of the aortic valve, the left ventricle is able, often for years, to maintain an adequate output of blood. The ventricle simply increases the amount of pressure needed to push blood through the narrowed aortic valve. Although this condition may persist without significant symptoms for many years, the gradual and marked thickening of the left ventricle wall increases the need for blood through the coronary arteries, which feed the heart tissue itself. When the coronary arteries are unable to supply heart tissue adequately, the patient may experience discomfort or pain. This condition, called angina pectoris (tightness in the chest), can develop in patients with severe narrowing of the aortic valve, even when the coronary arteries themselves are normal.

Stenosis of the aortic valve can also produce episodes of fainting or near fainting. These episodes, the result of inadequate blood supply to the brain, are most likely to occur with exertion. They may also happen if the heart experiences a sudden rapid change in rhythm, which, in the presence of a narrowed aortic valve, could significantly reduce the flow of blood. Stenosis of the aortic valve can, therefore, result in such symptoms as shortness of breath, fatigue, or faintness with exertion and angina pectoris and palpitations (awareness of the heartbeat or of disturbances of the rhythm of the heart). The nature of the symptoms as well as their severity depend on the nature of the valve lesions; in the most advanced condition, called congestive heart failure, fluid retention increases and swelling occurs in tissues of the lungs, liver, intestines, legs, and feet.

Occasionally, the first evidence of a narrowed valve is a clot that forms because of the stagnation of blood above the affected area. If the clot adheres to the wall of a heart chamber, there are no complications. But if the clot or part of it enters the circulatory system, it can cause serious damage, depending on where it comes to rest. Unfortunately, clots most commonly affect the circulation of the brain where arteries tend to be narrow and easily become blocked. Although many of these disturbances are minor and the symptoms clear after a few days, in other cases they can result in serious stroke symptoms. A clot that lodges in an eye vessel affects vision; one that lodges in a leg artery impairs circulation in that leg.

Valve disease, particularly of the mitral valve, can also lead to the development of an abnormal cardiac rhythm. Mitral valve disease also affects the size and shape of the left atrium. Any changes in enlargement of this chamber can lead to alterations in the normal rate of the heartbeat (60 to 100 impulses a minute). The normal pumping rate, under the control of the intrinsic pacemaker in the upper right chamber (the sinoatrial node) is replaced by a rapid irregular rhythm which fires 400 to 500 impulses a minute. Fortunately, specialized tissue between the upper and lower chambers allows only one in every three or four beats to get through to the pumping chambers. But even with this built-in control, a sudden change in rhythm that steps up the pumping chambers to 160 beats a minute or more can cause serious symptoms when valvular disease is present. Such an irregularity in rhythm, called atrial fibrillation, is commonly seen in patients with valvular heart disease.

DIAGNOSTIC CLUES

The progress of rheumatic mitral-valve disease is illustrated by the history of Mrs. S. She had suffered two attacks of acute rheumatic fever in childhood, one at the age of ten, the other at twelve. Both followed episodes of tonsilitis which had been treated with antibiotics for only a few days. In the first instance, although the symptoms of tonsilitis cleared, within a few weeks the child developed fever and general feelings of malaise. There was redness, swelling, and pain in her joints, which moved from one joint to another during many weeks. She was ill for three months and required an additional month of rest before being able to return to school. After the second attack of rheumatic fever, her doctor noted for the first time the existence of a heart murmur. However, the patient showed no other cardiac symptoms for twenty years, during which time she lived a normal life, married, and bore two children.

At the age of thirty, following an attack of influenza, Mrs. S became severely short of breath. The examining physician noted a rapid, irregular heart rhythm and lung congestion, the latter a result of flu infection and back pressure from the heart. Given the history of rheumatic fever, and abnormalities on exam of the mitral valve area, it was safe to conclude that Mrs. S was suffering the symptoms of a malfunctioning mitral valve.

The physician's conclusion was based on evidence gathered by means of several kinds of examinations. Despite the great advances in electronic testing equipment, the most important information on the condition of the heart valves comes from the simplest kind of examination: the doctor places his hand on the chest over the heart and feels the impulses transmitted through the chest wall. Applying the stethoscope, he carefully assesses the sounds and murmurs caused by the diseased valve. Experience teaches him to recognize the distinctive sounds of each malfunctioning valve.

In addition to such diagnostic tests as chest X rays, electrocardiograms, and blood tests, a doctor has at his disposal various kinds of special testing techniques. Fluoroscopy allows the radiologist to observe the size and movements of the heart chambers; it also reveals the presence of calcium deposits which stiffen the valve leaflets and reduce their mobility. Another technique is cardiac catheterization, in which a slender tube is passed from the groin or arm through the blood vessels and into the heart. This diagnostic technique provides valuable information on blood pressures, the level of oxygen in the heart chambers, and other conditions. A more recent technique called echocardiography has been very helpful in diagnosis. The instrument sends sonar beams (sound waves) into the chest, where they are then bounced back from the walls and valves of the heart. The recorded waves show the shape, texture, and movement of the valves, as well as the size and state of function of the chambers of the heart. This study is particularly helpful since it is noninvasive and can be done in the office without discomfort or risk to the patient.

MEDICAL TREATMENT   When mitral valve disease is first diagnosed, as with Mrs. S, the doctor will most likely advise the patient to avoid fatigue, unusual physical and emotional stress, and the possibility of infection. Anyone with mitral valve disease should have antibiotic protection before, during, and after any surgery, and particularly surgery that involves the nose, mouth, throat, bladder, vagina, or rectum. The patient should be put on a low-salt diet to reduce the likelihood of the kidneys' retaining salt and water.

The use of digitalis is an important part of the treatment of valvular dsease. Not only does the drug tend to slow down a fast-beating heart but also it increases the efficiency of the heart muscle and helps it to carry the burden created by the malfunctioning valve. In advanced stages of valvular disease, the patient will also require diuretic medicine, which makes the kidneys excrete salt and water. Because of the potent diuretics now available, it is often possible to keep patients with valvular lesions quite comfortable and free of excess fluid for many years.

SURGICAL REPAIR   As effective as such medical treatment can be, the disease often eventually progresses to such an extent and puts such an increased limitation on activity that surgical treatment becomes advisable. This was the decision in a case, again quite typical, of a middle-aged man with a congenitally defective aortic valve. The defect was actually not discovered until the patient, complaining of shortness of breath, was examined by a physician who observed the type of murmur associated with narrowing of the aortic valve. Further examinations revealed that the patient had been born with an aortic valve consisting of two instead of the normal three leaflets. Although an aortic valve with this defect may function normally for many years, it has a tendency to become narrowed or to develop regurgitation. At first, the patient improved with the usual treatment: digitalis, low-salt diet, restricted activity. But within five months, the shortness of breath returned, together with pressure pain in the middle of the chest and faintness on physical exertion. By then it was apparent that the patient's activity would have to be greatly curtailed and that he would continue to experience great discomfort. Fortunately, surgery offered a way to restore the patient to health and something close to his normal daily routine.

Surgical repair of valves and their replacement with prosthetic artificial valves have been among the major developments in medicine over the past twenty-five to thirty years. These operations, the culmination of many scientific, surgical, and technical advances, have restored thousands to improved or normal health. From an engineering point of view, this kind of heart surgery seems simplicity itself. After all, the heart is a pump, and the valves the mechanical devices that allow it to work effectively. Unlike medications, which have no direct healing effect on the valves but merely allow the heart muscle and the rest of the body to cope with a valve defect, an operation can attack the problem and solve it where it originates, in the faulty valve itself. Valvular heart disease and surgery, moreover, are ideally suited for each other, since surgery is in a sense a "mechanical" approach to disease, and valve disease is a "mechanical" problem.

Although surgeons had tried for generations to operate on heart valves, significant progress was not made until the late 1940s. Inadequate opening of the mitral valve (mitral stenosis) was the first abnormality to be repaired through surgery, most likely because the nature of the defect lent itself easily

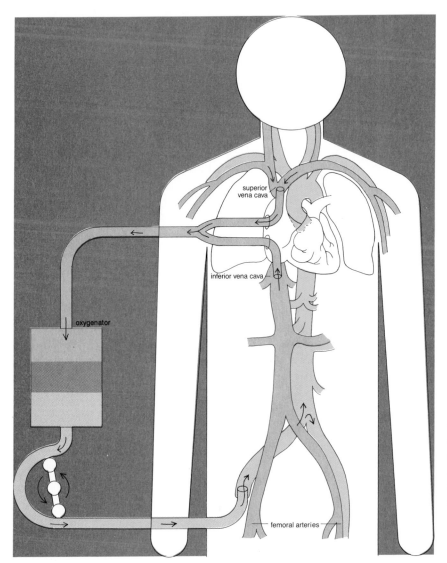

Venous blood returning to the heart is intercepted and passed through an oxygenator, where carbon dioxide is removed and oxygen is added. The oxygenated blood is then pumped into the arterial system.

to surgical intervention. As a result of rheumatic fever, the usual cause of the defect, the two leaflets of the mitral valve adhere to each other, although they may continue to be relatively flexible. The two leaflets need only be "unstuck" where they adhere, and the narrowing will be corrected. This can be accomplished in several ways by the surgeon's passing his finger into the beating heart and applying pressure by cutting any scar tissue which has formed, using a special knife fitted to the surgeon's finger; or by passing a dilating instrument through the valve. The operation, called mitral valvotomy (-tomy, cutting),was first performed on a beating heart in what is called "closed" heart surgery.

Since the development in the mid-1950s of the heart-lung machine, which assumes the functions of the patient's heart and lungs during an operation, surgeons have been able to see each of the valves as they work. This is the procedure called "open" heart surgery. With the heart stopped, dry, and visible to the surgeon, repairs can be made in other kinds of valve defects, including regurgitation of the mitral valve and either stenosis or regurgitation of the aortic or tricuspid valves. Congenital stenosis, one of the few disorders of the pulmonary valve, can also be repaired surgically.

The experience gained from open heart valve surgery convinced many surgeons that a number of valve diseases required more than repair. Often valve tissues were found to have such heavy deposits of calcium, or to have become so scarred and distorted, that simple reconstruction was not enough. Moreover, the calcium deposits and scar tissue were found to reappear within a few years after surgery. It became apparent that complete replacement would be the best remedy, especially with damaged aortic and mitral valves (diseased tricuspid valves do not often require replacement). But while the need for such replacement can be assumed from the patient's deteriorating condition and failure to respond to other treatment, the final decision regarding replacement (and often even reconstruction) is frequently not made until the surgeon actually sees the valve during open heart surgery.

The replacement of defective valves in human beings began in the 1950s, and many types of artificial valves have since been developed and inserted. At first, such operations were resorted to only in extreme cases, with patients who had no chance of survival without surgical replacement of totally defective valves. Although the artificial valves had been laboratory-tested, there was no certainty that they would perform well, and for long periods, in humans. To test the valves on animals for longevity, however, would have meant losing patients whose lives were in imminent danger, and the artificial valves were potential lifesavers. Experience fortunately proved that most of the artificial valves were quite durable, although some of the first patients to receive them returned for new and improved valves developed after their emergency surgery. Extensive monitoring and statistical analyses have continually been made of patients who have received all the various kinds of replacement valves. Much research has been devoted to the incidence, probable cause, and possible correction of the problems noted. Progress has been made, but research continues.

TYPES OF ARTIFICIAL VALVES There are three kinds of valves: ball, disk, and tissue. The ball valve, as the name implies, is basically a ball in a cage. When the ball is pushed by the forward flow of blood to the open end of the cage, blood passes freely through the valve. But when the heart's action would allow the blood to flow backward, the ball promptly falls into its closed position, preventing it. The ball rotates constantly in the bloodstream, minimizing wear. Very durable and long-lasting, the ball valve has been used so often and studied so extensively that medical science is aware of its advantages as well as its drawbacks.

The chief drawback of the ball valve is that blood clots occasionally form around the edges where it is sutured to the heart tissue. If such a clot breaks loose, it can be carried by the bloodstream. In a large artery the clot may be relatively harmless but in a small branch artery in the brain, kidneys, or heart, the clot could block the supply of oxygenated blood, resulting in significant or even serious damage. Because of this danger, patients take daily medication (an anticoagulant) to diminish the blood's clotting ability. Although such medication is not dangerous if carefully controlled by blood tests every three or four weeks, it is nevertheless not an ideal solution. It has been hoped that covering the metallic parts of the valve with a cloth meshwork would eliminate the need for anticoagulants. Subsequent studies have indicated, however, that such medication is needed even when "cloth-covered" valves have been used.

The disk valve was based initially on the same principle as the ball valve, except that instead of a ball that moved back and forth in a cage a flattened disk shifted back and forth. The disk offered no advantage over the ball valve, and it had a serious disadvantage: since it did not rotate about as freely as a ball, it showed a greater tendency to wear. Then a unique refinement was added: Instead of moving back and forth with the blood-stream, the disk was constructed to swing back and forth like a hingeless door. However, the free-floating and unhinged disk is restricted by the valve supports, so that it can only swing open and shut. The action of the valve, and therefore of the heart, is freer and more efficient because the blood does not have to detour when it passes through the valve. The disk valve has, how-ever, the same potential problem regarding the formation of blood clots, and anticoagulant medication is usually necessary after it has been implanted.

The tissue valve is made from donor tissues, such as an aortic valve taken from a human cadaver or from an animal, sometimes a pig. The tissue valve can also be constructed from strong flat membranes found in certain parts of the human body—the sturdy sheath that surrounds the brain (dura mater), the envelope in which the heart is encased (pericardium), and the fibrous layer protecting the muscles along the outside surface of the thigh (fascia lata). With the exception of those made from human membranes, all tissue valves are completely dead when inserted and thus do not stimulate the patient's body to reject them. Usually a tissue valve is mounted inside a special frame so that it can be properly fitted and securely attached.

The principal advantage of a tissue valve is that clot formation caused by it is minimal, and there is less need for long-term treatment with anti-coagulant medication. Although earlier methods for preserving tissue valves shortened their life span, making them dependable for only a few years, more sophisticated methods now in use seem likely to increase their dura-bility. Until this can be established, many surgeons continue to prefer an artificial, mechanical valve whose performance has already been tested.

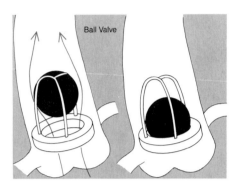

Ball valve replacing defective aortic valve rises under pressure of blood flow and falls into closed position when pressure drops.

PRINCIPLES

1. Each of the four chambers of the heart has a valve which permits blood to flow in only one direction. The

tricuspid valve lies between the upper chamber of the right side of the heart (right atrium) and the lower chamber (right ventricle). The pulmonary valve separates the right ventricle from the pulmonary artery, the vessel leading to the lungs. The mitral valve separates the left atrium from the left ventricle. The aortic valve is at the outlet of the left ventricular and the origin of the aorta.

2. *Valve malfunctioning has a number of causes, including rheumatic fever, bacterial infection, or congenital defects. Valves that do not close properly allow blood to leak back into the chamber from which it has just come. Valves may also not be able to open because of a narrowing of the opening. Both conditions force the heart to work harder and can result in serious cardiac conditions.*

3. *Symptoms of valve disease tend to appear gradually, usually fairly late in life. Victims of valve disease may notice that their hearts work harder during increased activity or emotional stress and that they suffer fatigue or shortness of breath. In some instances, valve disease causes symptoms of angina pectoris, particularly during physical exertion or emotional distress. Valve disease can also lead to the formation of blood clots and produce an abnormal heart rhythm.*

4. *Diagnosis of valve disease depends on examination with a stethoscope, chest X rays, electrocardiograms, blood tests, and in some instances cardiac catheterization and echocardiography.*

5. *Preferred treatment for severe cases of heart valve disease is surgical repair of the valve or replacement of the defective valve with an artificial valve or one constructed from tissue taken either from the patient or an animal. The prospect for an extended life after the operation is good, with the patient able to resume normal activity.*

In making the decision on when surgical replacement of a diseased valve is necessary, the cardiologist and the surgeon must consider the type of symptoms, heart size, severity of valve damage, findings from electrocardiograms, and other examination reports. If the decision is to defer surgery, careful re-evaluation at least yearly is usually necessary. The decision to replace a diseased valve is often actually made at the operating table, when the surgeon has had an opportunity to inspect the valve (or valves) at first hand. The safest time for surgery is before the heart and other organs have been so damaged that they can no longer return to normal even when the diseased valve has been repaired or replaced. On the other hand, it is not wise to proceed with surgery too early. Every type of replacement valve has some limitation. Even under the best of conditions, there is a definite although slight risk in the operation, and some patients can have valve malfunctions for prolonged periods before serious damage occurs.

If an operation seems desirable and even mandatory, great care will be taken to assure that the new valve will be securely and permanently attached and that the entire procedure will be conducted in a way that protects and preserves healthy heart muscle and other involved organs. After the operation, the patient will have the support of highly sophisticated intensive care units, where assistance can be provided to every vital organ of the body if there is evidence of fatigue or failure. After two or three days of such care, the patient may require another week or two in the hospital, although by the fifth or sixth day most of the discomfort will have eased and total bed rest is neither required nor desired. Most patients are eager to resume full activity by about the second month after the operation, but they are cautioned to avoid extended or unusual stress. They are also warned that antibiotic medication must be taken before and for a few days after any operation, including dental work and even routine instrumental dental cleaning. This holds true for the rest of their lives, since any germs that could get into the blood might lodge in the replacement valve and cause a potentially serious infection.

Heart surgery has made such remarkable advances in the last two decades that the risks from valve replacement are normally less than 5 percent with an experienced surgical team. (Certain cases, naturally, have a higher risk because of the nature and duration of the disease.) Although the life expectancy of a person with a replaced valve is somewhat lower than that for the general population, it is far better than it would be if the diseased valve had not been replaced. Heart valve surgery has given new prospects of health and long life to thousands, with the likelihood that thousands more will be helped as techniques and expertise continue to improve.

19

STROKE

Fletcher H. McDowell, M.D.

The modern computer is often compared to the brain, and in fact there has developed a whole popular mythology which imagines a world of supercomputers, outstripping the simple human brain in their ability to digest information, solve problems, and even feel emotions. In reality, however, the human brain far surpasses the capacity of the computer in most areas of information processing. The whole realm of emotions, imagination, and artistic creativity still remains distinctly "human." Nevertheless, it is helpful in understanding the brain to consider certain parallels between it and the computer. Both the brain and the computer are dependent on outside sources for the power to function properly, and any interruption in the source of power will have disastrous consequences. The computer requires energy and relies on electrical current, and any variation in the amount of current will seriously influence its working. The brain, too, requires energy, and the nourishment that energizes brain cells is produced by body chemistry through metabolism. The blood flow to the brain carries both oxygen, which all tissues require, and the elements that combine to produce minute but critical electrical impulses that are, in short, brain activity. Any interruption in that flow affects the functioning of the brain cells.

Medical science has long recognized the calamitous nature of a sudden break in the brain's energy supply, and as long ago as the beginning of the seventeenth century doctors used the word stroke to denote "an attack of disease, or an apoplectic seizure." Indeed, stroke is aptly named, for it is the third greatest disease threat to the lives of Americans. Although more people succumb to heart attacks and cancer, stroke claims 200,000 lives a year. Moreover, it has the dubious distinction of being the most expensive disease in the United States, costing about $1.2 billion a year exclusive of doctors' fees, nursing home costs, and nonhospital care and rehabilitation. Stroke is frequently called "cerebral vascular insult or accident," a term which implies that the disease strikes without warning and in random fashion. This notion is dangerously misleading, since there are many warning signs of impending stroke which, if heeded, can avert a disabling or fatal stroke. Moreover, some people are more prone to stroke than others, and its incidence can be reduced by proper health care, particularly control of high blood pressure. And while it is true that proper treatment after stroke can offer great potential for recovery, early detection and treatment are far more effective and less costly in money, time, and suffering.

CAUSES OF STROKE Stroke is usually the result of the death of brain tissue, either from a lack of blood supply or from bleeding into the tissues (cerebral hemorrhage). To understand how this happens, it is necessary to know how brain tissue utilizes and is sustained by the nutrients supplied by the bloodstream. The average adult brain weighs about 50 ounces (1417 grams) and requires about 1.5 ounces (45 milligrams) of oxygen per minute. To get this supply of oxygen to the brain, the lungs must exchange 4 gallons (6400 milliliters) of air, of which 20 percent is oxygen, and the heart must pump 1.5 quarts (750 milliliters) of blood per minute for the brain alone. Twenty percent of the total output of blood pumped from the heart goes to the brain, or in other words, the brain consumes about 20 percent of all the oxygen consumed by the body.

The brain not only demands a great deal of oxygen; it demands it constantly, being unable to tolerate loss of oxygen for more than a few seconds. As soon as oxygen delivery to the entire brain or any portion of it declines below critical levels or ceases altogether, the brain rapidly suffers damage. The resulting damage to nerve cells may be temporary, but it is more often permanent. If blood flow is not quickly restored, the brain tissue dies and cannot regenerate. If the tissue dies, there is no possibility of restored function. This brain tissue damage is ultimately reflected in failure of the part of the body controlled by the affected part of the brain.

Strokes manifest themselves in a variety of ways, and the clue to the nature of any specific kind of stroke lies in the anatomy of the cerebral circulation. The brain is supplied by four arteries; the right and left internal carotid arteries, and the right and left vertebral arteries. The left carotid artery rises directly from the aortic arch; the right carotid from the innominate artery, which itself rises from the aortic arch adjacent to the left carotid artery.

Both carotid arteries run in a parallel course to the head, following paths in the front part of the neck on each side of the esophagus. The two vertebral arteries arise from the subclavian arteries (the main arteries that supply the arms), travel up the back of the neck, then enter the head through a canal in the bony part of the spinal column. As is apparent from their position, the internal carotid arteries nourish the front (the largest) part of the brain, the right carotid artery feeding the right half and the left carotid the left half. The vertebral arteries supply the back of the brain, including the brain stem, the cerebellum, and the upper part of the spinal cord. The lower portion of the brain is supplied directly by the vertebral arteries; the upper part, however, is supplied by the basilar artery, which is formed by the juncture of the two vertebral arteries at the base of the brain. All these arteries are interconnected at the base of the brain by smaller communicating arteries in a system called the Circle of Willis.

An obstruction or block in the left carotid artery will cause tissue death in the left side of the brain but the symptoms of stroke will appear on the right side of the body, and the opposite occurs with the right carotid artery. Obstruction in the vertebral arteries causes tissue death in the brain stem; this kind of stroke can involve one or both sides of the body. An obstruction below the Circle of Willis can be compensated for by blood flow from the opposite side, since the Circle is the channel which allows blood to circulate from side to side. While this system protects the brain from reduced flow, any congenital defects in the Circle (connections that are too small or absent interconnections) make a stroke more likely.

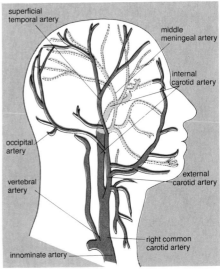

Arterial Route to the Brain

The intricate network bringing blood to all parts of the brain.

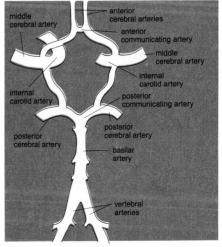

Circle of Willis

Smaller arteries in the Circle of Willis at the base of the brain link the main arteries, so that oxygenated blood can be delivered by alternate routes.

The symptoms of brain tissue death depend on the brain areas and arteries involved. For example, if tissue death occurs in the back (posterior) parts of the cerebral cortex, vision will be affected, since that part of the brain controls visual function. The front of the brain deals with motor function, and the area between it and the vision-controlling area is responsible for the reception and interpretation of sensation. Any tissue death in these control centers will manifest itself in the corresponding body function.

CONTROL CENTERS OF THE BRAIN

Other parts of the body are controlled by sections on the surface of the cortex, from the top of the brain to the lower edge of one hemisphere. At the top of the brain, the motor and sensory areas control the function of the foot, leg, and hip; the lateral surface from the top downward contains control areas for the motor function of trunk, shoulder, arm, hand, head, and neck. At various levels of the brain stem there are collections of cells which supply the musculature of such head and neck functions as eye movement, jaw and face movement, swallowing, vocalization, phonation, and tongue movement. Damage to these brain stem cells will produce disruption of some or all of these functions.

Cerebral injury (or infarction) may occur in the territory of the middle cerebral artery, the supply source for the side and the most central parts of the cerebral hemispheres. Infarction of this region causes paralysis and sensory loss on the opposite side of the body from the site of infarction, specifically the face, neck, arm, and hand. Both motor and sensory functions will be affected. Because the visual pathway goes through this section of the brain, there may be loss of half the vision field—that is, half the field of vision normally seen with the eyes fixed straight ahead. This usually encompasses about 90 degrees to each side and because of the limits imposed by brows and cheeks, about 80 degrees down and 60 degrees up. An infarction in the dominant hemisphere may result in loss of speech, loss of the ability to understand speech, or both. When the anterior cerebral artery is obstructed, the infarction results in paralysis and sensory loss in the hip, leg, and foot on the side of the body opposite that of the infarction. Obstruction of the posterior cerebral artery which supplies the visual cortex produces blindness in one field of vision (hemianopsia).

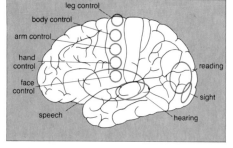

Different areas of the brain control bodily functions.

More varied clinical patterns occur when there is an obstruction of the arteries supplying the brain stem. Blockage of the arteries supplying the most posterior and most lateral parts (posterior inferior cerebellar arteries) causes difficulty in swallowing, tongue paralysis, loss of sensation on one side of the face and on the opposite side of the body, and difficulty in accurately coordinating movements on one side (ataxia). Obstruction of arteries supplying the upper portion of the brain stem leads to paralysis of eye movement, loss of sensation on one side of the body, and paralysis or weakness on one side with difficulty in performing accurate movements on the opposite side. When arteries supplying the base of the brain stem are obstructed, there may be bilateral paralysis, varying degrees of loss of the ability to communicate, and loss of consciousness. Patients with infarctions in the brain stem often appear to be awake but are unable to move or speak. Infarctions of this nature are less common but more serious than infarctions in the brain hemispheres.

CEREBRAL INFARCTION The most common cause of stroke death of brain tissues (infarction) is a result of reduction of loss of blood flow and oxygen to a part of the brain due to hardening of the arteries, or atherosclerosis. Atherosclerosis is one of the most common diseases of mankind, and while it is generally thought to be a problem of the aged, evidence of it can also be found in the blood vessels of children and adolescents. The disease does increase in extent and severity with age, however, so that only 4 percent of those aged eighty-five or over escape it. Atherosclerosis in the blood vessels of the heart is the most common cause of heart attack; in vessels leading to the head, it is the most common cause of stroke. The kind of disability suffered by a stroke victim is clearly related to the hardening and thickening of arteries supplying the area of the brain that controlled the body function impaired by the stroke.

Stroke is most common between the ages of sixty and eighty, and while it is more frequent in males until about the age of seventy-five, the incidence after that age is almost equal for males and females. Such factors as high blood pressure, diabetes, obesity, elevated blood lipids, smoking, and lack of exercise have been shown to increase the chance of developing atherosclerosis and its complications. Control or elimination of these factors is important in preventing stroke, although correcting them after a stroke has occurred has little effect on recovery or rehabilitation.

Cerebral embolism is another common cause of stroke due to infarction. An embolus (literally, a stopper) is a bit of clot or other material that has broken off from another site in the body (including heart valves or walls, blood clots in the heart, or materials on the walls of vessels affected by atherosclerosis). The material is caught in the bloodstream, and if it lodges in an artery feeding the brain, blood flow is reduced, brain tissue is injured or dies, and symptoms of stroke appear. The abrupt onset of symptoms, common with strokes, is most characteristic of cerebral embolus, usually beginning within a matter of minutes. (The onset for cerebral infarction from atherosclerotic obstruction may be spread over several hours.) Cerebral embolus is most common after heart attacks and in those with rheumatic heart disease and ulcerated atherosclerotic plaques.

While the onset of a stroke is usually abrupt and dramatic, there are frequent occasions when symptoms suggesting stroke appear and then fade in minutes or hours. These episodes are called transient ischemic attacks and are important signals, indicating the presence of serious cerebral atherosclerosis before infarction occurs. Weakness of one side, involving the face and arm and to a lesser extent the leg, may occur. If the left side of the brain is affected, there may be temporary difficulty in speaking. Temporary loss of vision in one eye, sometimes accompanied by weakness in the opposite arm and side of the face, is associated with obstruction and reduced blood flow in the internal carotid artery system. When the reduced blood flow is in the vertebral artery, symptoms include transient loss of vision in both eyes, double vision, vertigo, hearing loss, difficulty in swallowing, and difficulty in speaking. The symptoms of transient cerebral ischemia are often so brief and minor that they are ignored or forgotten, but they should be recognized as important advance warnings, giving the physician an opportunity to begin preventive treatment.

Transient Stroke Symptoms

The most common symptoms of cerebral infarction are weakness or complete paralysis on one side, with the lower part of the face and the arm more involved than the leg. Perception of pain, touch, temperature, sense of movement, and ability to determine the size, weight, and nature of objects may also be decreased or absent. Although the stroke victim is not aware of any loss of vision, examination may show that there is an actual loss of half the field of vision either to the right or to the left.

Cerebral infarction on the left side of the brain, the dominant hemisphere, may result in speech impairment, a condition called aphasia. There may be

Symptoms of Cerebral Infarction

total loss of the ability to speak or great difficulty in finding and expressing the correct word, great reduction in vocabulary, and difficulty in understanding what is being said by others. At times the victim may be able to speak, but the words uttered are without sense or completely trivial.

Cerebral infarction in the right hemisphere may result in loss of spatial orientation, so severe at times that the patient may not recognize the paralyzed limb as his own. Under these conditions, it is impossible to perform simple activities like dressing and eating.

Symptoms of brain-stem infarction are more varied, usually involving a combination of impaired eye movement, sensory loss, and difficulty in making accurate movements; or a combination of impaired eye movement and weakness of one side or both.

Examination and Diagnosis

The presence of the symptoms described indicates the existence of cerebral infarction. Further examination may also reveal evidence of heart disease, elevated blood pressure, and diabetes. The physician may detect murmurs or noises in the blood vessels of the neck. These sounds, called bruits, indicate turbulent blood flow at the site, and they point to the location of the arterial disease often outside the brain itself. Although X rays of the head are rarely helpful in diagnosis of stroke, they are routinely carried out to determine if the symptoms are the result of head injury rather than infarction. The record of brain impulses (electroencephalogram) taken after a cerebral infarction is usually abnormal and helps to localize the site of infarction. Normally rapid brain waves are greatly slowed in the region of infarction, returning to their customary rate with improvement of motor and sensory functions.

Brain scans (including computerized scans) are used to outline the area of infarction and to help identify any other causes of the symptoms, such as brain tumor and head injury. Examination of the suspected stroke victim may also involve arteriography, a diagnostic test whereby blood vessels to and within the brain are visualized. The test can be performed in two ways; either

A stroke on the right side of the brain causes paralysis on the left side of the body; a stroke on the left side of the brain causes paralysis on the right side of the body.

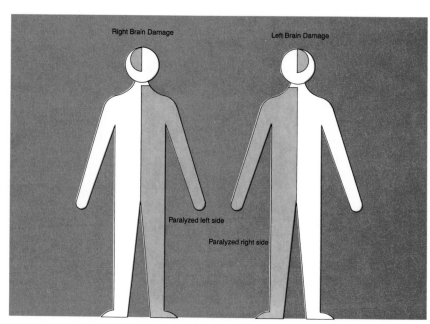

Right Brain Damage

Left Brain Damage

Paralyzed left side

Paralyzed right side

by injecting a radio-opaque contrast medium directly into the carotid arteries in the neck, or by inserting a catheter in the main artery of the leg in the region of the groin and threading it up the aorta to the point where the carotid arteries branch off. An injection of a contrast medium will outline all the cerebral arteries in the neck; with careful placement of the catheter, vessels can be visualized one at a time.

Arteriography helps to determine whether the symptoms are those of stroke or of another condition with a similar clinical picture. It also shows the condition of the cerebral arteries and the site, extent, and character of arterial obstruction and ulceration. Clear and precise information of this nature is essential in determining whether surgery is needed. The test is safe and largely without complication; reactions to the procedure occur no more frequently than one in a hundred and more serious problems at about half that rate. Some reactions are the result of problems at the site of injection, and there are rarer instances of reaction due either to sensitivity to iodine (in the radio-opaque contrast medium) or to the effects of injecting a concentrated solution into a cerebral artery.

Treatment of cerebral infarction is focused on prevention, acute care, and rehabilitation. Prevention, of course, must be stressed, because once stroke occurs there are usually severe losses in mental and body functions. Prevention is directed toward correcting the factors which hasten the development of atherosclerosis and its later complications. Hypertension is the most important of these factors and the one that is most amenable to correction. (See Hypertension, chapter 10.) A significant reduction in the chances of developing a stroke has been shown to be associated with the adoption of a program designed to produce sustained lowering of blood pressure in those identified with hypertension.

Treatment of Cerebral Infarction

Another preventive measure is the identification and treatment of individuals with transient ischemic attacks. Evaluation by cerebral angiography may reveal surgically accessible lesions which, if removed, would reduce the chances of a stroke. (Only lesions in the cerebral arteries in the neck can be treated in this manner.) It is also possible to prevent transient ischemic attacks by administering anticoagulants over periods of six months or less, but there are drawbacks to this kind of treatment. Some conditions are aggravated by anticoagulants, and there must be close, at least monthly, monitoring to prevent overdoses or underdoses.

The realization that many transient ischemic attacks are caused by emboli from ulcerated areas of atherosclerosis in cerebral arteries has opened a new approach to stroke prevention. The platelets which make up the emboli function as circulating "tire patches," plugging holes in the lining of arteries. If the wall of an artery is damaged, certain chemical changes cause platelets to adhere to one another and to the damaged arterial wall surface. Emboli capable of blocking cerebral circulation occur when the platelets break off and enter the bloodstream. Most often the emboli are small and the blockage they cause is transient, giving rise to transient symptoms, but larger ones can cause permanent obstruction and result in cerebral infarction. It is now known that a number of chemical agents, including simple aspirin, prevent platelets from adhering to arterial ulcers. The chemicals have been effective in stop-

Surgical Methods for Reducing Risk of Stroke

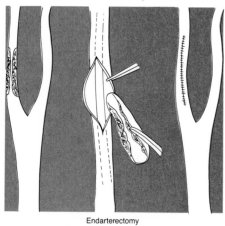

Endarterectomy

Plaques obstructing blood flow are removed from the arterial wall to restore normal blood supply to the brain.

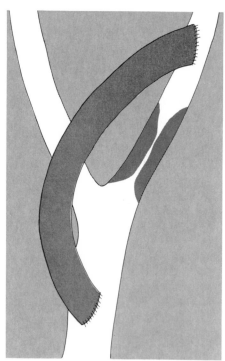

Bypass Graft

In large occlusive lesions, blood flow to the brain is restored by grafting arterial routes around the occlusive lesion.

ping transient ischemic attacks and are now being evaluated in the United States and Canada to test their effectiveness in preventing stroke.

Acute care for a patient with cerebral infarction involves maintaining respiration, blood pressure, and fluid intake if these functions are failing. This usually happens only in the case of very severe infarctions, where the mortality rate is high and disability in survivors frequent. In cases of moderate or mild infarction, acute care is mainly concerned with accuracy of diagnosis and a program of physical therapy. The latter is important to avoid such complications as joint fixation and tendon and muscle shortening in paralyzed limbs. As the acute effects of a stroke wear off, most patients show some spontaneous improvement. This natural recovery generally continues for about three months. Recovery occurring in the following six to eighteen months involves the learning of new skills with parts of the body not affected by the stroke. There is no treatment yet known that can speed natural recovery, regenerate brain tissue, or reduce the extent of an infarction.

Treatment of cerebral infarction that has resulted from a cerebral embolus centers on determining the source of the embolus and treating it, since further episodes are likely to occur if the causes of the emboli are not removed. Cardiac surgery or treatment with anticoagulants may be required in cases of rheumatic heart disease or damaged heart valves. In the case of narrowing of the mitral valve opening (mitral stenosis), anticoagulants will reduce the chance of clot formation and hence of recurrent cerebral emboli. Such conditions are lifelong and therefore require continued treatment. Anticoagulants have also been found effective in reducing the chances of subsequent stroke when administered for from thirty to sixty days (the period of greatest danger of recurrence) after a cerebral embolus has followed a heart attack.

Rehabilitation therapy is designed to teach new skills and new ways of functioning by circumventing the motor and sensory defects of a stroke. Although these skills are often learned spontaneously and with little outside help, more often a formal program is needed. Well-planned programs, adequately staffed with trained personnel, can take as little as forty to sixty days. The initial therapy should be conducted by trained professionals, but the stroke victim's family and friends can and should learn the basic approach to the therapy and how to help the victim. For example, although there may be no sensation in a paralyzed arm, there can be pain in the shoulder joint from the steady weight of the immobilized arm. This can be relieved by the use of a simple sling or by propping the arm on a pillow. If the paralyzed hand is clenched tight, it is important to keep the fingernails trimmed short to avoid cutting the palm.

Following a stroke, muscles in paralyzed arms and legs shrink, often causing soreness. A program of physical exercise can help to restore muscle length and also help the patient learn ways to use the muscles again. Neurological loss may require learning to walk with leg braces, canes, or walkers. There are many special devices that make living with the aftermath of stroke more comfortable and more dignified: table utensils that can be used with one hand alone, shoes that do not have to be laced, seats and protective handles that make it possible to take baths and showers, and toilet seats with adjustable levels.

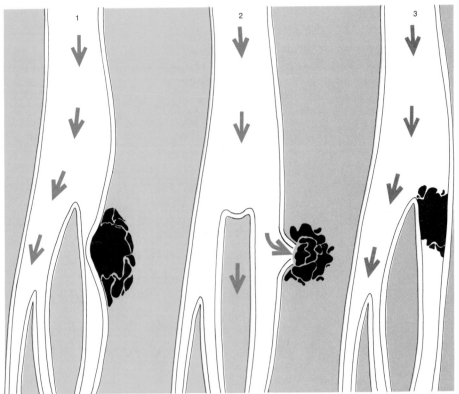

1. Blood clot lodged in an artery in the neck or the brain obstructs blood flow, depriving tissues of essential oxygen.

2. Blood flowing into brain tissue through a ruptured arterial wall destroys brain tissue directly or indirectly by compression.

3. Compression of an artery by pooling of blood in brain tissue or a tumor compresses blood vessels, cutting off or reducing blood supply.

Principal Causes of Stroke

CEREBRAL HEMORRHAGE

Cerebral hemorrhage, the other principal cause of stroke, results when an artery ruptures and bleeds into the substance of the brain or into the fluid-filled spaces over the surface of the brain. While the several different causes of cerebral hemorrhage produce similar symptoms, the differences in their basic mechanism mean that the treatment will vary.

Bleeding into the substance of the brain tissue either destroys tissue directly or forms pools of blood (hematoma) which compress brain tissue. This blood and the ensuing swelling (edema) cause the brain to expand and to become distorted in parts and compressed in others, thus compromising the blood supply. The complications of hemorrhage can be serious enough to result in impairment of vital functions, loss of consciousness, and death. The effects of bleeding over the surface of the brain are not as serious, for while the increase of pressure in the head may result in intense headache and loss of consciousness, the neurological loss is not great.

Bleeding within the brain substance, primary intracerebral hemorrhage, is associated with severe high blood pressure and with the presence of small defects on artery walls deep inside the brain. Elevated blood pressure causes the walls in these areas to thin and bulge and eventually to burst. Blood spurting from the rupture distorts nearby tissue, destroying some and causing swelling. In a massive hemorrhage, the fluid-filled spaces in the brain (ventricles) fill with blood, and internal brain pressure increases. The cerebral hemispheres are forced through a narrow gap into the posterior parts of the skull, with resultant compression of the brain stem. The results are sudden loss of consciousness and death.

Primary Intracerebral Hemorrhage Primary intracerebral hemorrhage is the second most common kind of intracranial hemorrhage and is clearly associated with high blood pressure, being more prevalent among those who have a history of high blood pressure. (The incidence is highest among the black population and seems to be greater in the southeastern sections of the United States.) The characteristic symptoms are sudden severe headache, nausea, and vomiting, followed by loss of consciousness. At times the onset may seem indistinguishable from that of cerebral infarction, with sudden weakness or paralysis on one side of the body without loss of consciousness. A minor hemorrhage usually results in headache and neurological deficit without loss of consciousness; but in a massive attack headache is usually followed by coma, with death the usual result.

Examination of a victim of primary intracerebral hemorrhage almost invariably reveals high blood pressure, narrowing of the retinal arteries, and other pathological changes in the eye visible through an ophthalmoscope. These eye changes, together with enlargement of the heart, suggest that the victim has had elevated blood pressure for a long time. At times the patient is able to respond to stimuli, in which case the kind of paralysis and sensory loss may give some indication of which side of the brain is involved. But as a rule the victim is deeply unconscious or in a coma, unresponsive to any form of stimulation and showing no evidence of spontaneous movement of the extremities. Respiration may fail, making artificial ventilation necessary. The mortality rate is extremely high—up to 90 percent—and major disabilities are suffered by the few who survive.

Diagnosis of intracranial hemorrhage is confirmed by the presence of blood in the cerebral spinal fluid, obtained by means of a spinal tap. More sophisticated forms of examination may be used, but since the information gained rarely changes the victim's condition or treatment, such tests are usually deferred. One of these procedures, computerized brain scannings, is useful in demonstrating the existence of hemorrhage in the brain and, more important, eliminating as causes such less serious and at times more easily treatable conditions as brain tumor and subdural hematoma, a pool of blood between the outer membrane of the brain and the skull. X rays are not useful, except to eliminate the possibility of head injury; arteriograms, however, are often needed to help establish the site of hemorrhage and to eliminate such causes as a ruptured aneurysm and ruptured arteriovenous anomalies. An electroencephalogram will reveal slowing of brain impulses over the area of damage; if the patient is unconscious, the entire recording of brain waves will show marked slowing of wave frequency.

Treatment of primary intracerebral hemorrhage is largely concerned with keeping the patient alive in the hope that some functions may recover spontaneously. Breathing is assisted and blood pressure maintained; if pressure is extremely high, antihypertensive drugs are administered to reduce it to normal levels.

If the patient survives the initial attack, and there is continued and severe loss of neurological function, arteriograms or computerized brain scanning are used to locate a possible blood clot or hematoma within the brain. Surgical removal of a clot often hastens improvement and lessens disability. Long-term treatment of elevated blood pressure, together with a rehabilitation program for neurological disability, are essential in continuing care.

The most common kind of intracranial hemorrhage is subarachnoid hemorrhage, the result of a ruptured berry aneurysm in a blood vessel that lies beneath the arachnoid membrane, the middle of three membranes covering the brain. Aneurysms are blood-filled pouches that balloon out from a weak spot in an artery wall and are usually found where the artery branches. Berry aneurysms are most often found on the large arteries at the base of the brain around the Circle of Willis. Bleeding from a ruptured berry aneurysm may be confined to the fluid-filled surface of the brain or may penetrate into the brain substance.

Symptoms, determined by the areas of the brain involved, almost invariably include severe headache, beginning abruptly either on one side of the head or behind the eye. The pain, described by victims as the most intense ever experienced, may cause brief loss of consciousness at first and then may become generalized over the entire head. If bleeding has occurred only over the surface of the brain, there will be no paralysis or sensory loss. Bleeding into the brain is likely to produce neurological deficit and other symptoms, depending on the areas involved. For example, aneurysms on the middle cerebral artery often cause motor and sensory abnormalities on the opposite side of the body. Aneurysms on the anterior cerebral artery can cause damage in the frontal lobes of both sides, causing such changes in personality as apathy and indifference. Aneurysms on the posterior cerebral artery can cause defects in visual fields.

On examination, the victim of a subarachnoid hemorrhage usually shows some elevation of blood pressure, lethargy and drowsiness, a stiff neck, and headache if moved. Neurologic deficits may include paralysis on one side of the body, sensory loss, defects in vision fields, and symptoms related to the local effects of the aneurysm rather than to its impact on the brain; among these are ocular palsy or dilatation of a pupil. Some degree of one-sided paralysis is usual, and there may be hemorrhage around the optic nerve under the retina and even into the posterior chamber of the eye.

Laboratory examination includes a lumbar puncture to demonstrate the presence of blood in the subarachnoid space. Since blood in the spinal fluid is often caused by the spinal puncture itself, special care must be taken to exclude this as the cause of bleeding. Skull X rays are necessary to rule out unrecognized head injury as a cause of bleeding. While computerized scans can detect bleeding in the brain, aneurysms are too small to be detected by brain scans. Arteriography is the only available diagnostic technique useful for this purpose, with an accuracy rate of almost 90 percent. All the intracranial vessels must be visualized, because aneurysms are frequently multiple and those that have ruptured must be identified before surgical treatment can be given.

Immediate treatment is designed to preserve and assist vital functions and to relieve headache pain and stiff neck. Long-range treatment is aimed at preventing recurrence by removing the aneurysm from the cerebral circulatory system, by promoting clotting within the aneurysm, and by eliminating factors associated with recurrent bleeding, among them high blood pressure.

Prevention is especially important in subarachnoid hemorrhage, not only because little can be done after hemorrhage takes place, but because each recurrence carries a risk almost as great as the first—there is a mortality rate

Subarachnoid Hemorrhage

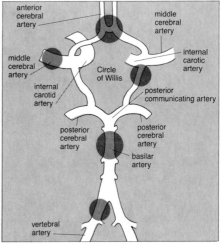

Common Sites of Aneurysm

PRINCIPLES

1. *Strokes are due to obstructions in, or hemorrhages of, blood vessels in and around the brain. These vessels (and the carotid and vertebral arteries as well) are subject to atherosclerosis, with subsequent narrowing of the passageway for blood flow. They may also be obstructed by a clot formed at the narrowed segment, or by a clot that formed elsewhere in the cardiovascular system and drifted to the narrowed artery.*

2. *In stroke, brain tissue is injured or dies because of lack of blood supply or because bleeding from a blood vessel in the brain has destroyed brain cells.*

3. *The left and right internal carotid arteries and the left and right vertebral arteries are the major sources of blood supply to the brain. These four arteries feed into a series of smaller vessels inside the head.*

4. *Obstruction of blood flow through the left carotid artery affects tissue in the left side of the brain. (The left side of the brain controls the right side of the body and vice versa.) Blockage in the right carotid affects the right side of the brain. Obstructions in the vertebal arteries cause strokes that affect either one or both sides of the brain.*

5. *A stroke caused by a clot is indicated by sudden symptoms of weakness or loss of power over limbs, loss of speech, dizziness, and unconsciousness. The symptoms may also be spread over hours. Strokes due to hemorrhage often show progressive symptoms and may be accompanied by headache. Transient strokes are episodes in which the blood supply to brain tissue is interrupted only momentarily. Symptoms usually pass after several minutes, or hours, but these warning signals should be reported at once to the physician.*

6. *Diagnosis of stroke is made by examination of blood vessels, brain scans, and electroencephalograms. These locate the area of damage. Arteriography, the visualization of blood vessels, can indicate whether the problem is in the carotid or vertebral arteries. Hemorrhage is detected by the presence of blood in the spinal fluid.*

7. *Preventive measures include lowering blood pressure if elevated and lessening the threat of atherosclerosis. For those who have already suffered transient attacks, surgery may be necessary to open up narrowed segments of the major arteries to the head. Drugs, including aspirin, may prevent the formation of embolisms which can block blood vessels in the brain.*

8. *Stroke patients require careful care. Respiration, blood pressure, and fluid intake must be maintained and steps taken to prevent recurrence of stroke. Rehabilitative therapy should be instituted as quickly as possible to restore control over muscles and to teach ways of compensation for lost motor and sensory control.*

of almost 50 percent associated with the first episode. There is, moreover, some evidence that this kind of hemorrhage is an important cause of sudden death. Nearly one-half of afflicted individuals die before reaching a hospital, and although a wide age group is affected, younger victims predominate. Standard preventive treatment of a ruptured aneurysm is surgical removal of the aneurysm itself, or its removal from the cerebral circulation. Success of surgery depends on the shape and size of the aneurysm and its position in the cerebral vascular system. A small aneurysm without a neck is very difficult to treat surgically, nor is surgery desirable if it will cause damage to the brain. In these cases, aneurysms can be removed only by blocking the flow in the parent artery (aneurysms of the anterior cerebral artery are particularly difficult to treat).

Because patients in coma or in a lethargic state do not respond well to surgery, the operation is usually delayed until such effects have passed, usually several days and up to ten days after hemorrhage. Since this is also the period when the chance of recurrence is greatest, the physician must weigh the risk of surgery against the possibility of renewed hemorrhage. Surgery that must be delayed into the second or third week is often of dubious value, since the danger of complications from the surgery itself are by then almost equal to the chance of rebleeding.

Surgical treatments are designed to reduce arterial pressure in the blood vessels feeding the aneurysm or to clip the neck of the aneurysm or remove it entirely. Surgery is least successful for aneurysms of the middle cerebral artery and the anterior cerebral artery.

Although careful control of blood pressure with antihypertensive medication can prevent recurrence of bleeding, the problems of maintaining the controls are such that few physicians or patients are willing to use this treatment. Another medication, amino-caproic (Amicar R), used in treating subarachnoid hemorrhage, has as yet yielded only equivocal results. Its use reduces the chances that the normal body mechanism might dissolve a clot in the ruptured aneurysm and cause bleeding.

20

CARDIOVASCULAR SURGERY

Russell M. Nelson, M.D.

The renowned nineteenth-century German physician, Theodore Billroth, who pioneered in the field of abdominal surgery, insisted that the heart itself was beyond the reach of the scalpel. "Any surgeon who wishes to preserve the respect of his colleagues would never attempt to suture the heart" was one of his admonitions, and in the context of his time it was well founded. It would be seventy-five years before technology and knowledge equipped surgeons to invade the sacred precincts of the heart with any hope of success. And even today, most people feel qualms at the notion of a surgeon working inside one's own heart. Such feelings are perfectly natural, for the heart is, as all instinctively know, what the great William Harvey called "the first principle of life." Heart surgery is a major operation requiring great skill of the doctor and his assisting technicians, as well as complex life-supporting machinery. Yet tens of thousands of heart operations are performed annually in the United States and the rate of success is extremely high.

The decision for cardiovascular surgery is made by the patient and the patient's family in consultation with the family doctor and the cardiovascular surgeon. Every individual is unique, and so is every heart condition. The medical team that conducts heart surgery operations is trained to respect this uniqueness; the patient need not hesitate to make his own feelings and needs known in the preoperative period. He should also be supported by the knowledge that even in the most radical type of cardiovascular surgery, open-heart surgery, thousands of operations are performed every year with a remarkably high degree of success.

Cardiovascular surgery is designed to repair congenital and acquired defects of the heart or the major vessels, thereby improving body function and prolonging life. The kinds of patients that need cardiovascular surgery are as diverse as the operations themselves, ranging from the newborn "blue baby," to the young mother with a narrowing of her mitral valve, the middle-aged executive on the verge of a massive heart attack, and the grandmother awakened in the night by a severe pain in her right leg caused by the shutting off of blood supply in a major artery. Each requires a special kind of cardiovascular surgery and therefore special care, and yet some aspects of treatment before, during, and after surgery are the same for all patients.

PREOPERATIVE CARE The preoperative care of all candidates for cardiovascular surgery is critically important. The patient must enter the operating room in the best possible physiological and psychological state. The first step in achieving that goal is to record the patient's medical history, as a guide to treatment. The history documents when and how the illness began, the medications that have been taken, individual sensitivity or allergic reactions to drugs or antibiotics, and any tendency to excessive bleeding. It is important to know which medications the patient is taking, because some must be stopped before surgery; among these are digitalis, diuretics, aspirin, and anticoagulants (blood thinners).

A complete physical examination is the next essential, because an incidental discovery of infection—respiratory, urinary, teeth, or skin—can sometimes postpone the decision to undertake cardiovascular surgery. The examination may also uncover a previously undiagnosed condition which could affect the outcome of surgery if not taken into consideration.

Cardiac patients are usually admitted to the hospital two days before surgery, although some may require longer preoperative care for control of heart failure and disorders of cardiac rhythm. During the period of bed rest before the operation, the patient is given antibiotics to protect against possible infection, and special soap is provided to reduce the number of skin bacteria. Blood and urine are evaluated by laboratory tests, chest X rays assess the condition of the heart and lungs, and an electrocardiogram records the electrical activity of the heart. The results of all these tests provide a basis for comparison with subsequent changes before, during, and after the operation. In addition, special diagnostic studies, such as angiography, cardiac catheterization, or echocardiography, may be needed.

ANGIOGRAPHY This technique is used to examine the condition of blood vessels. A solution that is visible on X rays is injected into the vessel, outlining it for study. The procedure is done most frequently on arterial blood vessels (arteriography), but it is also done on venous blood vessels (phlebography). Several kinds of arteriograms may be taken, including one that examines the aorta, the main artery leading from the heart, and its immediate branches (aortogram). Other arteriograms visualize the arteries leading to the brain, the coronary arteries, the kidneys, the legs and other areas. In these procedures, the patient is given a local anesthetic and an opaque dye solution is injected through a needle or small tube inserted in the artery. The X-ray film reveals the location of an obstruction to the flow of blood and helps the surgeon decide whether an operation would be helpful.

CARDIAC CATHERIZATION This is accomplished by passing a long, narrow hollow tube through a blood vessel in an arm or a leg and into the chambers of the heart. The catheter allows the doctor to measure pressure, take samples of blood, and make other studies to determine the presence of obstructions or impairments in valve function and the structure of the heart. Angiographic procedures may be included as part of this examination.

ECHOCARDIOGRAPHY In this procedure a small instrument called a transducer is placed on the patient's chest. It emits high-frequency sound waves across the heart, and the reflection of these waves is recorded on the surface of the instrument at the same time that an electrocardiogram is being taken. The two tests give information about the motion and anatomy of the structures in and around the heart, much as sonar techniques (also reflected sound waves) give information on the movement of a school of fish.

The patient's stay in the hospital before an operation allows time for staff members to answer his questions and to allay the inevitable anxieties that are felt before any major operation. The psychological state of the patient may be improved if he is informed about the functions and responsibilities of the members of the cardiac operating team, which includes the chief surgeon, the first assistant, an anesthesiologist, circulating and instrument nurses, a perfusionist, a computer technician, and an orderly.

The chief surgeon, assisted by another qualified surgeon, controls and directs THE OPERATION the entire operating procedure. The anesthesiologist, a doctor who has specialized in the administration of anesthesia, is responsible for initiating and continuing anesthetic "sleep" and for supportive care during the operation. Preparation of the operating room is the responsibility of the circulating and instrument nurses, who also record data and dispense sterile equipment and instruments to the surgeons. The perfusionist operates the heart-lung machine during open-heart surgery. The computer technician connects the patient to a computer which monitors the patient's responses, and these are relayed to the surgeon. The orderly helps transport the patient to and from the operating room. All operating room personnel wear special cotton suits, masks, hats, and shoes to minimize the risk of infection. Those actually participating in the operation scrub thoroughly and wear sterile gowns and gloves. When the operation is about to begin, the anesthesiologist gives the anesthetic compounds that put the patient to sleep, and during the operation, he continuously monitors arterial and venous blood pressure, electrocardiograms, urinary output, and other data which indicate the patient's condition.

Heart Surgery

Heart surgery can be closed or open. Closed-heart surgery is performed without halting the pumping action of the heart and without exposing the interior of the heart. In open heart surgery, the pumping action is halted, the interior of the heart is visible, and the surgeon works in a "dry field"—that is, where there is no blood circulating.

Because of its position in the chest, the heart may be approached from the right, left, or front. (The heart lies in the lower mid-central portion of the chest, is protected by the breastbone and the ribs, and is completely enveloped in a tough protective membrane called the pericardial sac.) When the heart is approached from the right or left side, an incision is made (a lateral thoracotomy), the ribs are spread gently apart, the pericardial sac is opened, and the heart is exposed. When cardiac repairs have been made, the surgeon closes the opening in the chest by passing strong sutures about the ribs, to bring them back together. When the heart is approached from the front (a median sternotomy) the sternum (breastbone) is severed by a power saw and the pericardial sac is opened. Afterward, the sternum is brought together and held in place by stainless steel wires or other strong suture material. The wires provide complete immobilization of the two parts of the sternum while it heals and do not have to be removed because they are tolerated by the body as easily as a filling in a tooth.

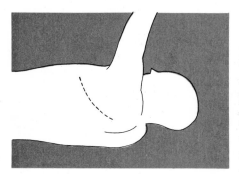

Posterior Lateral Thoracic Incision. When the heart is approached from the side, an incision is made, the ribs are spread gently apart, the pericardial sac is opened, and the heart is exposed.

The Heart-Lung Machine

The heart-lung (cardiopulmonary bypass) machine supplies oxygenated blood to the body while the heart is undergoing repairs. This machine intercepts blood before it enters the heart (from the venous or right side), aerates it (as the lungs would do), and then returns it to the arterial system by way of the aorta, keeping the tissues provided with life-sustaining blood. While the blood is circulating in the machine, the natural clotting mechanism is temporarily suspended by the use of heparin, an anticoagulant. When natural circulation is restored, the effect of the heparin is reversed by protamine sulfate, which restores normal coagulation.

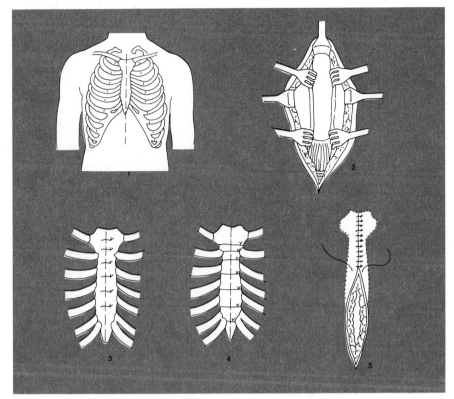

Median Sternotomy Incision. When the heart is approached from the front, the sternum (breastbone) (1) is cut and spread apart, and the pericardial sac is opened (2). After surgery, the sternum is closed and held in place by stainless steel wires or other strong suture material (4, 5, 6). These do not have to be removed, but are tolerated by the body as easily as a filling in a tooth.

POSTOPERATIVE CARE

Regardless of the kind of heart surgery, the postoperative care of all patients follows the same general pattern. Convalescence begins in the intensive care unit to which the patient is transferred immediately after the operation. Specially trained nurses, respiratory therapists, and other skilled professionals are at hand. A mechanical ventilator supports the lungs until the patient is awake and able to breathe satisfactorily. The staff, with the aid of electronic monitors, watches arterial blood pressure and electrocardiograms. Precautionary measures, including the use of antibiotics, are taken to minimize the possibility of infection. The patient is encouraged to breathe deeply and to cough in order to clear away any secretions which may have accumulated in the lungs. Drainage tubes gently suction off oozing blood in the chest. If the oozing is significant, blood is replaced in equivalent amounts by transfusion.

Cardiovascular surgery rarely interferes with the organs of digestion, therefore patients can return to normal eating and drinking somewhat sooner than abdominal surgery allows. Fluid intake and output are carefully measured, and the patient is weighed daily to detect any accumulation of fluid in the body. If anticoagulants are required, the proper dosage is monitored by frequent blood tests. When all monitoring and drainage tubes have been removed, the patient is allowed to get out of bed, use the bathroom, and gradually resume a pattern of activity tailored to the specific requirements of his condition.

VALVE DISEASE

Because of the phenomenal advances made in cardiovascular surgery in recent decades, many forms of acquired and congenital defects are now

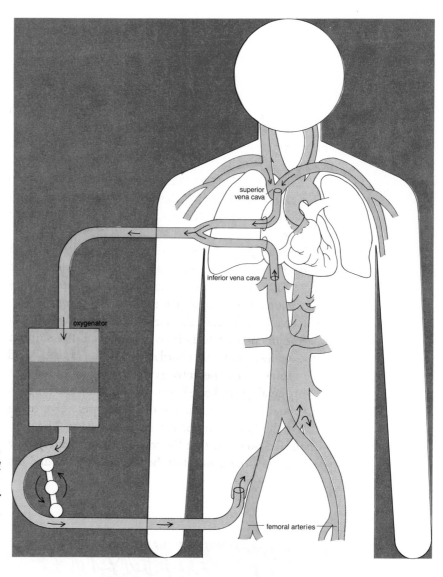

Total Cardiopulmonary Bypass. Venous blood is drained from the superior and inferior vena cavas to the machine where it is oxygenated and then returned under systemic pressure to the femoral artery.

amenable to surgical treatment. Among the acquired diseases are those that affect the heart valves. Rheumatic fever and other kinds of infection can damage previously normal heart valves so that they no longer open and close properly. The valves most often affected are the mitral, the aortic, and the tricuspid; the fourth heart valve, the pulmonary, is rarely damaged.

THE MITRAL VALVE   Situated between the left atrium and the left ventricle, this valve is named because of its resemblance to a bishop's miter—pointed at the top, with sides that flare out like ballooning sails. The two sails, called leaflets, open and close with each beat of the heart, allowing blood to enter the ventricle but preventing it from flowing back into the atrium. The leaflets are normally soft and supple, yet very strong. They are anchored to the muscle below by delicate sinews called chordae tendineae.

If rheumatic fever attacks the mitral valve, the leaflets can become thickened and fused, obstructing the flow of blood. The result can be likened to a dam across a river: behind the dam the water forms pools, while below it the flow of water drops off. Narrowing of the mitral valve (stenosis) causes pooled blood to back up into the lungs, creating congestion which the patient experiences as shortness of breath. At the same time, the reduced flow below the valve means that the body's nourishment is restricted, and fatigue results. Disease may cause the closing of the mitral valve to become defective, allowing seepage or leakage of blood backward through the valve. This happens when one or more of the supporting sinews breaks or when disease causes a hole in one of the leaflets. Leakage also results when the two leaflets have become distorted or have lost flexibility and no longer meet properly. A leaky or improperly functioning mitral valve can expose the delicately structured lungs to a surge of blood propelled by the powerful contraction of the left ventricle. As the regurgitated blood moves back and forth between the lungs and the heart, the cardiovascular system's efficiency and the patient's well-being are seriously reduced.

Either closed or open heart surgery can be used in correcting mitral valve defects. When the closed technique is used for stenosis, the surgeon inserts his finger or an instrument through a small opening made in the heart to separate the fused leaflets. The heart-lung machine is not used in this surgical procedure but is kept on a standby basis in case the surgeon decides to switch to open-heart surgery. When the open-heart technique is employed, the surgeon is able to inspect the two leaflets and the chordae tendineae directly and remodel them if possible. In some cases, the valve is so severely damaged that it must be replaced by an artificial (prosthetic) one. In that case, the surgeon removes the destroyed valve and leaves a small rim of the natural valve tissue as a base onto which he sews the fabric ring of the synthetic valve. The multiple strong stitches are then tied down so that the valve is held securely. The body's natural healing process seals the connection between the tissue and the artificial valve.

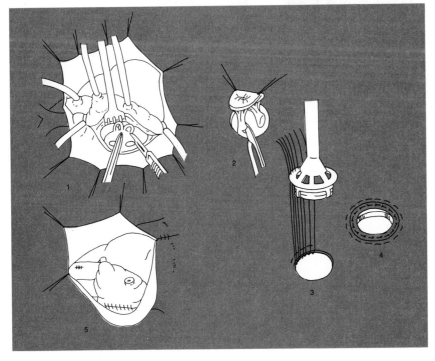

Mitral Valve Replacement. When the mitral valve is severely damaged by disease, it may be replaced by a prosthetic one. The process, which requires open-heart surgery (1), consists of removing the defective valve (2, 3), and sewing the fabric ring of the artificial valve to a small rim of the natural valve tissue with multiple stitches (4). The body's natural healing process seals the connection between the tissue and the artificial valve. The incisions in the heart are then closed with stitches.

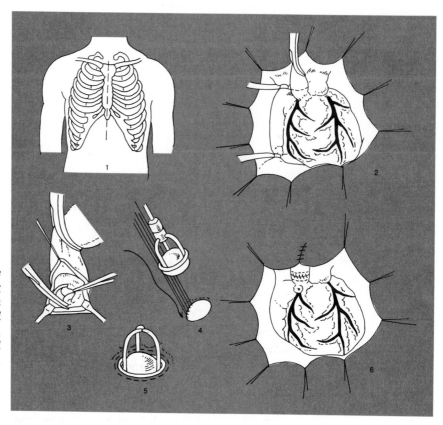

Aortic Valve Replacement. With the patient connected to a heart-lung machine, the heart is exposed by a midline incision (1), the aorta is opened (2), the diseased leaflets are removed (3), and the prosthetic valve is installed (4, 5, 6).

THE AORTIC VALVE   This valve, situated between the left ventricle and the aorta, normally has three cup-shaped leaflets. The surge of blood from the ventricle causes these leaflets to fold upward toward the wall of the aorta. As the ventricle sucks in the next load of blood from the left atrium, the pressure in the ventricle falls and the aortic valve closes. However, when calcified material accumulates on the leaflets, either as a result of rheumatic fever or a degenerative process, the valve becomes rigid. This condition in the valve, somewhat similar to tightening a nozzle on a watering hose, narrows the stream of blood and increases the work load of the ventricle. Leakage at the aortic valve occurs when the leaflets do not close properly as a result of rheumatic fever, infection, or a splitting or stretching of the aorta wall. The leakage causes the blood to flow back into the ventricle, creating an additional strain which can result in an enlarged heart.

Surgical repair for damaged aortic valves is only rarely possible; therefore in most cases the diseased valve is replaced by an artificial one. With the patient on a heart-lung machine, the heart is exposed by a midline incision, the aorta is opened, the diseased leaflets are removed, and the artificial valve is installed just as in the replacement of the mitral valve.

THE TRICUSPID VALVE   Resembling the mitral valve in structure except that it has three leaflets instead of two, this valve is located between the right atrium and the right ventricle. The valve's delicate tissue is held in place by cords attached to the muscle structure within the ventricle. Like the mitral valve, it may become obstructed or incompetent. When the valve narrows, there is a decrease in the amount of blood flowing from the right atrium into the right ventricle. This reduces the volume of blood that can be delivered to the lungs and causes pooling of blood in the peripheral veins of the body and sometimes edema (swelling) of the legs, liver, or other organs. A leaky or incompetent valve causes blood to flow back into the right atrium from the right ventricle. The tricuspid valve may be repaired or replaced by techniques similar to those used in mitral valve surgery.

Prosthetic Valves

Surgical treatment of valve disease was at first directed at the repair of malfunctioning valves; there was little that medical treatment alone could offer to those whose valves were severely damaged. The picture has changed dramatically with the development of the two categories of prosthetic valves, mechanical and tissue valves.

Among the mechanical prosthetic valves available is a caged ball or disk type. When such a valve is in a closed position, the ball or disk rests on a ring at the base of the valve. When the valve is open, the ball or disk moves to the end of the retaining mechanism, thus allowing the blood to flow through the valve. These valves all open and close as a result of the hydraulic pressure changes created by the contracting and filling cycles of the ventricles.

Although mechanical prosethetic valves are made from very durable, inert materials, such as noncorrosive metals, hard carbon, Teflon, Silastic, and Dacron, their ultimate longevity has yet to be determined because they have been in widespread use only since the early 1960s. One potential danger from mechanical valves, the possibility of clots forming on the hardware of the valve, is guarded against by administering anticoagulants after valves are implanted.

In addition to mechanical valves, there are tissue valves derived from a variety of sources. The most frequently used is a natural heart valve taken from a pig. How long the tissue valves will last is also not yet known. One advantage of tissue valves over mechanical devices is that anticoagulants are not generally required. Even though the duration of neither type of artificial valve is as yet known, surgeons use them because the probability is that valve replacement will give the patient a better chance for longevity than will reliance on a natural valve that is known to be defective and life-threatening.

CORONARY ARTERY DISEASE

The most common acquired heart disease is segmental obstruction or narrowing of the coronary arteries. In the normal heart, the right and left coronary arteries deliver the blood which nourishes the powerful pumping muscles of the heart. In the disease known as atherosclerosis, segments of the coronary arteries become narrow or obstructed, diminishing the flow of blood to the heart muscle. When this happens, the reduced flow of blood and oxygen to the heart may cause chest pain with exertion (angina pectoris), or a complete blockage may cause a heart attack or myocardial infarction.

Surgical treatment of severely narrowed coronary arteries is often possible because there are clear passages on either side of the blockage. This segmental distribution of blocks fortunately enables the surgeon to build a bypassing "artery," connecting clear passages above and below the block. Generally, a bypass graft is constructed by use of vein taken from the patient's own thigh.

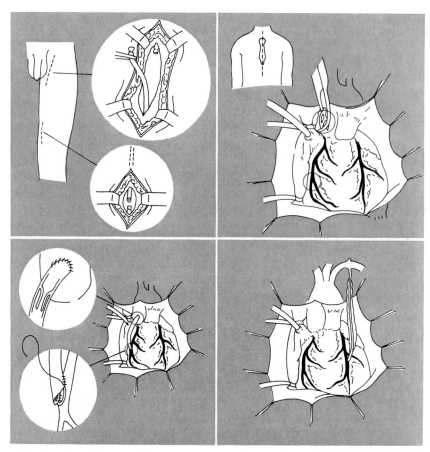

Coronary Bypass. Generally, a bypass graft is constructed by use of a vein taken from inside the patient's own thigh. The internal mammary artery from inside the chest wall may also be used. The graft is sewn to the aorta and attached to the diseased artery distole to the site of obstruction. This results in an increased flow of blood to the heart muscle.

The internal mammary artery from the inside of the chest wall may also be used. In the latter case, the artery is separated from the chest wall so that the flow from it may be redirected to a coronary artery. During graft surgery the patient's circulation is supported by a heart-lung machine. Special instruments and tiny sutures have been developed to sew the grafts to the coronary artery and the aorta. The surgeon's view of the delicate, minute coronary arteries is facilitated by the use of special headlights and magnifying glasses.

Surgical relief may also be offered for certain complications from coronary artery disease. A severe heart attack may leave scar tissue which bulges under the strain of continuing pressure in the heart. If this bulge, known as an aneurysm, is large, it diminishes the effective force of the heartbeat. Surgical removal of the aneurysm thereby improves the efficiency of the heart. Severe heart attacks may also cause malfunctioning of the mitral valve or a hole in the wall that separates the two ventricles. These complications may be relieved by surgical repair.

HEART BLOCK The heart is a pump made of special muscle whose contractions are triggered and synchronized by electrical impulses produced by its own natural pacemaker. Impulses travel from the pacemaker along a specific path, causing the muscle walls to contract and thus to pump blood. As long as these electrical impulses are transmitted normally, the heart pumps and beats at a regular pace.

In disorders of the cardiac electrical conduction system surgery can be a vital tool. A complete block of this electrical conduction may occur, which leaves the patient with a very slow heartbeat, inadequate to sustain normal life. Disease processes can also interfere with the impulses by causing the heart to pump too fast, too slowly, or erratically. When the natural pacemaker falters, an artificial pacemaker, using batteries and timers, can be used to produce electrical impulses which are transmitted along tiny wires secured to the heart. The heart, responding to these stimuli, pumps at a rate determined by the artificial pacemaker's timer.

Congenital heart disease occurs in approximately 10 out of every 1,000 babies. **CONGENITAL HEART** Although the cause of faulty development of the heart is unknown in most **DISEASE** instances, viral infections or drugs taken by the mother may disturb the development of the heart during the fifth to eighth weeks of intrauterine life. There are many types of congenital defects, appearing singly or in combination, and these are discussed in chapter 16, Congenital Heart Defects. In general, congenital defects include incorrectly formed valves, holes in the walls (septa) that separate the two sides of the heart, and abnormalities in the blood vessels leading in and out of the heart. These fall into two broad categories: conditions in which the baby is "blue" (cyanotic heart disease) and those in which the baby's color is normal (acyanotic heart disease).

A "blue" baby is born with a blockage in the pathway which normally carries blood from the heart to the lungs and also with a hole in the partition between the two ventricles. The unoxygenated (blue) blood is unable to reach its normal destination and is shunted through the hole into the left side of the heart and subsequently delivered to the tissues. Surgery can be performed to the obstructed pathway from the right ventricle to the lungs (pulmonary artery) and to close the hole in the partition of the ventricle.

The most common cause of the blue baby condition is transposition of the great arteries; that is, the aorta arises from the right ventricle instead of the left, and the pulmonary artery comes from the left ventricle, rather than the right. The abnormality prevents a normal mixing of the circulation to the lungs and to the body. For immediate though partial relief, the doctor uses a balloon-tipped catheter to make a hole in the partition between the upper two receiving chambers of the heart, thus allowing the two circulations to mix. At a later time, the upper chambers can be repartitioned surgically to establish a more normal circulation.

Another blue baby abnormality is a condition in which all the blood coming from the lungs enters the right atrium instead of the left. This is called total anomalous pulmonary venous connection. Surgery is necessary to reroute the blood from the lungs to the left atrium and to close the abnormal connections to the right side of the heart.

A baby may be born with only one large artery coming from the heart instead of the two (aorta and pulmonary artery) that are normal. This condition is called truncus arteriosus. The single trunk may have either large branches going to the lung, which are subjected to excessive pressure or flow, or very small branches, inadequate for delivery of blood to the lungs.

Many other abnormalities are characterized by the alarming blue tint to the newborn infant's skin—a sign that serious defects exist in the circulatory

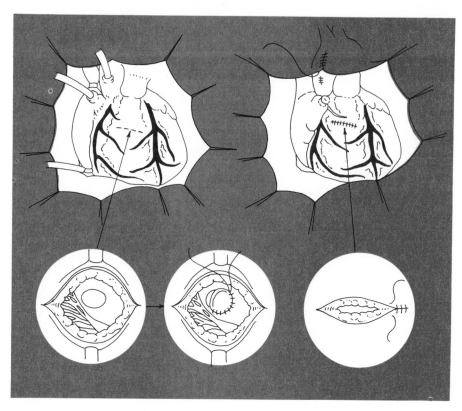

Among congenital malformations of the heart is an abnormal opening between the ventricles, caused by a ventrical septal defect. It can be closed by surgery by sewing a patch of dacron to the septum.

system of the heart and lungs. The pediatric cardiologist and the surgeon must determine the precise nature of the abnormality in order to decide what kind of surgical procedure to follow and what relief may be possible.

Acyanotic congenital defects are those which do not result in a bluish tint. In the normal heart, the circuit to the body and that to the lungs are securely partitioned off from each other. The separation is important because arterial circulation to the body is a high-pressure circuit, while that to the lungs is a low-pressure circuit. Abnormal connections allow leakage of blood from one side to the other. If there is a shunt between the aorta and the pulmonary artery, blood spills from the high-pressure aorta into the low-pressure pulmonary artery, causing an overload in the pulmonary circuit. The same situation occurs if there is an opening between the two ventricles (caused by a ventricular septal defect) or communication between the two atria (caused by an atrial septal defect). In each case, blood destined to nourish the entire body leaks through the hole into the right side of the heart and returns to the pulmonary circuit from which it has just come. This inefficient use of the heart's power is something like trying to heat a house with the doors and windows wide open—it can be done, but at an extravagant waste of fuel and at the certain risk of wearing out the furnace sooner than necessary. Fortunately, these abnormal channels can be corrected surgically.

Other acyanotic congenital defects are those that obstruct the flow of blood through the pulmonary valve or the aortic valve. When there is an obstruction to the outlet of blood from a pumping chamber, the muscle in the ventricle obstructed by the narrowed valve overdevelops. Surgical relief is afforded by enlarging the narrowed aperture in the valve. Congenital malformations also include nonvalvular obstructions. One common defect is a severe narrowing or hourglass constriction of the aorta (coarctation of the aorta) as it makes its major turn downward in the chest on its way toward the abdomen. The result is high blood pressure above the obstruction and low blood pressure below. The narrowed segment can be removed surgically and the two ends of the aorta reconnected by splicing them together.

VASCULAR SURGERY

In addition to surgery on the heart itself and on its valves and arteries, a related branch of surgery known as vascular surgery is concerned with the major blood vessels beyond the heart. Vascular surgery is used to correct congenital malformations or to repair damage due to injury, acquired disease, or the aging process. The problems encountered can be broadly classified as conditions that affect the arterial (or delivery) system and those that affect the venous (or collecting) system. Arterial problems requiring operation are usually related to obstruction or to leakage. The obstructions are caused by clots or by an accumulation of material in the artery most often associated with aging (atherosclerosis). An obstruction that involves only a short segment of an artery can be satisfactorily removed. This type of operation is frequently used on the carotid artery. A longer obstruction usually requires bypassing the obstructed area with a graft, which then becomes a new pathway. The graft is constructed either from the saphenous vein in the patient's thigh or from tubing made of Dacron. In either case, the healing process secures the graft and allows blood to flow smoothly through the bypass and into the artery below the obstruction. Arterial leakage may be actual or potential, the latter being the case when the wall of the artery becomes so weakened that it develops a bulging enlargement, or aneurysm. The weakened segment is removed by surgery and a graft is implanted, restoring the blood flow. Ideally the surgical repairs are done before the weakened area bulges excessively, because a bursting aneurysm leaks blood with a rapidity that can be catastrophic. In some cases, however, the leakage is slow enough to allow blood transfusions to be given, and the patient is able to undergo lifesaving surgery.

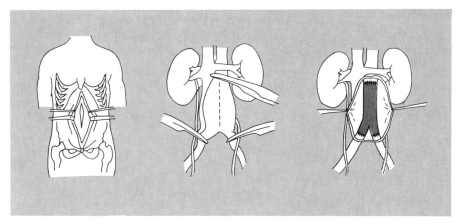

Atherosclerosis of the aortic wall may cause a weakening and bulging of the aorta, called an aneurysm. Such aneurysms are most common in the abdomen and may be surgically replaced by opening the abdomen (1), removing the entire aorta and the adjoining major leg branches (the first part of the iliac arteries) (2), and replaced with a Y–shaped synthetic graft (3).

The venous system, like the arterial system, can be affected by obstruction, weakness, and stretching of the walls, as well as leakage. Obstruction in the venous system is usually due to a blood clot. If a clot forms and remains in place, the venous drainage system will become impaired and swelling will occur. If the clot breaks loose, it will travel throughout the venous system,

PRINCIPLES

1. *Before any cardiovascular surgery is performed, the patient must undergo a complete examination that includes a medical history as well as a physical examination. Some special diagnostic studies may be performed in order to evaluate specific aspects of the individual's cardiovascular system.*

2. *Closed-heart surgery is done without interrupting the work of the heart pumping blood to the body. In open-heart surgery, the heart itself is opened. During this operation a heart-lung machine does the work of the heart by pumping oxygenated blood to the rest of the body. The heart-lung machine enables the physician to see the heart as he works.*

3. *Surgically correctible heart defects are either acquired or congenital. Acquired heart defects include damage to the major valves of the heart (mitral, aortic, and tricuspid valves). In most instances the defective valve is replaced either by an artificial valve or one fashioned out of animal tissue. Coronary artery disease may be surgically treated by means of a bypass that detours blood around the afflicted area. Disorders of the natural pacemaker system of the heart may be treated surgically through implantation of an artificial pacemaker. Congenital heart disease is present at birth. Many types of congenital heart abnormalities can be surgically corrected.*

4. *Vascular surgery is repair work on major blood vessels beyond the heart itself. Blood clots or other obstructions in arteries may be removed surgically or corrected by a bypass operation. Aneurysms (bulges in an artery wall caused by weakness or leakage) may be treated surgically. In addition to work on arteries, surgical repairs may also be done on veins that become enlarged or weak (varicose veins).*

enter the right side of the heart, and lodge in the pulmonary artery. This is called pulmonary embolism and it can have disastrous consequences if the clot is large enough to block the main pulmonary artery. Most clots are small, however, and lodge in the smaller branches of the pulmonary artery. They are nevertheless capable of causing trouble, especially if a number of them together block major portions of the pulmonary vascular system. Venous clotting can be treated surgically by removal of the clot or entrapment of the clot by the use of clips or netting, and medically by the administration of anticoagulant drugs to minimize further clot formation.

Venous enlargement or a weakening of vein walls is most commonly seen as varicose veins in the legs and arms. If varicosities are severe, surgical removal of the damaged veins is sometimes advisable. Usually, however, the weakened venous system is simply supported by elastic stockings which help return blood from the extremities to the heart. Elevating the leg or arm periodically also brings relief. Dilated veins do not ordinarily rupture and relatively little blood is lost if they do because the pressure in the venous circulation is low. The consequences are therefore not as severe as those resulting when an artery ruptures. When a vein ruptures, blood oozes into the tissues, causing pressure to build up there, and this in turn compresses the hole in the vein, thereby retarding further leakage.

21

CARDIOVASCULAR DRUGS

Lewis B. Sheiner, M.D.

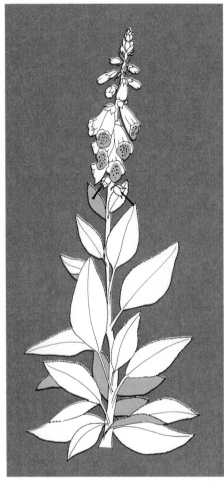

Digitalis

Long before medical science discovered its ability to increase the strength of the heart's contraction, digitalis—found in the foxglove plant—was used in folk medicine to aid the heart patient.

Drugs are used extensively in treating patients with diseases of the heart and blood vessels, but, as in drug therapy for any other kind of disease, the potential danger must be weighed against the known benefits. Since every useful drug can also have toxic effects, a decision must be made as to whether probable good will exceed possible harm. The doctor and the patient together must make this judgment. The patient's part is to let the doctor know how much trouble the symptoms are causing and, if drugs are being taken, how unacceptable certain side effects have become. Not only is no drug completely safe, but there is no clearly defined dosage for any particular drug. Each patient's body will absorb or eliminate a drug at its own rate, and each patient will have a particular level of sensitivity to a drug. Because of these individual responses, what may be an effective dose for one person may be a toxic dose for another. In a certain sense, therefore, every use of a drug is an experiment to discover the right kind of drug and the correct dosage. If the patient with cardiovascular disease realizes this, he will be in a position to help the doctor arrive at a drug treatment program tailored to his own particular needs.

Drugs are basically of two kinds: curative drugs, which correct the cause of an illness, and symptomatic drugs, which modify the effects, or symptoms. Obviously, curative drugs are preferable, but in spite of the popular belief in "miracle" drugs, they are available for only a few conditions. An example of a curative drug is penicillin. When used to treat a streptococcal infection ("strep" throat is a leading cause of rheumatic fever and subsequent rheumatic heart disease), penicillin helps the body's defenses to fight the germ causing the disease. The disease is then cured, and the symptoms are relieved. In contrast, aspirin is a symptomatic drug which can relieve the pain and fever of the strep throat (its main symptoms) but does not deal with its cause. Aspirin also lowers fever and reduces the inflammation of arthritis but again leaves the basic causes largely uncured. A symptomatic drug must be continued as long as the disease producing the symptoms is still present. Arthritis is a chronic condition, an example of a disease that does not spontaneously correct itself. That is why many arthritis sufferers are put on a lifetime program of daily doses of aspirin.

Certain kinds of high blood pressure (hypertension) are also chronic conditions, and many patients require long-term drug treatment to avoid the serious complications that can result from these conditions. (See Hypertension, chapter 10.) For conditions in which the body corrects the problems in a relatively short time—a common cold or even a broken limb—symptomatic treatment is relatively brief. Almost all cardiovascular diseases are chronic, and almost all drugs currently in use for their treatment are symptomatic rather than curative. Taking the drugs, therefore, becomes part of the patient's daily routine for long periods of time—even, in some cases, for the rest of his life. Long-range drug treatment not only relieves immediate symptoms of cardiovascular disease but also may stabilize the condition, where this is possible, and prolong the period of normal activity.

CONGESTIVE HEART FAILURE

Congestive heart failure is the end result of many diseases affecting the heart. (For a more complete discussion, see Congestive Heart Failure, chapter 13.) The heart is said to "fail" when its pumping action is impaired, rendering it unable to deliver an adequate supply of blood and nutrients to the organs of the body. To compensate for the diminished flow of blood and the diminished oxygen supply, the heart increases its rate of beating. At the same time, the kidneys conserve water and salts, thereby increasing the volume of blood. Some of the excess fluid leaks through the small vessels into the tissues, causing swelling, or edema, of the ankle and legs. The excess fluid also collects in the lungs, making them "stiff" and resulting in shortness of breath (dyspnea), particularly after exertion or when lying down.

Drug treatment for congestive heart failure is directed either toward increasing the ability of the heart to pump and thus enabling it to deliver the needed blood supply, or toward relieving the symptoms arising from the body's attempts to compensate for the impaired heart function, the edema, and the stiff lungs. Three types of medication are therefore helpful: drugs that increase the strength of the heart's contraction (digitalis is the most important of these); drugs that cause the kidneys to excrete more salt, and therefore more water, to lessen edema (diuretics); and drugs that relax blood vessels (vasodilators) and thereby decrease the pressure against which the weakened heart must pump.

Digitalis was first introduced to formal medicine in 1785 by the English physician William Withering, but its use in folk medicine preceded that date by many years. In fact, Dr. Withering discovered that the common garden flower, the foxglove, was being used by an old woman to treat persons suffering from what was at the time called dropsy (now identified as edema), and many showed marked improvement. Dr. Withering's knowledge of botany enabled him to extract the substance in foxglove responsible for the improvement, digitalis, which can also be extracted from a variety of other plants. Subsequent research showed that digitalis increases the strength of the heart's contraction, making it beat more forcefully, even though it does not affect the cause of the heart's failure to pump adequately.

Digitalis

Digitalis belongs to a group of drugs called the cardiac glycosides. Glycosides vary in the way they are administered (orally or intravenously), in the level of daily maintenance dose necessary, and in the length of time it takes for the action to start, peak, regress, and finally disappear. The two most commonly used glycosides are digoxin and digitoxin. Both of these need be taken only once a day, because both are eliminated slowly from the body. This is obviously a convenience for the patient, but it also indicates certain built-in drawbacks. Chief among these is the danger that excessive amounts will accumulate in the body, leading possibly to digitalis toxicity. The most serious toxic effect is a dangerous irregularity of the heartbeat, but the patient may also suffer nausea, vomiting, and various symptoms of brain involvement, including drowsiness, headache, and blurred or strangely colored vision. Fortunately, the remedy is generally very simple: discontinuance of the drug for a period of time. Special care is required in determining the proper dosage for a patient who has other complications of congestive heart failure (cor pulmonale, for example) or for one who is also taking a diuretic. The same precaution is necessary for those who are advanced in years. In all these cases, toxicity tends to occur with lower doses than usual. In many patients, the amount of digitalis needed to strengthen the heartbeat is very close to the amount that is likely to cause toxicity. The doctor must monitor treatment, therefore, and be alert for any signs of sensitivity or toxicity. The patient, too, must always be aware of the danger of overdosing and never take more than the amount prescribed for daily maintenance.

Diuretics Because diuretics prevent the reabsorption of salt and water by the kidneys, they lessen edema and thus diminish some of the symptoms of congestive heart failure. There are many kinds of diuretics, and the mechanics of their operation are not always fully understood, but all have the same objective: to increase the output of salt and water in urine. The major problem they present is an excess of their benefit; that is, an excessive loss of salt and other minerals, especially potassium. Potassium loss, most common with the widely used thiazide class of diuretics (chlorothiazide and hydrochlorothiazide), can result in feelings of weakness and if digitalis is being taken can make toxicity more likely. A loss of potassium can be counteracted by potassium supplements or by adding a second diuretic—one that does not cause potassium loss —to the thiazide. However, the combination of diuretics introduces another danger: diuretics which prevent potassium loss do so by interfering with the ability of the kidneys to excrete the mineral. This can lead to a dangerously high level of potassium in the body. Tests to determine the potassium level in the blood are usually made while the thiazides are being taken, and therapy is adjusted accordingly. Thiazides can also reduce the elimination of uric acid and thus aggravate an existing case of gout, an arthritic condition caused by an excess of uric acid, although these drugs rarely cause the disease.

Vasodilators Vasodilators, drugs that are used to relax blood vessels, are discussed in detail in the following sections on angina pectoris and hypertension, conditions in which they are more commonly used. Their use for heart failure is relatively new, still somewhat controversial and applicable only to certain cases of congestive heart failure. When blood vessels are relaxed, resistance to the flow of blood is decreased; the heart works no harder than before, but more blood reaches the tissues.

ANGINA PECTORIS When the coronary arteries, the vessels that supply the heart muscle itself, become inefficient because of deposits of fatty tissue in their walls (atherosclerosis), the blood supply to the heart may become insufficient. The patient feels this loss as chest pain on exertion or even at times during rest. (See Coronary Artery Disease, chapter 11.) The angina is likely to be intensified by conditions which either decrease the heart muscle's oxygen supply or increase its demand for oxygen. For example, the oxygen supply to the heart is decreased by cigarette smoking, because it reduces the oxygen-carrying capacity of the blood. The heart's demand for oxygen increases with elevated blood pressure because more work must be done to pump blood at higher pressures, and with physical exertion, because that increases the tissues' demand for oxygen. To meet such demands, blood flow, heart rate, and the speed of contractions increase.

Drug treatment for angina is symptomatic, not curative. Certain cases of angina are caused by spasm of the heart's blood vessels. In these cases angina usually occurs when the patient is at rest, and drugs can increase blood supply to the heart because the spasm is not a permanent narrowing. In most cases of angina, however, permanent narrowing is the problem, and no drug can even temporarily reverse the alterations in the heart's blood vessels which result in narrowed or obstructed arteries. In most cases then, blood supply to the heart cannot be altered. Because this is so, most anti-angina medications are aimed at reducing the heart's demand for oxygen.

Drugs that relax blood vessels, causing them to dilate, are of two kinds: the **Vasodilators** nitrates and the nonnitrate vasodilators. None of these drugs dilates diseased coronary arteries that have undergone permanent changes. However, when spasm is the problem vasodilators can relieve this, and even with permanent narrowing, they act on other blood vessels throughout the body, causing them to dilate and retain more blood, which would normally go to the heart. This reduction in the amount of blood within the heart decreases the over-all size of the heart itself, because it does not have to expand as much as with a normal volume. With less blood to pump, the heart has less work per beat and therefore needs less oxygen. This decreased demand prevents or relieves the pain that comes when heart muscles poorly supplied with blood are called upon to perform beyond their capacity.

The action of vasodilators can further decrease the demand for oxygen by reducing blood pressure. However, the body's natural compensatory mechanisms are then activated to reverse this effect by accelerating the heart rate and the speed of the contraction of the heart muscle. Thus, the effectiveness of the vasodilators is somewhat offset by the body's own self-regulators.

NITRATES   The vasodilators longest in use (more than one hundred years) are the nitrates, and they are still the most effective drugs for angina, because they work particularly well on the large arteries and the veins. Nitroglycerin is the most frequently used, usually taken in tablets which are placed under the tongue and allowed to dissolve. Nitrates can be effective when swallowed, but they are also well absorbed through the membranes of the mouth and even through the skin and therefore can also be used as a tablet under the tongue or as a paste rubbed onto the skin at night. Their action is short-lived, lasting for a few hours at most. They are usually taken when angina occurs or when the patient is about to undertake an activity which is likely to cause angina.

The side effects and toxicity of the nitrates follow upon their dilating action: dilated blood vessels and lowered blood pressure can result in faintness or dizziness. Headache is the most common side effect, probably caused by dilation of blood vessels in the head. The side effects are usually of short duration, however, and most patients develop a tolerance to the headaches. Palpitations are another possible side effect, resulting from the compensatory increase in heart rate and the speed of heart contraction.

NONNITRATE VASODILATORS   These drugs have little or no effect on the veins, acting primarily on the arteries by relaxing them. They can, therefore, be of some aid in angina caused by spasm. When spasm is not the problem, because the compensatory mechanisms of the body oppose the blood-pressure-lowering action of these drugs, their net effect is not to change the blood pressure very much, but to increase the heart rate and the speed of the heart's contraction. In short, since oxygen demand is increased, angina is likely to be aggravated, rather than relieved. For this reason the use of nonnitrate vasodilators is no longer recommended except for angina caused by spasm or in the unusual situation where heart failure is caused by the large volume of blood within the heart. In that case, when angina is present, a nonnitrate vasodilator can relieve heart failure and reduce the size of the heart, thereby decreasing oxygen demand.

Propranolol   Propranolol (Inderal) is a drug that blocks some of the sympathetic nerves to the heart. These nerves (the beta-sympathetic or beta-andrenergic nerves) carry messages from the brain that cause the heart to increase its rate and the speed of its contraction. By blocking these messages, propranolol slows the heart rate, decreases the speed of contraction, and thus decreases the heart's demand for oxygen. The drug is quite effective in preventing angina. Unlike the nitrates, it is used continuously to prevent rather than relieve episodes of pain. Used in combination with nitrate vasodilators, propranolol prevents the compensatory increase in heart rate and the speed of contraction that limit the effectiveness of nitrates.

However, propranolol has certain hazards. One of the possible dangers is the development of congestive heart failure because the speed and the force of the heart's contraction are reduced. This poses two problems: the congestive failure itself, with its disturbing symptoms, and the consequent expanded volume of blood in the heart, which increases its size and may make the angina worse. The problem, when it occurs, is usually met by adding digitalis, alone or with a diuretic, to the propranolol regime. Another toxicity results from propranolol's basic function of blocking beta-sympathetic nerves. Unfortunately, this action affects the beta-sympathetic nerves throughout the body, not just those of the heart. Since these nerves are responsible for dilating the blood vessels of the skin, propranolol can cause constriction of these vessels, leading to pale, cold hands and feet. The same nerves also cause the body's air tubes to dilate, and when propranolol blocks that dilation, the air tubes become constricted. A patient with asthma can find this condition aggravated, although the drug will not cause asthma in a person who does not already have it. Patients who are taking insulin for diabetes should be warned about another possible side effect of propranolol. Beta-sympathetic nerves cause an increase in blood sugar when the level drops too low. In a diabetic person who is taking insulin a low-sugar level can be aggravated or prolonged when propranolol is also being taken. Propranolol can also cause depression, difficulty in sleeping, and sometimes, though rarely, impotence. The side effects are not permanent; all disappear when the drug is stopped. It is important, however, that the drug be gradually discontinued, rather than suddenly withdrawn. An abrupt halt of propranolol can worsen the angina condition and may result in a heart attack. The beta-sympathetic nerves also may help dilate the heart's own arteries, and in angina caused by spasm propranolol may not be advisable.

Digitalis   Digitalis is useful in angina only when combined with propranolol or when congestive heart failure from some cause not related to angina is present. In the presence of both congestive heart failure and angina, digitalis reduces the volume of blood in the heart, thus relieving the angina. When congestive heart failure is not present, however, the effect of digitalis (to increase the strength and speed of the heart's contraction) may aggravate rather than relieve angina because of the heart's increased need for oxygen.

Millions of Americans have hypertension, but despite such widespread incidence, the cause of the disease is largely unknown. An unknown cause cannot, of course, be treated curatively; therefore drug therapy must be symptomatic, not curative, in most cases of hypertension. There is an essential distinction, however, between the therapy for hypertension and that for angina and congestive heart failure. In the latter two instances, drugs are prescribed to relieve symptoms that are either actually painful or unmistakably present. In high blood pressure, distressful symptoms are usually absent, and the person is unaware of the condition until it is discovered by a doctor measuring blood pressure. In spite of the absence of symptoms, the condition must be treated once it is discovered, because persistent, long-term hypertension can cause permanent damage, including stroke, kidney failure, blindness, congestive heart failure, or heart attack. These disastrous consequences can often be prevented if blood pressure is lowered and kept low by drugs.

Ideally, treatment begins before damage to a vital organ takes place. Realistically, the patient must recognize that treatment can often be a lifelong matter. It is particularly difficult to convince persons who feel perfectly well that they must take medications routinely every day, especially when the medication produces some unpleasant side effects. Patients must be warned about the dangers of forgetting or deliberately suddenly stopping medication because blood pressure can increase to very high levels, often higher than those that prompted the treatment program. Such extremely high blood pressures have been known to cause strokes.

Drugs used to lower blood pressure work in different ways, and often several are taken at the same time. Various combinations with different actions are selected, so that no one of them acts excessively, yet the over-all pressure-lowering effect of the combination is good. Except in extreme cases, high pressures can be lowered gradually, giving the doctor and the patient time to discover the most comfortable and effective combination of drugs.

To understand how various drugs work in lowering pressure, it may be useful to recall that blood pressure is determined by the flow of blood through the vessels and the resistance to that flow offered by the vessels. Blood flow itself is determined by the amount of blood pumped by the heart with each beat and the number of beats a minute. The amount of blood pumped with each beat is in turn dependent on the force and speed of the heart's contraction and on the amount of blood returning to the heart via the veins. The resistance of the blood vessels to the blood flow depends on the diameter or "tightness" of the vessels. Most persons with hypertension have greater than normal resistance, rather than increased blood volume or heart rate.

Diuretics

Diuretics lower blood pressure in two ways. First, by causing loss of fluid, they reduce the volume of blood and the amount returning to the heart. Second, they also act as vasodilators, relaxing blood vessels and thereby lowering resistance to the flow of blood. Diuretics are usually the first drugs used in the treatment of high blood pressure and in mild cases are often effective by themselves.

Vasodilators

On first thought, vasodilators would seem to be the best drugs for high blood pressure, because they lower resistance. In reality, when used alone, they produce only a slight fall in pressure. This is because their effects are counterbalanced by the body's compensatory efforts, and the heart rate and the force and speed of the heart's contraction are increased. The compensations not only overcome the effect of the drug on the heart action, but the kidneys retain more salt and water, and blood volume is increased. Vasodilators alone are of little use, then, in the treatment of hypertension, but when combined with a diuretic and with propranolol (to block beta-sympathetic nerve reaction), they are very effective. This combination is becoming the mainstay of **drug treatment of high blood pressure.**

Hydralazine is the major vasodilator used for long-term treatment of high blood pressure in the United States. When used alone, its side effects are similar to those of the nitrates: headache and faintness. Moreover, if the patient also has angina, the drug may aggravate the condition by speeding up the heart rate and the force and speed of heart contractions. However, when used with propranolol and a diuretic, hydralazine has very few side effects. In a few patients, and usually those on high doses, it produces an arthritislike condition, with pain and redness in the joints, rashes, and other manifestations. These effects usually disappear when the drug is stopped.

A newer vasodilator, prazosin, is coming into wider use. Perhaps because it may actually work by blocking certain special kinds of sympathetic nerve responses, it does not cause the body to compensate as strenuously as does hydralazine. It may therefore be used alone, or in combination with only a diuretic.

Sympathetic Nerve Inhibitors

Certain drugs act on the brain to inhibit the instructions it sends to the body to tighten the arteries and thereby maintain a high blood pressure. Among these drugs are alphamethyl-DOPA, clonidine, and reserpine. The drugs are often effective when used alone, but because they do not inhibit the compensatory mechanism that retains fluid and increases blood volume, they are best used with a diuretic. Used in combination with vasodilators, these sympathetic-nerve blockers increase the effectiveness of the former by preventing the body's compensatory actions from canceling out their effects.

Because these drugs act on the brain, they can cause such brain-related side effects as drowsiness and depression. Impotence may also occur, but this, like the other side effects, is not permanent and disappears when the drugs are stopped. Alphamethyl-DOPA is more likely than the other drugs to cause a moderate degree of allergy in susceptible patients, leading possibly to anemia, liver reactions, and fever. The side effects cease when the patient stops taking the drug.

Propranolol, described in the section on angina, acts only on the beta-sympathetic nerves to the heart. It seems to have an additional property of lowering high blood pressure and is particularly useful because it also increases the effectiveness of vasodilators. Other drugs, guanethedine in particular, act on the entire sympathetic nervous system. Guanethedine dilates the small veins, causing pooling of blood in those vessels and a reduction of the amount of blood returning to the heart. This action, which lowers blood pressure, is only prominent when the patient is standing, a position which allows gravity to favor the pooling of blood in the veins of the lower part of the body.

Because of their many toxicities, drugs like guanethedine are never used alone. As is the case with many drugs, the toxicities are excesses of beneficial actions; if pressure is lowered too much, the patient may feel tired or weak or even faint when standing. Fluid retention is common, and a diuretic is almost always required. Guanethedine, and other drugs like it, also decrease the functions of other parts of the sympathetic nervous system. Because the sympathetic nerves act on the bowels, the drugs can cause diarrhea. Although guanethedine does not cause impotence, it may inhibit ejaculation or cause sperm to flow into the bladder. Another problem is that the action of guanethedine can be short-circuited by drugs which prevent its entry into the nerve cells. Certain antidepressant drugs totally and rapidly prevent guanethedine from acting (and also decrease the effectiveness of clonidine) and can cause a severe and dangerous return of high blood pressure if the two kinds of drugs are taken together. Guanethedine is eliminated from the body slowly, and sudden stoppage of the drug does not present any particular danger. The drug's effects take place gradually and persist for a long time after the drug is stopped.

A number of other drugs, either vasodilators or those that act on the sympathetic nervous system, have been used in the treatment of high blood pressure. Some of these are extremely potent and are used only in severe cases and under close supervision, usually when the patient is in a hospital.

ARRHYTHMIAS

Arrhythmias, abnormalities in the heart rate or rhythm, usually result in disturbances of the impulse which starts each heartbeat or in the conduction of this impulse to the rest of the heart. (See Arrhythmias, chapter 12.) Certain drugs act to correct these disturbances either by blocking the abnormal conduction of impulses or by restoring normal conduction. These drugs are symptomatic; they may decrease or eliminate the abnormal rhythm but they do not correct the basic cause. Fortunately, many arrhythmia conditions are not chronic, and the underlying cause may correct itself in time. Some arrhythmias are, however, chronic or recurrent, requiring prolonged therapy.

Abnormal Conduction of Impulses

The most important drugs used to block abnormal conduction of impulses in the heart are quinidine and procainamide and a relatively new drug, disopyramide. All three are similar in action, so that if one is not effective in any given case, the others are unlikely to be. However, some exceptions to this rule have been reported. All are eliminated somewhat rapidly from the body, requiring frequent doses to achieve a sustained effect. The major toxicity of these drugs again comes from an excess of their beneficial action. In excess, they can begin to decrease or block conduction of normal heart impulses and may themselves cause the arrhythmias they are meant to treat. In such cases, it is difficult to determine whether the condition itself has deteriorated, requiring further treatment with the drug, or an excess of the drug is the problem. In ordinary practice, however, modest doses are prescribed to prevent the recurrence of certain arrhythmias. These doses are well within the tolerance of most patients.

Quinidine and procainamide each have other kinds of toxicities. Quinidine may produce allergic reactions affecting the platelets, the small blood cells responsible in part for blood clotting. If, as a reaction to the drug, the number of platelets decreases, bleeding may result. More commonly, quinidine causes nausea, vomiting, or diarrhea. Procainamide may also, though rarely, cause an allergic reaction in the blood that results in fewer white cells, thus diminishing the patient's protection against infection. Procainamide may also produce an arthritis-like reaction similar to that associated with hydralazine. The reaction is usually reversible on stopping the drug.

Restoring Conduction to Normal Phenytoin, used primarily in the treatment of epilepsy, is the only drug given orally to patients outside a hospital in the attempt to restore conduction to normal. The drug is effective only in certain arrhythmias and is generally less effective than quinidine, procainamide, or disopyramide. Excessive doses can cause drowsiness, dizziness, and poor coordination of physical movements. Occasionally, average doses, through processes not fully understood, can cause excess growth of the gums and various allergic reactions affecting the blood or skin.

Digitalis Digitalis neither blocks abnormal conduction nor acts to restore conduction to normal. Through a complex process, it acts to modify the conduction of impulses in the heart. It is sometimes used in long-term therapy to prevent certain recurring arrhythmias, and it is also used to slow the heart rate in certain arrhythmias that cause very rapid heart rates. In the latter case, the required dose is even greater than for heart failure. Great caution is necessary, therefore, because the dose required is very close to that which can cause toxicity.

Propranolol Like digitalis, propranolol does not work directly on the abnormal conduction of impulses or restoration of normal conduction. The drug's ability to slow the pulse is useful in treating certain kinds of arrhythmias.

VASCULAR DISEASES The diseases of the blood vessels—arteriosclerosis and peripheral arterial and peripheral venous diseases—are discussed elsewhere (see chapters 14 and 15). All these are chronic conditions on which drugs act symptomatically and not curatively. The major problem in arterial disease is the narrowing or blockage of the arteries, decreasing their capacity to supply body organs with oxygen and nutrients. The result may be stroke, angina, or heart attack. The major problem in venous disease is the formation of blood clots that can cause inflammation and swelling or, if the clots break loose, can travel to the lungs and block vital blood vessels. Drug treatment of these conditions is directed toward preventing the formation of atherosclerotic deposits in the arteries or preventing formation of blood clots. Therapy directed toward dissolving already formed clots is still in the experimental stage.

Lipid-Lowering Drugs Persons who have large amounts of lipids (fats) in the blood have been found to develop arteriosclerosis earlier and more seriously than do those who have less of these fats. A theory based on this fact is that arteriosclerosis may be prevented or at least arrested by lowering the fats in the blood. This is still speculation, and the usefulness of lowering blood fats has not yet been totally proved. In the light of present knowledge, many doctors believe that it is prudent, and certainly not harmful, to attempt to lower blood fats. Drugs used for this purpose either lower blood fats, particularly cholesterol, by a mechanism that has not yet been identified, or they lower the level of cholesterol by preventing its absorption from food and by encouraging its elimination through the bowel.

Two drugs moderately effective in lowering cholesterol and other fats in a way that is not yet understood are clofibrate and nicotinic acid. Although both are relatively well tolerated, clofibrate can cause nausea and drowsiness and on rare occasions cramps and stiff muscles. It can also interfere with the action of some anticoagulants, and if these are used together, special precautions must be taken. Nicotinic acid is both a lipid-lowering agent and a vasodilator. Its major side effect is that it sometimes causes dilation of the blood vessels of the skin, causing a flushing of the face.

Cholestyramine is the major drug used in the United States to lower lipids by changing fat absorption and promoting fat elimination. The drug acts by binding bile in the bowel. Bile is a necessary substance in the body's absorption of fat, and when it is inactivated by the drug, fat is less readily absorbed. Bile is largely composed of cholesterol and is normally broken down in the bowel, where the cholesterol is reabsorbed. Cholestyramine prevents the breakdown of bile, therefore more cholesterol is used to make bile, and this cholesterol is then lost in the feces along with the drug. Because the drug must be taken in large doses to be effective, nausea and gastrointestinal upset may result. It has a distinctly unpleasant taste and may cause constipation and also bind other drugs (including digitalis preparations and some of the anticoagulants), preventing their absorption and decreasing their effectiveness.

Anticoagulants are used in diseases of the arteries and veins to prevent clotting. The clotting of blood is due to a complicated interaction of a series of proteins and small cells (platelets) normally present in blood. The anticoagulant drugs either decrease the amount of proteins or inhibit the clotting tendency of the platelets. Anticoagulants that act on the proteins are of unquestioned value in the treatment of venous clots but of less certain value in arterial disease. Warfarin and bishydroxycoumarin are the most common long-term drugs of this kind. (Another drug, heparin, is of limited use because it must be given by injection.) Both drugs block the body's ability to use vitamin K, an agent necessary in the production of the clotting proteins.

A danger in using these drugs is that they may interfere too drastically with clotting, possibly resulting in serious bleeding, either externally or internally, which is more serious, particularly when it occurs in the brain. The effect of the drugs can be reversed with an excess of vitamin K, however. Most patients on coumarin drugs therefore carry vitamin K tablets which can be taken at the first sign of serious bleeding. Careful supervision and frequent testing of clotting ability are essential in managing patients on this kind of drug therapy. Another problem is that the anticlotting effect of these drugs can be augmented by other medications. Aspirin, for example, which has only a slight ability to decrease clotting when taken alone, can have a marked increase in this ability when taken with an anticoagulant. Any patient who takes an anticoagulant drug should consult a doctor before taking a new drug or stopping an already-prescribed one. Certain sedatives are known to decrease the effectiveness of anticoagulants, while other drugs increase it.

Anticoagulants

PRINCIPLES

1. There is no "miracle" drug that can cure cardiovascular disease, but there are many drugs that can modify the effects and relieve the distressful symptoms of a malfunctioning heart or damaged blood vessels.

2. Two kinds of drugs are beneficial in treating congestive heart failure (the inability of the heart to pump sufficient oxygenated blood); digitalis, which causes the heart to contract more strongly with each beat and thus brings the rate closer to a normal level; and diuretics, which increase the output of salt and water in urine, thereby reducing the characteristic swelling of heart failure. Vasodilators are also sometimes used.

3. *The drugs used to treat angina pectoris usually relieve pain by reducing the heart's demand for oxygen. Principal among these are the nitrates, especially nitroglycerin.*

Other Drugs

Propranolol also reduces oxygen demand by slowing the heart rate and decreasing the speed of contraction. Digitalis is sometimes used in conjunction with propanolol to offset some of propanolol's toxicities or when heart failure aggravates the angina. When angina is caused by spasm of the heart's arteries, nitrates are especially useful.

4. *Unlike congestive heart failure and angina pectoris, hypertension often presents no symptoms. Drug treatment is designed to lower blood pressure and prevent the serious complications that may result from persistent high blood pressure. Diuretics lower blood pressure by reducing the amount of fluid in the body and by relaxing blood vessels. Vasodilators also relax blood vessels but must be combined with other drugs because the body's compensatory mechanisms cancel out some of their benefits. Drugs used in combination with vasodilators to prevent the compensation block some of the messages from the brain and the sympathetic nerves to the heart.*

5. *Abnormalities in the heart rate or rhythm can be corrected by drugs that block the conduction of abnormal impulses in the heart or by drugs that restore normal conduction.*

6. *Treatment for blood vessel diseases is primarily directed toward preventing the formation of atherosclerotic deposits, which block arteries, or the formation of clots, a major problem in venous disease. Several drugs are moderately effective in lowering levels of cholesterol by preventing its absorption or by a mechanism that is unknown. Anticoagulant drugs are effective in preventing the formation of clots in the veins but are of less certain value in arterial disease.*

Drugs that act on the platelets may somewhat reduce clot formation in both veins and arteries. Although their effectiveness has not yet been proved, they are far less dangerous than the other anticoagulants and by themselves almost never cause bleeding. Aspirin, dipyridimole (also a vasodilator), and anturane (an anti-gout medicine) are the major drugs in this category.

Vasodilators have been tried in the treatment of arterial disease, but the efforts were abandoned when it was discovered that permanently diseased vessels cannot dilate. Indeed, the effort to dilate them may actually be harmful to the body. Because vasodilators promote blood flow preferentially through normal vessels, these normal vessels would, in effect, "steal" blood from the diseased vessels, making their diminished flow even less. In certain conditions, however, vasodilators or drugs blocking the sympathetic nerves may be useful; for example, when decreased blood supply to such areas as the hands and feet (or heart) is due to spasm of the small arteries, rather than to arteriosclerosis or blood clots.

Recently there have been some efforts toward dissolving blood clots in cases of stroke or heart attack, on the assumption that if blood supply can be restored quickly, the degree of damage can be lessened. Drugs used in these experiments augment and intensify the body's own mechanism for dissolving blood clots, but there is to date no clear evidence that they are of any use in minimizing the damage from stroke or heart attack. Since such drugs can cause severe bleeding, they require careful supervision, and patients receiving them must be hospitalized.

22

OTHER FORMS OF HEART DISEASE

Walter H. Abelmann, M.D.

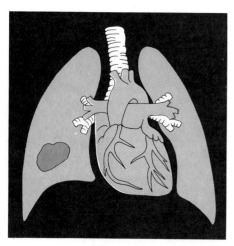

Pneumonia. Acute inflammation of an area of the lung resulting from bacterial invasion may have serious side effects on the heart, particularly if there is an underlying heart disease. The body attempts to combat the infection by increasing the demand for blood, which in turn places an added burden on the heart, forcing it to pump more blood with each beat.

The systems and organs of the body are so interrelated that disease or malfunction of one can have serious consequences for the others. That interdependence is particularly important to the closed-circuit cardiovascular system when there is decreased function of the lungs and kidneys, the organs of exchange with the external environment, or of the endocrine system, the group of ductless glands which helps regulate the internal and external environments. Fortunately, the body is equipped with an almost miraculous ability to detect failure in one system or organ and to compensate by adjustments in another system or organ. The cardiovascular system has its own process of compensation and adjustment, enabling it to deal with the burden of weakened or diseased lungs, kidneys, glands, and other parts of the body. The compensation can fail, however, when disease in a related system is severe or prolonged or when the compensating organ is itself weakened by disease or malfunction.

Although the heart can make a prodigious effort to compensate for the failure of other systems and organs, it too is vulnerable to a variety of diseases and malfunctions. Diseases of the coronary arteries and hypertension are well known in the United States and other industrialized countries because of their prevalence. However, other less-known and equally dangerous diseases can affect the heart, either directly or through its compensatory role, and these, in fact, constitute the principal forms of heart disease in many parts of the world. To understand the workings of the heart, it is necessary to know something about the origins, course, and cure of these diseases, many of which are entirely preventable, and many treatable with specific measures.

SYSTEMIC DISEASES
Lung Diseases

PNEUMONIA   An acute infection and inflammation of the lungs, pneumonia is still a leading cause of disability and death. Even though most bacterial pneumonias are amenable to antibiotic treatment and most viral pneumonias are self-limiting and not in themselves life-threatening, the disease remains a threat because of its potentially serious side effects on the circulatory system. The fever and heightened metabolism that are characteristic of pneumonia create a demand for a greater blood supply to the organs of the body, which can only be met by an accelerated heart rate and an increased volume. A healthy heart can tolerate the increased demand, but if the heart is impaired by disease or congenital defect, even of a previously unrecognized nature, the extra stress could result in heart failure. Such a chain of events lies behind the high death rate seen among persons with chronic heart disease during outbreaks of influenza.

Many systemic infections besides pneumonia increase body temperature and metabolic demands, but an infection of the lungs puts particular stress on the cardiovascular system. The parts of the lung that are affected by the disease cannot be ventilated adequately, and because these areas contain less oxygen, the blood flowing through them receives a less than normal supply. The resultant lower concentration of oxygen in the blood reaching the left ventricle and ultimately the heart muscle itself, may in turn impair the functioning of the already overworked heart. The problem is compounded by the fact that local irritation of a lung stimulates the respiratory center in the brain to increase the rate of breathing. Moreover, if the lung has become hardened and stiffened by the disease, the respiratory muscles must work harder to overcome the resistance, thereby increasing the demand for energy and blood flow. The extraordinary demand for blood in the pulmonary circulation can only be met by a great volume of blood in the right ventricle. Unfortunately, the demand is made at a time when perspiration and increased respiration result in loss of water (exhaled air is saturated with water vapor) and thus a decrease in blood volume. Under the circumstances, the blood returning to the heart actually decreases in volume, the heart does not pump the required amounts of blood, and blood pressure may fall.

In addition to the burden of lung infection on the work load of the heart, there is a risk of direct invasion of either the muscle of the heart (myocardium) or the thin membrane which surrounds it (pericardium). The infection may result in irregularities of the heartbeat, especially premature beats or contractions of the atria, or in some cases completely erratic and uncoordinated contractions, called atrial fibrillation. A pneumonia virus sometimes invades the heart muscle, producing an inflammatory condition called myocarditis. Pneumonia bacteria may create acute inflammation of the inner layer of the heart (endocardium), a condition called bacterial endocarditis. Both complications are discussed in detail later in this chapter.

The cardiovascular effects of pneumonia range from palpitation, weakness, fatigue, and dizziness to the full symptomatic picture of congestive heart failure. (See Congestive Heart Failure, chapter 13.) It is imperative that pneumonia in a cardiac patient be promptly recognized and treated, not only with appropriate antibiotics but also with adequate fluids and oxygen. Digitalis and cardiac drugs may be needed if heart failure or atrial fibrillation develops. Patients with chronic heart disease should also be protected by vaccines, especially the influenza and pneumococcal vaccines, to prevent at least some forms of potentially dangerous pneumonia.

PULMONARY EMBOLI Blood clots or thrombi which have formed in the veins of the legs or abdomen, or within the right atrium and ventricle, are sometimes dislodged and carried by the bloodstream to the lungs. Such emboli can be due to a number of conditions and are frequently associated with the sluggish circulation of chronic heart failure and with surgical procedures following which blood has a greater tendency to clot. When a significant part of the pulmonary arterial system becomes plugged by emboli, pulmonary arterial pressure rises. The right ventricle must then pump harder at a time when the blood nourishing it may be deficient in oxygen (because the lungs have failed to oxygenate the blood adequately). When pulmonary circulation is seriously blocked or when heart function is impaired, the right ventricle becomes enlarged and begins to fail, producing the symptoms of congestive heart failure. The condition is called acute cor pulmonale, or "heart disease due to lung disease."

Pulmonary emboli sometimes result in damage to the lung tissue supplied by the blocked artery (pulmonary infarction). The condition can produce chest pains which are aggravated by breathing, and blood-stained sputum; both symptoms alert the physician to the possible existence of emboli. The

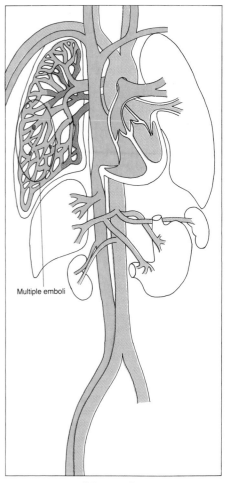

Multiple emboli

Pulmonary emboli

Blood clots formed in various parts of the body—the veins of the legs or abdomen or within the heart itself —are carried to the lung, where they may become trapped in the pulmonary arteries. The clogged arteries cause a rise in pressure within the lung, forcing the heart to work harder.

diagnosis can be confirmed by physical examination, chest X ray, and inspection of the lungs by means of lung scans or pulmonary angiograms (a process similar to cardioangiography).

Treatment of acute cor pulmonale is designed to dissolve clots and prevent their further formation, usually by injections of heparin, an anticoagulant, which may be supplemented by urokinase or streptokinase. The patient is then put on a long-term program of oral anticoagulant drugs such as warfarin (Coumadin), to prevent recurrence of the clots. On occasion, surgery is necessary to remove clots or to prevent additional clots, particularly those formed in the legs, from reaching the lungs.

CHRONIC LUNG DISEASE Long-term disease of the lungs results in increased pressure in the pulmonary arteries (pulmonary hypertension) and an additional burden of work on the right ventricle. Eventually, the right ventricle becomes enlarged and may ultimately fail, particularly if chronic lung disease impairs the supply of oxygen. One effect of decreased oxygen in the blood is cyanosis, a bluish discoloration of the skin. The syndrome, called chronic cor pulmonale, is most often seen in patients with emphysema, a chronic obstructive lung disease, which is sometimes a late complication of chronic bronchial asthma. Cor pulmonale may also be a complication of severe tuberculosis, as well as of fibrosis of the lung, a condition in which there is an abnormal increase in connective tissue. But whatever the underlying cause, the manifestations are almost always overshadowed by the symptoms of advanced lung disease, which has reached the stage of significant shortness of breath and disability. The treatment of congestive heart failure associated with cor pulmonale, though similar to that for other forms of heart failure, is not effective if the underlying lung disease is not recognized and its progress reversed.

Endocrine Diseases Virtually all hormones secreted by the glands of the endocrine system (the adrenal, thyroid, and pituitary glands, for example) directly or indirectly affect the cardiovascular system. The thyroid, which produces two hormones, thyroxine and triiodothyronine, is frequently associated with heart disease related to overproduction of a hormone.

HYPERTHYROIDISM The disease resulting from overaction of the thyroid gland is characterized by an accelerated rate of metabolism. The disorder demands increased intake and transport of oxygen, which is met by more rapid breathing and blood flow, brought about by an increase in heart rate and stroke volume. Since an augmented stroke volume results in a full and bounding pulse, as well as increased systolic blood pressure, heart palpitations are a common symptom. The normal heart can tolerate the extra work, providing the heart muscle itself does not become diseased and atrial fibrillation does not develop. In addition to palpitations, the symptoms of hyperthyroidism may include restlessness and overactivity, sweating, nausea, nervousness, and diarrhea. Specific biochemical blood tests facilitate an accurate diagnosis, and medical and, occasionally, surgical therapy are effective in curing the disease.

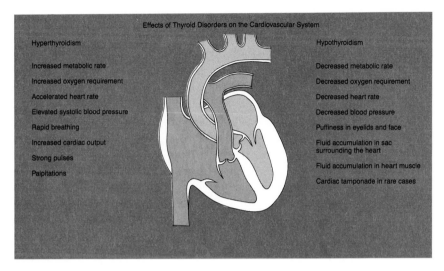

Effects of Thyroid Disorders on the Cardiovascular System

Hyperthyroidism

Increased metabolic rate

Increased oxygen requirement

Accelerated heart rate

Elevated systolic blood pressure

Rapid breathing

Increased cardiac output

Strong pulses

Palpitations

Hypothyroidism

Decreased metabolic rate

Decreased oxygen requirement

Decreased heart rate

Decreased blood pressure

Puffiness in eyelids and face

Fluid accumulation in sac surrounding the heart

Fluid accumulation in heart muscle

Cardiac tamponade in rare cases

Thyroid Gland Diseases

HYPOTHYROIDISM   Underaction of the thyroid gland results in a decreased rate of metabolism and a decreased oxygen requirement. The heart beats slowly, and blood pressure tends to be low. A particular form of edema, most noticeable in the eyelids and face (myxedema), sometimes accompanies hypothyroidism. Fluid also accumulates in the pericardial sac about the heart and even in the heart muscle itself, producing an enlarged cardiac silhouette on X-ray examination. Hypothyroidism often coexists with arteriosclerotic heart disease and may predispose a person to that disease. In exceptional cases, cardiac tamponade may also develop. In this life-threatening situation, the heart is compressed by fluid filling the pericardial sac. Hypothyroidism is treatable and curable by providing a substitute for the missing thyroid hormone. Treatment must proceed cautiously, however, because a too sudden increase in the heart's work load may bring out manifestations of an underlying coronary artery disease such as angina pectoris.

Chronic Failure of the Kidneys

Chronic kidney failure is frequently accompanied by circulatory congestion, even in the absence of significant hypertension. (The association between kidney disease and hypertension is discussed in Hypertension, chapter 10.) The condition closely resembles congestive heart failure, but it is not necessarily identical with or closely related to it. The increased circulating blood volume and edema of chronic failure are largely the result of failure of severely diseased kidneys to regulate body water and essential minerals. Because sodium is retained rather than excreted, less water is eliminated. The accumulation of acid metabolites, which are waste products of the metabolic process, tends to intensify the condition and may also indirectly impair cardiac function. If hypertension and anemia accompany cardiac overload, circulatory congestion may degenerate into true congestive heart failure. Although diuresis (increased excretion of urine) and correction of acidosis may bring some relief, normal circulation will not be restored until the underlying renal failure is corrected. Some disorders resulting in renal failure are self-limiting, running their course in a more or less definite time pattern. Others may require repeated kidney dialysis (mechanical removal of fluid wastes) or kidney transplants.

Blood Diseases

ANEMIA   This condition is characterized by a decreased number of red blood cells and a decreased amount of hemoglobin circulating in the blood. Since hemoglobin is the pigment which binds oxygen, the result is a decreased concentration of oxygen in the blood and therefore a less than normal supply to the tissues. Oxygen for the tissues may in part be obtained by a compensatory process which extracts more oxygen than normal from the blood. The main compensatory mechanism, however, is an increase in the amount of blood pumped, thus bringing the delivery of oxygen up to a normal level. Anemia, therefore, is accompanied by increased cardiac output, brought about by both a greater stroke volume and an accelerated heart rate. The result is more work for the heart. The usual evidences of high cardiac output are a bounding pulse and high systolic and low diastolic blood pressure. A healthy heart functions well under the increased work load, but weakness and fatigue may become evident on exertion. However, in cases of severe chronic anemia in physically active individuals, especially children, or cases in which anemia develops rapidly as a result of disease or hemorrhage, even the normal heart may fail. When the heart is impaired by disease, heart failure may develop with an even less severe decrease in red cells. Finding the cause of the anemia and correcting it are therefore major considerations in treatment.

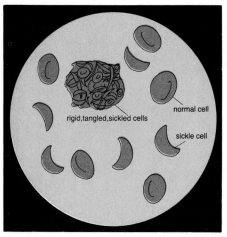

Sickle Cell Anemia

Crescent-shaped red cells, distorted by an inherited abnormality in the structure of hemoglobin, are removed from the blood more quickly than normal red cells, decreasing the oxygen content of blood. Sickle cells tend to form clots which obstruct the flow of blood through small vessels.

SICKLE CELL ANEMIA   A special type of anemia is found almost exclusively among black persons. In this inherited ailment, the normally disk-shaped red blood cells become sickle or crescent in shape. Sickle cells are removed from the blood more quickly than normal red cells, and therefore the blood carries less oxygen than normal. Under conditions of low oxygen or low blood flow, sickle cells tend to aggregate and form plugs which may block blood flow in small blood vessels. Some sickle cell anemia patients have inherited two genes for the abnormal cell formation; this condition is both rarer and much more severe than the one that occurs when a single abnormal gene is balanced by a normal one. In the latter case, anemia is mild or nonexistent. Sickling of red blood cells in the coronary circulation may impair heart muscle function directly, and sickling in the pulmonary circulation may, on rare occasions, cause cor pulmonale. The main cardiovascular complications of sickle cell disease, however, are the anemia itself, thrombosis, and myocardial infarction.

POLYCYTHEMIA   An abnormal increase in the number of circulating red blood cells results in increased viscosity or thickening of the blood. This increases both the resistance to flow and the work demand on the heart. Severe polycythemia may lead to heart failure if the heart is already weakened by other disease. Polycythemia may develop as a compensatory mechanism, as in the case of a congenital heart defect with a right-to-left shunt (see Congenital Heart Defects, chapter 16), but even this kind of secondary polycythemia may eventually become damaging to the circulation. In severe polycythemia, it may be necessary to reduce the number of red blood cells by removing blood from a vein, a treatment procedure called phlebotomy. Reduction in blood volume offsets the problem of viscosity, but only for a while and must be repeated at regular intervals.

LEUKEMIA   The malignant proliferation of white blood cells in leukemia eventually leads to infiltration of tissues with these cells. The heart muscle tissue may ultimately be invaded, resulting in decreased heart function or disturbances in the conduction of the electrical impulses that regulate contraction (arrhythmias). Leukemia is one of the causes of secondary cardiomyopathy, discussed later. Treatment is aimed at controlling the leukemia by administration of therapeutic agents, which unfortunately are sometimes themselves toxic to the heart.

A generalized infection caused by the spirochete *Treponema pallidum* and acquired as a venereal disease through sexual contact—the disease syphilis— can have a disastrous effect on the cardiovascular system. The damage caused by the organism often does not become apparent until many years after initial, untreated symptoms appear. The late complications are leaking of the aortic valve resulting from dilatation of the valve ring, and formation of aneurysms in the ascending aorta. The aneurysms or outpouchings of the aorta may impinge on neighboring tissues and nerves, causing pain or discomfort. The most feared complication is a life-threatening rupture of an aneurysm. Surgical resection and replacement of the affected portion of the aorta is the preferred treatment. Aortic leaking or insufficiency results in a backward flow of blood from the ascending aorta into the left ventricle during each diastole. The left ventricle must therefore pump a much larger volume of blood with each contraction, and the extra load results in both dilatation and hypertrophy of the heart, which may reach great size. The clinical manifestations of syphilitic aortic insufficiency are almost identical with those of rheumatic aortic insufficiency. (See Rheumatic Fever, chapter 17.) In cases of severe valve damage, surgical intervention and replacement of the aortic valve may be necessary.

Syphilis is a preventable disease, but if the infection has been acquired, prompt recognition and effective treatment, usually with penicillin, will prevent later cardiovascular complications.

Syphilis

The most common forms of cardiovascular disease in the Western world are coronary artery disease, hypertension, and stroke, and these are discussed in separate chapters. However, a number of other diseases can afflict the heart muscle, as well as its inner and outer membranes, causing damage through infection and inflammation, and these are reviewed here.

INFLAMMATORY DISEASES OF THE HEART

Inflammation of the inner lining of the heart, the endocardium, results in wart-like growths on this smooth, thin membrane, usually on a heart valve. The condition is called endocarditis. The growths, which usually contain a mixture of bacteria, blood cells, and fibrin (a protein in a blood clot), seed the bloodstream with bacteria and can deform and even destroy heart valves. The growths may also break off, enter the circulation as emboli, and clog peripheral arteries. If an artery in the brain becomes clogged, a stroke may result; a myocardial infarction may follow if the blockage is in a coronary artery. (See Coronary Artery Disease, chapter 11.) If the aortic valve is affected, the result can be severe aortic regurgitation, or backward flow of blood through the

Endocarditis

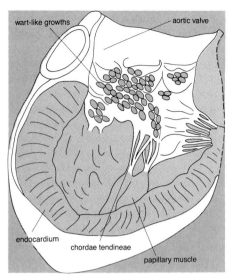

Advanced Bacterial Endocarditis

Cross-section of the heart shows clusters of bacterial growth in the cusps of the aortic valve extending to the chordae tendineae. Unable to close completely, the valve permits severe backward flow of blood from the aorta into the left ventricle.

valve. Impairment of the aortic valve usually leads to failure of the left ventricle, with symptoms of shortness of breath.

Bacterial endocarditis is most likely to occur on a valve already scarred by rheumatic fever or syphilis. Some congenital heart abnormalities also predispose a person to endocarditis; among these are ventricular septal defect, coarctation of the aorta, and patent ductus arteriosus (see Congenital Heart Defects, chapter 16). Introduction of an artificial valve increases the risk of the disease. The most common infecting agents are streptococcus, pneumococcus, and staphylococcus. The disease was once almost invariably fatal, but since the advent of antibiotics early recognition and treatment have led to a 70 to 80 percent survival rate. Unfortunately, the more dangerous staphylococcal endocarditis has increased in frequency, as has endocarditis caused by bacteria other than those listed and even by fungi and rickettsiae. Rickettsiae are small organisms (cocci or coccobacilli) which occupy a position in life form between viruses and bacteria and require the presence of living cells to grow.

Acute endocarditis occurs when a large number of bacteria enter the bloodstream, producing fever, chills, rapid destruction of a heart valve, and heart failure. More often, however, the process of the infection is slow, or subacute, resulting in weakness, fatigue, slight fever, sweating, and sometimes aching joints. Physical examination often detects anemia and heart murmur. The existence of the disease is proved by blood cultures, and multiple blood samples are often required to identify the invading microorganism. Identification of the type of bacteria involved is important, since it permits selection of the most appropriate antibiotic treatment.

Alertness to the possibility of bacterial endocarditis on the part of the patient and the physician is the first step in early recognition. Persons with known rheumatic or congenital heart abnormalities are most frequently affected, and prevention is critical in their case. Preventive antibiotic treatment should be undertaken before, during, and after any procedure that could result in bacteria entering the bloodstream. Such procedures include dental and oral surgery (and even routine dental work, such as cleaning the teeth), gastrointestinal and genitourinary tract surgery, and surgery of the upper respiratory tract.

Pericarditis Inflammation of the pericardium, or outer covering of the heart, results in a roughening and thickening of the membrane and an outpouring of fluid into the pericardial sac surrounding the heart. Acute pericarditis, the most frequent kind, is caused by a viral infection (coxsackie, echo, or influenza virus). Viral pericarditis is especially frequent in young patients. More rarely, the disease is caused by a bacterium such as staphylococcus, streptococcus, or even tubercle bacillus. The pericardium is sometimes also affected by fungi such as histoplasma or actinomyces, or by parasites such as amoeba or toxoplasma. Noninfectious pericarditis may be caused by irritation stemming from disease of the underlying heart muscle, such as acute myocardial infarction; by injury, such as a stab wound or heart operation; by tumors; or by radiation. Rheumatic fever, rheumatoid arthritis, lupus erythematosus, and other connective tissue disorders are known to involve the pericardium. The accumulation of waste products in the blood and tissues resulting from kidney failure can also lead to a severe inflammatory reaction in the pericardium, known as uremic pericarditis.

Acute pericarditis stimulates the pain receptors in the pericardium, resulting in pain under the breastbone, over the left side of the front of the chest, and often in the left shoulder. The pain is usually made worse by deep breathing and relieved when the patient sits up and leans forward. A stethoscope applied to the front of the chest may detect a grating sound with each heartbeat, produced by the rough surfaces of the pericardium rubbing against each other. Several days of laboratory tests may be necessary before the disease can be accurately diagnosed. The difficulty arises from the fact that the electrocardiogram and the chest pains can at times be confused with the manifestations of myocardial infarction.

Acute viral pericarditis is also referred to as acute benign pericarditis because in most cases it follows a self-limiting course without complications. It may, however, be associated with the more serious inflammation of the underlying heart muscle (myocarditis) and may recur.

CONSTRICTIVE PERICARDITIS In a late complication of bacterial pericarditis, associated with pus formation as well as with chronic pericardial disease, a thickening and stiffening of the pericardium constricts the heart, preventing adequate filling and emptying of the ventricles, and culminates in congestive heart failure. The complication is especially associated with tuberculous pericarditis. Eventually, it may require surgical removal of a section of the pericardium (pericardiectomy) to allow the heart to function normally again. Fortunately, the heart can function quite well after being deprived of some of the protection the pericardium offers. Early detection and diagnosis of bacterial pericarditis is important so that appropriate antibiotic therapy may be instituted, both to contain the process and to prevent acute and late complications.

CARDIAC TAMPONADE An early and especially life-threatening complication of pericarditis is known as cardiac tamponade. In this condition, fluid accumulates in the pericardial sac, making the membrane tense, and the resultant pressure on the heart prevents adequate filling of the ventricles and decreases cardiac output. The initial result is a rise in venous pressure, followed by a fall in arterial blood pressure, creating a medical emergency that requires prompt treatment. A puncture of the pericardial sac (pericardiocentesis) is performed to remove the fluid and relieve the pressure. Cardiac tamponade rarely accompanies viral pericarditis but is frequently seen in bacterial pericarditis, in pericardial disease secondary to tumors, and after chest injury.

Myocarditis

Inflammation of the heart muscle, myocarditis, may accompany almost any infectious, toxic, or inflammatory disease which is blood-borne or generalized. The reason for this is easily understood; about 20 percent of the systemic blood flow is pumped through the coronary arteries, perfusing the heart muscle with some 380 quarts (360 liters) of blood a day in the case of a sedentary person. Fortunately, there is great protection from any disease carried by the blood because of the wealth of vessels in the heart muscle, its generous lymphatic drainage, and its natural resistance. Since an inflammatory reaction is likely to be localized and spotty, the large reserve of the heart muscle prevents impairment of its pumping action. Thus, although some involvement of heart muscle in generalized infections is not uncommon, there are usually no clinical cardiac symptoms, disability, or complications. However, if the conduction system is affected by myocarditis, arrhythmias may occur. And when a large portion of the heart muscle is affected by the disease, the pumping action of the ventricles can be severely impaired, which may result in collapse and sudden death. If the progress of the disease is more gradual, the weakening of the heart muscle will eventually result in congestive heart failure.

Acute myocarditis may follow infection by certain types of virus, such as coxsackie, echo, or influenza, as well as mumps, measles, rubella, or psittacosis (parrot fever). Or it may be caused by bacterial infections, rickettsial infections (typhus or Rocky Mountain spotted fever) fungal infections (histoplasmosis or actinomycosis), or parasitic infections (trichinosis or toxoplasmosis). Toxic myocarditis is seen in diphtheria and in phosphorus or arsenic poisoning. Inflammatory lesions in the myocardium are also associated with systemic diseases (rheumatoid arthritis, lupus erythematosus, and rheumatic fever) and with hypersensitivity reactions to drugs and other substances.

As with pericarditis, most cases of myocarditis in the United States are due to viral infections, occur most frequently among young people, and tend to run a benign course. Pericarditis and myocarditis so often occur simultaneously that the condition has been given the name myopericarditis.

The clinical manifestations of myocarditis are related either to cardiac arrhythmias or to conduction disturbances caused by small, localized areas of damage or disease. At times the symptoms are those of heart failure and heart muscle weakness, conditions which are secondary to widespread and severe infection of the heart muscle. Excessively slow or fast heart rates, cardiac irregularities or enlargement, symptoms of heart failure, and an abnormal electrocardiogram for a patient with an acute infection should lead to a presumptive diagnosis of myocarditis, especially when there is no previous history of heart disease or abnormality. However, the diagnosis is at times obscured by prominent manifestations of the infection in other areas.

Treatment consists of specific medication, where available, for the underlying infection. All substances potentially toxic to the heart—alcohol, for example—must be avoided, and the patient must rest in order to reduce the work load of the heart. Digitalis is often prescribed for congestive heart failure, and anti-arrhythmic agents for cases of arrhythmia. Heart block may occasionally occur and become life-threatening, in which case a temporary pacemaker may be needed. When arrhythmias and conduction disturbances are pronounced, close supervision in an intensive care or coronary care unit is often desirable.

Although the vast majority of cases of myocarditis are self-limiting and permit full recovery, some are followed by residual impairment, recurrent attacks, or chronic heart disease and some are fatal. Some cases of chronic cardiomyopathy, described in the next section, may be a late complication of acute myocarditis. There is a remote possibility that an acute respiratory or gastrointestinal infection may result in myocarditis, and that is why excessive physical effort during such illness is inadvisable.

The medical term for acute, subacute, or chronic disease of heart muscle is cardiomyopathy. The endocardium and pericardium are not ordinarily affected, but the conduction system may be. Strictly speaking, acute myocarditis may be included among the cardiomyopathies, which are categorized as primary, or of unknown cause, and secondary, due to specific causes, often associated with diseases involving other organs as well as the heart.

HEART MUSCLE DISEASE (CARDIOMYOPATHY)

Changes in myocardial structure and function which cannot be attributed to a specific cause are called primary cardiomyopathies. Two principal types are distinguished—hypertrophic and congestive.

Primary Cardiomyopathy

HYPERTROPHIC CARDIOMYOPATHY   In this condition the muscle mass of the left and occasionally also the right ventricle is larger than normal. The increase is primarily in the size rather than the number of fibers. In one form of the disease, the wall between the two ventricles (septum) becomes enlarged and obstructs the flow of blood out of the left ventricle. The syndrome is known as hypertrophic obstructive cardiomyopathy or asymmetrical septal hypertrophy. (It is also termed idiopathic hypertrophic subaortic stenosis—IHSS.) In addition to obstructing blood flow, the thickened wall sometimes distorts one leaflet of the mitral valve, causing it to become leaky. In over half the cases, the disease is hereditary. Blood relatives of such persons are often found to have nonobstructive hypertrophic cardiomyopathy, in which the enlarged muscle does not obstruct blood flow. The disease is most common in young persons, primarily young adults.

The symptoms of obstructive cardiomyopathy are shortness of breath on exertion, dizziness, fainting, and angina pectoris. Some patients experience cardiac arrhythmias which, in some instances, lead to sudden death. The obstruction to the flow of blood from the left ventricle produces an added burden of work on the ventricle; a murmur may be heard during contraction. The murmur resembles that found in patients with narrowing of the aortic valve (aortic stenosis). When the mitral valve is involved, an additional murmur of mitral insufficiency or incompetence may be heard. The electrocardiogram may sometimes resemble that seen in patients with old myocardial infarction.

Diagnosis may be made on the basis of characteristic physical findings, electrocardiograms, and echocardiograms and may be confirmed by cardiac catheterization and angiocardiography. Treatment is usually with the drug propranolol, which, in proper doses, can reduce or eliminate the obstruction. Certain drugs, among them digitalis and isoproterenol, increase the obstruction and should not be taken. Surgical treatment is possible if the drug treatment fails.

CONGESTIVE CARDIOMYOPATHY   This is by far the most frequent form. In it the cavity of the heart is enlarged and stretched (cardiac dilatation), in contrast to the thickening of the walls in the hypertrophic form. In some cases, the myocardium shows evidence of degenerative changes and loss of muscle cells, which are replaced by fibrous tissue; in other cases, microscopic examination reveals little evidence of the disease. However, the heart is weak and does not pump normally, and most patients develop congestive heart failure. The condition may at first respond to conventional treatment for heart failure but it **tends** to recur at shorter and shorter intervals, becoming increasingly resistant to therapy. Arrhythmias and conduction disturbances may also occur.

Since blood flows more slowly through a heart that has become enlarged, blood clots are easily formed. Clots that stick to the endocardium are called mural thrombi. If the thrombotic material breaks off the right ventricle, it can be carried into the pulmonary circulation, forming pulmonary emboli. Mural thrombi formed in the left atrium or left ventricle may be dislodged and carried into the systemic circulation to form cerebral, renal, peripheral, **or even coronary** emboli. A patient with cardiomyopathy may suffer a major embolus before any other manifestation of cardiomyopathy appears, and anticoagulant therapy may be indicated. Arrhythmias may require anti-arrhythmic drugs, and, more rarely, a heart block may develop, requiring an artificial **pacemaker.** Therapy for congestive cardiomyopathy is often disappointing, however, and because the disease is so relentlessly progressive and the patients are often young and otherwise healthy, cardiac transplantation is sometimes considered. Although the basic scientific problem of tissue rejection has not been solved, transplantation has had some success.

Diagnosis of congestive cardiomyopathy is made on the basis of positive clinical findings on the one hand and the elimination of other known forms of heart disease on the other. (Coronary disease, valvular disease, hypertensive disease, and congenital heart disease may present similar symptoms.) Echocardiography, radionuclide imaging, cardiac catheterization, and biopsy of the heart muscle, which permits microscopic study of the tissue, may be helpful in diagnosis. When cardiomyopathy results in marked cardiac dilatation, the leaflets of the mitral and tricuspid valves may be unable to close, resulting in murmurs which are identical to those heard in patients with rheumatic valvular disease. True anginal pain is not typical of congestive cardiomyopathy, but the patient may feel nonspecific chest pain. Blood pressure may be increased in response to increased sympathetic nerve activity. This compensatory mechanism evoked by congestive heart failure is a condition which simulates hypertensive heart disease. Some patients therefore have high (or high normal) blood pressure readings, even though the typical patient with congestive cardiomyopathy and low cardiac output has a low or low normal pressure. Inasmuch as the level of blood pressure determines the work load and oxygen needs of the heart, one new approach in treatment is

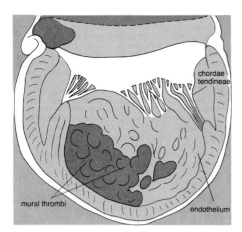

Congestive Cardiomyopathy

Cross-section of an enlarged heart cavity with clots adhering to the endothelium (mural thrombi). Dislodged particles of the thrombi may be carried by the blood to other areas of the body, causing blockage of cerebral, renal, peripheral, or coronary arteries.

the use of vasodilating agents to lower blood pressure and thereby decrease the work load on the left ventricle.

No specific cause of primary cardiomyopathy has thus far been identified by medical research. The condition may possibly be due to several factors, among them viral infections, hyperimmune responses, genetic abnormality of heart muscle, nutritional deficiency, lack of oxygen, toxins, and drugs. Careful study of patients reveals that at times cardiac involvement is actually secondary to a systemic process. Nevertheless, a large majority of patients with clinical manifestations of cardiomyopathy, and particularly patients with the congestive form, show no evidence of a specific cause. Some medical researchers believe that there are specific causes for the disease which have not yet been discovered. Others contend that the heart muscle becomes damaged by several processes which singly might be relatively innocuous but which collectively produce cardiomyopathy as the end result. In any case, prompt treatment of infection is essential for patients who have some evidence of existing heart muscle damage, as are a well-balanced diet and avoidance of alcohol and cardiotoxic drugs. Obesity, cigarette smoking, and anything that might increase blood pressure should also be avoided, since all these increase cardiac work and hence the burden on the damaged heart muscle.

Secondary Cardiomyopathy

Heart muscle dysfunction associated with generalized diseases is called secondary cardiomyopathy. The involvement of the heart often does not show significant clinical manifestations or symptoms, and even if these are significant, they may be overshadowed by other manifestations of the basic disease or disorder. Since cardiac involvement is generally not specific, the diagnosis is made from the noncardiac manifestations and characteristics. Therapy for the basic disease often reduces the cardiac involvement.

Cardiomyopathies, secondary to such systemic conditions as hyperthyroidism, leukemia, tumors, and thiamine deficiency, are possible. In addition, diseases of skeletal muscle, and neuromuscular disorders, such as the different forms of muscular dystrophy and Friedreich's ataxia (an inherited disease of the nervous system), especially in the more advanced stages, tend to involve the heart muscle, often resulting in arrhythmias, conduction disturbances, and heart failure.

Sarcoidosis is an inflammatory disease that can affect many tissues, most frequently those of the lungs. The condition may also involve heart muscle and is known to produce arrhythmias and heart block. An artificial pacemaker is often the best therapy and a protection against further complications.

In amyloidosis, a poorly understood generalized disease, particularly of the elderly, the heart muscle may be penetrated by amyloid, a fibrous, extracellular protein. The resulting stiffening of the heart prevents complete filling of the ventricles, as in hypertrophic cardiomyopathy. The condition mimics constrictive pericarditis and is an example of restrictive cardiomyopathy. It is often accompanied by arrhythmias.

Hemochromatosis is a condition in which excessive amounts of iron are deposited in tissues, creating a characteristic change in the pigmentation of the skin and resulting in liver disease and diabetes. The cause for this disorder of iron storage is unknown, except when it occurs in patients who have received excessive iron from multiple blood transfusions. Iron deposits in the heart may impair ventricular function and result in heart failure, arrhythmias, and conduction disturbances. Diagnosis is confirmed by detecting elevated blood iron levels or by biopsy. Removal of blood by phlebotomy may lower the iron level and relieve some symptoms, but the process must be repeated frequently.

Rheumatoid arthritis, lupus erythmatosus, scleroderma (a disease characterized by patchy hardening of the skin), and other connective tissue disorders may involve the heart muscle, valves, pericardium, and endocarium. Although the valves are rarely damaged or their function impaired, these diseases can give rise to heart murmurs. Lupus is particularly known for its tendency to produce pericarditis.

Toxic Cardiomyopathies

A number of drugs and chemicals, especially phosphorus, lead, and mercury, have a poisonous effect on the heart. Even some drugs used in the treatment of cardiovascular diseases can have toxic effects (see Cardiovascular Drugs, chapter 21). Among the therapeutic agents used in noncardiac disease, certain drugs commonly taken for emotional or psychiatric disturbances deserve special consideration.

PRINCIPLES

Many diseases besides coronary artery disease, valvular defects, strokes, and hypertension affect heart function, either directly by invasion of its tissues or secondarily by the extra stress they put upon the heart.

1. *Lung disease, particularly pneumonia, adds strain to the heart—a dangerous complication when its function is already impaired by a defect or disease. Lung disease reduces the oxygen level in the blood, thereby making the heart work harder to meet the demands of the body tissue, and presents the additional hazard of a possible spread of infectious agents to the heart itself, causing inflammation of the muscle and its membranes. Pulmonary emboli, originating in the legs and abdomen, can become lodged in the arteries of the lungs, and this too forces the heart to work harder. When lung disease is chronic, as in emphysema, the constant low level of oxygen in the blood causes cyanosis, a bluish discoloration of the skin. Heart failure may result.*

2. *An overactive thyroid gland speeds metabolism and demands a greater consumption of oxygen, which can*

DRUGS Phenothiazine drugs such as chlorpromazine and thioridazine (Mellaril) have been associated with degenerative changes in heart muscle, as well as with electrocardiographic abnormalities and with arrhythmias.

Tricyclic antidepressant drugs, such as imipramine and amitryptyline may also induce arrhythmias and abnormalities in electrocardiogams. In high doses they may decrease the heart muscle's force of contraction.

Adriamycin and daunorubicin, chemotherapeutic agents effective in the treatment of some forms of leukemia and malignant tumors, are known to be toxic to the heart muscle if large doses are given.

Emetine, chloroquine, and antimony drugs, used mainly in the treatment of such tropical diseases as amoebiasis, malaria, and schistosomiasis, have long been known to be potentially toxic to the heart.

None of these drugs is usually prescribed for patients with a history of significant heart disease. If any are taken continuously or in large doses, periodic heart examinations are advisable. Electrocardiographic and, in some instances, echocardiographic follow-up examinations can detect early toxic effects, and the drugs should generally be discontinued upon such findings.

ALCOHOL The most common substance known to be toxic to the heart is alcohol. The amount of alcohol contained in one or two standard-sized drinks is known to be sufficient to produce significant, if transient, impairment of heart muscle function. In larger doses, alcohol may also induce cardiac arrhythmias such as premature beats or even atrial fibrillation. Regular use of alcohol over long periods of time may also be accompanied by chronic congestive cardiomyopathy. Although the condition may be improved by abstention, it may often reach a state where it is not reversible—a form of heart disease called alcoholic cardiomyopathy. Excessive use of alcohol may be especially damaging to anyone with an already existing heart disease.

only be met by an accelerated heart rate and an increased stroke volume. An underactive thyroid, on the other hand, slows metabolism and the use of oxygen, and blood pressure falls. Edema may follow, but clinical heart disease is rare.

3. Circulatory congestion often

Tumors of the Heart

A few benign and some malignant tumors may originate in the heart; in addition, a larger number of malignant tumors may involve the heart either by direct extension, or by spreading from elsewhere in the body (metastases). Primary tumors of the heart are exceedingly rare, but one type should be mentioned. This is atrial myxoma, a benign tumor which forms in the left atrium (in three out of four cases) or in the right atrium. It may produce steady or intermittent obstruction, mimicking mitral or tricuspid stenosis. If obstruction is intermittent, there may be episodes of dizziness or syncope, often specifically related to changes in body position. Surgery is effective in treating this kind of tumor. Secondary tumors may involve the pericardium or myocardium, giving rise to pericarditis and cardiac tamponade, arrhythmias, or conduction disturbances. Cancers of the lung are among the tumors most frequently involving the heart.

accompanies chronic kidney failure, even when there is no significant hypertension. The condition closely resembles heart failure.

4. Blood diseases directly affect the heart's work. Anemia, a shortage of red blood cells, means that less oxygentated blood is supplied to body tissues. Polycythemia, an excess of red blood cells, slows blood flow because of increased viscosity, and

EATING HABITS

MALNUTRITION   Although many electrocardiograph abnormalities have been recorded in generally malnourished patients or in those with specific nutritional deficiencies, only one nutritional deficiency has been associated with a specific form of heart disease. This is a deficiency of thiamine or vitamin B_1 which has been linked with beriberi heart disease, a rare form of cardiac output failure. The disease is seen mainly in the Orient among active individuals whose diet consists primarily of polished rice. It is, however, occasionally seen in the West, especially in chronic alcoholic subjects. Heart failure results from the combination of dilation of peripheral blood vessels and impaired function of heart muscle and is largely reversible by administration of vitamin B_1 in the form of thiamine hydrochloride.

Kwashiorkor, a rare form of heart disease seen primarily in children in tropical climates, is associated with protein malnutrition. Proper nutrition can restore health.

the heart must pump harder. Leukemia, the malignant proliferation of white cells, may ultimately infiltrate heart muscle tissues.

5. Syphilis, if untreated, can attack the aortic valve and cause aortic insufficiency as well as aneurysms many years after the intial infection.

6. Bacterial infections sometimes inflame the inner lining of the heart, a condition known as endocarditis. Antibiotics are used to treat these potentially dangerous infections. Inflammation of the outer covering of the heart, the pericardium, may be caused by bacteria or viruses. There is also a noninfectious form of pericarditis due to irritation of the heart muscle, wounds, or other injuries, as well as some kinds of tissue disorders. Occasionally, pericarditis causes fluid to accumulate in the pericardial sac,

OBESITY   Severe obesity is associated with increased over-all metabolic requirements, blood volume, and cardiac output. Because of the increased work load, the heart may eventually become dangerously enlarged. In persons weighing 300 pounds or more, congestive heart failure has been observed in the absence of other heart disease or hypertension, although the latter is also found in such obese individuals. In the presence of other cardiovascular disease, the excessive burden obesity places on the heart can cause cardiac symptoms to appear *stiffening it. This dangerous complication is called cardiac tamponade. Myocarditis is an inflammation of the heart muscle itself caused by bacterial or viral infection. The mild, localized inflammation of heart muscle accompanying common infectious diseases is not a serious threat, but widespread infection can impair heart function.*

7. *Cardiomyopathy is the medical term for heart muscle disease. One form of the disease, hypertrophic cardiomyopathy, results in increased muscle mass of the left or right ventricle, or both. The hypertrophic tissue may also block blood flow through the heart. Congestive cardiomyopathy is a condition in which the heart's chambers enlarge and the normal pumping function is impaired. Neither of these conditions has any known cause. Because congestive cardiomyopathy may grow progressively worse, heart transplantation is sometimes considered. Secondary cardiomyopathies are associated with a number of specific causes or generalized diseases. Heart involvement is often not significant and may be overshadowed by symptoms of the underlying disease.*

8. *Many chemicals are toxic to the heart, as are a number of drugs used in treatment of emotional or psychiatric problems. Alcohol, in large doses or on a regular basis for many years, can also damage the heart.*

9. *Tumors of the heart are extremely rare. A benign tumor, atrial myxoma, may form in either the left or the right atrium, causing varying degrees of obstruction.*

10. *Eating habits may affect the heart. Deficiency of vitamin B$_1$ has been associated with the rare condition called beriberi heart disease. Excessive overweight leads to increased effort by the heart, and a high rate of congestive heart failure has been observed in persons weighing more than 300 pounds.*

earlier than they otherwise would. In either situation, weight reduction reverses the cardiovascular manifestations. The role of obesity in precipitating cardiac symptoms due to other heart disease, and the beneficial effects of weight reduction, cannot be overemphasized.

23

PREGNANCY AND THE CARDIOVASCULAR SYSTEM

Jay M. Sullivan, M.D.

The capacity of the body to adapt to stress is nowhere more dramatically evident than in the response of the cardiovascular system to the demands of
pregnancy. The exact process whereby the body, after conception has taken
place, begins to respond to the presence of life is not fully understood, but
medical science does have a good knowledge of the overall changes that take
place in the mother's body and the implication of some of these changes for
women with cardiovascular problems.

Shortly after conception, the series of changes that begin in the mother's
body result in an abundant supply of oxygen-rich blood for the developing
fetus. These changes in the mechanics of circulation involve the amount of

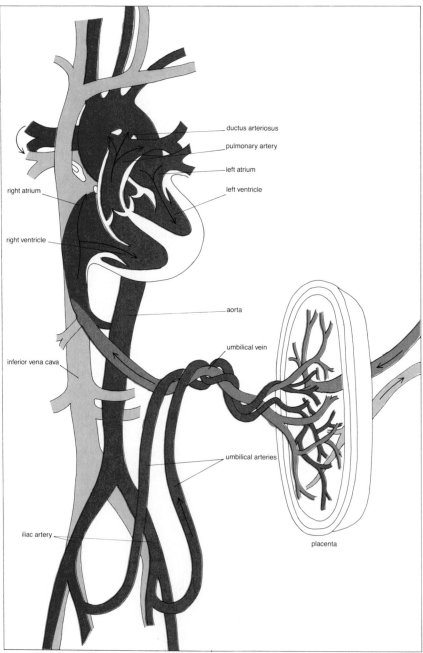

*Until the moment of birth, the
mother's placenta will supply
oxygen and blood to the fetal heart
and remove all waste as well. Thus
the mother both nourishes and
breathes for the fetus.*

ductus arteriosus

pulmonary artery

left atrium

left ventricle

right atrium

right ventricle

aorta

umbilical vein

inferior vena cava

umbilical arteries

iliac artery

placenta

Circulation in the Unborn Child

blood within the mother's vascular system (total blood volume), the volume of blood pumped every minute (cardiac output), and the degree of constriction or relaxation of the smallest arterial vessels, the arterioles (peripheral vascular resistance).

CARDIOVASCULAR CHANGES DURING PREGNANCY

Although the sequence of changes in the cardiovascular system and their interrelationship are not fully understood, it is clear that early in pregnancy the vascular resistance of the blood vessels in the uterus decreases, allowing a greater flow of blood to the uterus. This drop in resistance may be due to hormonal changes. Experiments have shown that estrogens, which are normally elevated in pregnancy, will cause a drop in vascular resistance in non-pregnant animals. Decreased resistance may also be the result of another hormone, prolactin, which is released from the pituitary gland during pregnancy. Prolactin lowers blood pressure, even with an augmented blood volume, which suggests a fall in resistance. The fall in vascular resistance is not limited to the blood vessels in the uterus, however, for the kidneys, hands, arms, and legs are similarly affected. Blood flow to the kidneys and the hands rises early in pregnancy but falls as term approaches. Flow to the arms and legs increases in the second half of pregnancy.

Blood volume begins to increase during the first three months. (Blood volume increases proportionally in multiple pregnancies; a woman carrying twins has a greater increase than does one carrying a single child.) By the thirtieth week of gestation the volume reaches a level about 40 percent above that before pregnancy and thereafter remains about the same until term, or may even fall slightly. The increase is due to a greater volume of plasma (the liquid part of blood) and a greater number of red blood cells (from 20 to 40 percent more). The increase in plasma volume occurs first, reaching a level about 50 percent higher by the thirty-second week. This is believed to be the result of

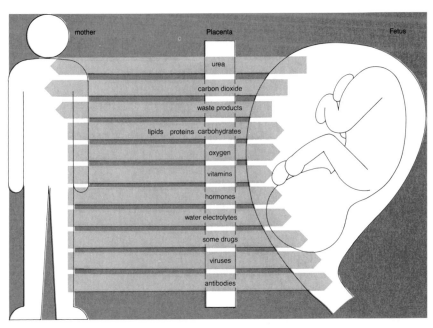

Until birth, blood rich in oxygen and nutrients is transported from the mother's circulatory system to the developing fetus via the umbilical vein. A branch of the umbilical vein, the ductus venosus, is connected to the inferior vena cava, which carries the blood to the right atrium. Two openings in the fetal heart —the foramen ovale between the atria and the ductus arteriosus connecting the pulmonary artery and the aorta—cause most of the blood to bypass the uninflated lungs and to enter the aorta. After supplying fetal tissue needs, the blood returns by way of the umbilical arteries to the placenta, where waste products are given off and nutrients and oxygen are picked up in the capillary exchange between mother and fetus.

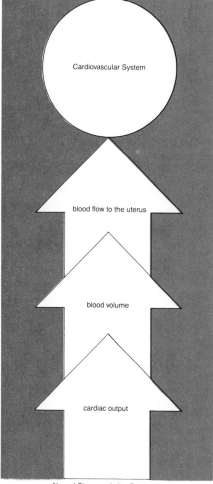

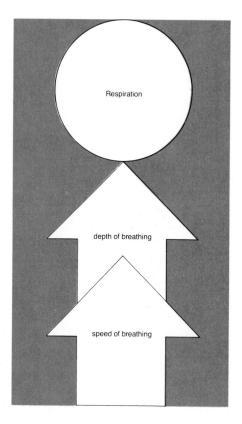

Normal Changes during Pregnancy

chemical changes in the body that cause retention of salt and water. The increase in plasma dilutes the blood, producing the physiologic anemia typical of pregnancy. Plasma volume stabilizes as pregnancy continues, but if sufficient iron is available the number of red cells in circulation will increase steadily. Many healthy women are, nevertheless, slightly anemic at term.

Cardiac output begins to rise early in pregnancy, reaching a peak (from 30 to 45 percent above resting nonpregnant levels) about the twentieth week and either remaining elevated or falling slightly until delivery. As the uterus enlarges, it compresses the large vein in the abdomen that returns venous blood from the legs to the heart (inferior vena cava). Changes in body position during pregnancy result in different degrees of compression of this vein, and thus in changes in cardiac output. Cardiac output is in fact very sensitive to changes in position, the effect being most pronounced while the woman is lying face up and least marked while she is lying on her left side.

Even though cardiac output rises, the changes that occur in the vessels leading away from the heart do not produce changes in blood pressure except for, in some instances, a drop in average pressure levels. Any rise in blood pressure during pregnancy must therefore be considered a warning signal and a cause for concern.

In addition to adaptation in the cardiovascular system, important changes in the mother's breathing also occur during pregnancy. Female sex hormones act upon the brain to make her breathe more deeply and more rapidly (hyperventilation), causing an increase in the quantity of air breathed. Thus from early pregnancy, the respiratory system, like the cardiovascular system, works hard to provide an optimal environment for the developing fetus. There is, however, a disproportionate increase in the work involved in breathing, since the respiration must be accomplished against the handicap of the enlarged uterus, which must be displaced downward with every inspired breath. As a result, many pregnant women are aware of their breathing even when they are at rest. This condition is perfectly normal during pregnancy and should not be confused with the shortness of breath (dyspnea) that is often an early sign of fluid congestion in the lungs of patients with heart disease.

Respiration

Although certain sudden and dramatic changes take place in the mother's circulation during labor and delivery, the magnitude of these changes is often less than that of those which occur during the final weeks of pregnancy. In labor, cardiac output increases about 20 percent with each uterine contraction (although pulse rate slows somewhat), but since labor is intermittent, the heart has a chance to rest between contractions. A rise in the mother's cardiac output immediately after delivery is a natural response which is often augmented by pain and anxiety. The increase in maternal blood volume that has gradually taken place during pregnancy is greater than any blood loss in normal labor. Even the greater average loss in Caesarean section delivery no longer constitutes a serious threat. An ample margin of safety is assured by modern blood replacement and operative techniques, as well as anesthesia. It can be said that pregnancy itself is the long testing period during which the mother's heart is prepared to withstand the stress of labor and delivery. The hazards of delivery, except for women with certain forms of heart disease, are amply prepared for and present no threat to the average healthy woman.

Labor and Delivery

In the first and second weeks after delivery, the mother's cardiovascular system gradually returns to its normal prepregnancy condition. Any additional stress on the circulatory system at this time is the result of blood loss during delivery, the beginning of lactation and the reabsorption and excretion of the expanded extravascular volume.

Although significant cardiovascular disease imposes an increased risk on the health of both mother and child during pregnancy and immediately after, most women with such problems are able to tolerate pregnancy quite well. Careful evaluation and follow up by both obstetrician and cardiologist are essential, since many authorities are convinced that early detection and proper care of cardiovascular problems would greatly reduce the mortality rate among such patients. Studies have found that from 0.4 percent to 4.1 percent of pregnant women show evidence of heart disease; of these 0.4 to 22 percent die from complications of pregnancy, usually at the time of delivery.

HEART DISEASE AND PREGNANCY

A careful cardiovascular examination is thus an essential part of every woman's medical evaluation during every pregnancy. The reason for this lies in the fact that pregnancy is accompanied by radical changes in the circulatory system; in this hyperdynamic state, heart lesions which previously had not been evident may become detectable on physical examination. Similarly, a mild or moderately severe cardiac problem which had not showed symptoms before pregnancy becomes a potential hazard when the heart is called upon to increase its work load. In addition, a damaged heart valve may worsen with time, and although a first pregnancy may not necessarily cause serious problems, subsequent pregnancies may very well aggravate the condition.

Medical examination during pregnancy is vital for another reason, which might be considered the reverse of the one just given: the patient may *not* have a heart condition, although recurring symptoms cause her to fear that she has. This kind of situation is not at all unusual, since the overactive circulation occurring in pregnancy can produce physical signs that mimic those of cardiovascular disease. Various innocent cardiac murmurs can be produced by increased blood flow through the heart or through the vessels of the chest wall and the breasts; rapid, but harmless, breathing can be caused by elevated hormone levels; unusual sounds within the lungs (pulmonary rales) suggesting heart failure may result when the enlarged uterus displaces the diaphragm upward; ankle swelling (edema) develops in as many as 50 percent of pregnant women as a result of added plasma volume. The pregnant woman should be reassured that such signs do not indicate a cardiac condition. It is important, however, that the progress of any symptom be checked regularly during pregnancy and immediately after. If the signs have not disappeared, further examination must be undertaken to determine whether they do point to an underlying heart disease.

Rheumatic Diseases Worldwide surveys indicate that most pregnant women with cardiovascular disease have either rheumatic heart disease or some form of congenital heart disease. Rheumatic heart disease (see Rheumatic Fever, chapter 17) is most commonly caused by a clinical or subclinical attack of acute rheumatic fever in childhood or early adulthood, which leaves the patient with a damaged mitral valve, e.g., mitral stenosis. This potentially hazardous condition involves progressive narrowing of the mitral valve, which regulates the flow of blood between the left atrium and the left ventricle. Because blood from the lungs cannot flow freely into the ventricle, it backs up in the atrium and then into the pulmonary vessels. When pressure on the pulmonary vessels rises to a critical point, fluid accumulates in the lung tissue (pulmonary edema) and interferes with the transfer of oxygen into the bloodstream.

Pulmonary edema can result from the increased work load on the heart handicapped by mitral stenosis or from other factors which increase the heart rate significantly. The treatment consists of adequate rest, salt restriction in diet, cautious use of diuretics to relieve congestion, digitalis to control any abnormalities in heart rhythm, and precautions against infection, which would put added demands on the damaged heart and valve. Patients who fail to respond to this kind of medical treatment can undergo corrective surgery to repair the defective valve or replace it completely. The best time for such surgery is between the twentieth and the twenty-fourth week of pregnancy, and the results have been encouraging.

Many patients with rheumatic heart disease are already on a regime of regular penicillin. The medication is continued during pregnancy, and at the time of delivery penicillin and streptomycin (or appropriate alternative antibiotics for allergic patients) should be taken as a precaution against bacterial endocarditis, an infection and inflammation of the lining of the heart.

Some patients with mild heart valve diseases do not show any symptoms prior to pregnancy and ordinarily tolerate without difficulty the added strains of pregnancy and delivery. Other patients—those, for example, with seriously damaged mitral or aortic valves—need careful medical management and possibly corrective surgery either before or early in pregnancy.

Women who have previously had valve replacement usually do not experience complications with pregnancy. The risk is further lessened if the artificial valve is one of the more recently developed kinds. Unlike the earlier types, these do not require the use of anticoagulants because the danger of clot formation is less. The constant use of anticoagulants to prevent clotting does pose a risk to the fetus. Some studies reveal a fetal mortality rate as high as 30 percent when the mother has regularly taken anticoagulants. (See Heart Valve Disease, chapter 18.)

Congenital Heart Disease

In most instances, congenital heart disease is not a threat to normal pregnancy and delivery. Medical centers have reported low maternal and fetal mortality rates in association with such common congenital defects as patent ductus arteriosus, tetralogy of Fallot, and atrial septal defects (see Congenital Heart Defects, chapter 16). Coarctation of the aorta, although usually well tolerated during pregnancy, poses the risks of aortic aneurysm and infection. However, in certain cases pregnancy is not advised. Patients with congenitally defective blood vessels often develop lasting changes in their pulmonary blood vessels that result in pulmonary hypertension. The death rate among these patients, and among those patients with "primary" pulmonary hypertension, is significantly elevated. Therapeutic abortion in these and other instances of congenital heart defects must be performed before the twelfth week of pregnancy; thereafter the abortion carries as great a risk as does the continuation of the pregnancy.

Other Cardiovascular Complications

PERIPARTAL CARDIOMYOPATHY This disorder, the cause of which is unknown, results in a gradual softening, thickening, and dilatation of the heart muscle (myocardium). As a result, congestive heart failure develops in the last month of pregnancy or in the first five months after delivery. The disease seems to occur primarily among black women and may be the result of poor nutrition. Many exceptions to these general findings have been shown, and both the cause and the prevalence of the disease in particular groups of the overall population are still subjects for speculation. Treatment of peripartal cardiomyopathy consists of rest, improved diet, salt restriction, diuretics, and digitalis. The treatment is successful in about half the cases. Other patients develop recurrent episodes of congestive heart failure, with serious consequences. Subsequent pregnancies may be dangerous, even with patients who respond well to therapy.

PRE-ECLAMPSIA This complication of pregnancy is extremely serious. The term "toxemia of pregnancy" is often used to describe this disorder because it was once thought to be a condition in which the blood is infested with poisonous products. Pre-eclampsia develops in about one out of twenty pregnant women, and usually begins in the twentieth week of pregnancy, with elevated blood pressure, edema, and protein in the urine. If it is not treated, eclampsia may follow, leading to generalized seizures, coma, and death. Although there are many theories about the causes of pre-eclampsia, they are still not clearly understood. Microscopic studies of the kidneys of patients reveal a characteristic lesion which consists of a thickening of the capillary endothelial cells so that blood flow through the filtering units of the kidneys is impaired. Blood platelets have been implicated in the production of this lesion.

No effective way has yet been found to prevent the development of pre-eclampsia, although prophylactic use of diuretic agents was once thought to be beneficial. Women in their first pregnancy, or with a history of complications in previous pregnancies, are more likely to develop the condition. Delivery of the fetus usually halts the progress of pre-eclampsia. If term has not been reached, control of the condition and additional time for fetal growth can sometimes be gained by bed rest, sedatives, and cautious use of diuretics, preferably in a hospital. A further rise in blood pressure and the development of neurological symptoms require the use of anticonvulsants, magnesium sulfate, and other agents to reduce hypertension. Delivery should follow as quickly as possible. With close medical attention, the chances of the mother's survival are excellent, although a favorable outcome for the infant is less likely. Early recognition of pre-eclampsia is essential, with regular checkups to determine that neither blood pressure nor weight show excessive increases.

THROMBOPHLEBITIS. This condition develops in the weeks after delivery rather than during pregnancy. Blood clots (thrombi) form in association with inflammation in the wall of a vein (phlebitis). An associated condition is pulmonary embolism, the escape of a portion of a blood clot (embolus) in a vein and its movement to the lungs. Study of both of these thromboembolic complications reveal that neither condition is significantly higher in pregnant women than in nonpregnant women of comparable age. In the first four weeks after delivery, however, the incidence of both superficial and deep phlebitis of the leg veins may be as much as forty-nine times as great as in nonpregnant women. Those most likely to develop these complications are patients in the older age groups, those who have had difficult deliveries, and those with a prior history of thrombophlebitis.

The classical signs of thrombophlebitis in pregnancy are pain in the calf of the leg, together with redness, swelling, tenderness, or warmth in the area. Nineteen percent of patients with deep vein thromobophlebitis develop pulmonary embolism, which was fatal in 28 percent of the cases shown in one study. It is essential that patients with such symptoms be treated with bed rest, heat, and anticoagulants.

Another, but fortunately low, risk associated with this complication is that of stroke. An increased frequency of strokes has been noted during pregnancy and in the immediate postpartum period. Arteriographic and autopsy studies have found that most of these attacks are due to thrombotic blocking of an artery within the brain.

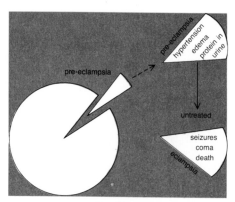

Pre-eclampsia

Pre-eclampsia is a serious complication that can lead to death of the fetus and, more rarely, the mother if it is not brought under control.

Finally, the incidence of phlebitis is greater in women who do not breast-feed their babies. Since this higher rate has been attributed to the relatively large doses of estrogen given to suppress lactation, the use of lower doses is being studied.

Women who use oral contraceptives appear to suffer from a wide range of disorders, including gall bladder disease, benign liver tumors, hypertension, myocardial infarction, and thromboembolism. A British study of 46,000 women showed that deep vein thrombosis occurred five times as frequently and cerebrovascular disease four times as frequently in those who used oral contraceptives as in women who did not use them. These conclusions have been supported by other studies. Further investigation indicates that thromboembolism occurs less frequently when oral contraceptives with lower doses of estrogen are used, but the rate is still higher than for patients who do not use oral contraceptives.

Studies made of women who have been hospitalized with nonfatal myocardial infarctions show a relatively high use of oral contraceptives as compared to control subjects. In addition, studies which take into consideration other risk factors—hypertension, diabetes, elevated blood lipids, and cigarette smoking—indicate that oral contraceptives add to the risk of myocardial infarction independently of these other risk factors. It has been estimated that with women who are currently using oral contraceptives, the risk of infarction is increased 2.8 times for those between the ages of thirty and thirty-nine and about 4.7 times for those between forty and forty-four years old. Every woman must weigh these risks against the risks that are normal in pregnancy.

A statistically significant rise in blood pressure occurs in women who take oral contraceptives, although this is of major significance only in less than 8 percent of the cases. The elevation is almost always reversible if the contraceptive is discontinued, but the reversal may take as long as six months. Women likely to develop hypertension while taking oral contraceptives are those most likely to develop it for other reasons—women who are older, excessively overweight or obese, have a family history of hypertension, or have a past history of blood-pressure elevation during pregnancy. Since hypertension may be aggravated by oral contraceptives, these agents are not the preferred method of contraception for patients with hypertension. Women taking oral contraceptives should have blood pressure readings at least every six months, particularly since symptoms may not always be evident to the individual. Severe, although infrequent, incidents of hypertension following the use of oral contraceptives have been reported. Patients who do have hypertension should inform their physicians if they are taking these contraceptives.

Alternative methods of birth control are preferred for many women. These may include the "rhythm" method, contraceptive diaphragms, or condoms. In cases where these are unacceptable, an intrauterine device (IUD) inserted with antibiotic protection to avoid infection appears to be less potentially dangerous than oral contraceptives. Particular care must be taken so that the IUD does not cause infections. The usual symptoms of such an

BIRTH CONTROL AND CARDIOVASCULAR PROBLEMS

PRINCIPLES

1. *Pregnancy increases the work load on the heart as the developing fetus and the mother's uterus require added blood flow. The heart's output may rise as much as 45 percent above normal prepregnancy rest states, reaching a peak about the twentieth week and either remaining elevated or dropping slightly after that. Labor and delivery place additional demands on the heart, but the mother's cardiovascular system returns to normal within a week or two after delivery.*

2. *Cardiovascular disease adds a risk during pregnancy, but it is often well tolerated. Close medical supervision is required before, during, and after pregnancy.*

3. *Because the cardiovascular system is under stress, heart disease which was not observed before pregnancy may become obvious and possibly be hazardous to health. Pregnancy may also cause symptoms that mimic those of heart disease.*

4. *Damaged heart valves, the result of prior rheumatic fever, constitute one of the commonest cardiovascular problems in pregnancy. If the defective valves cause such symptoms as accumulation of fluid in the lungs, treatment is necessary, either by drugs, diet restrictions, and bed rest or by surgical repair or replacement of the valves. Victims of rheumatic fever are usually on a program of antibiotics to prevent recurrence of the disorder.*

5. *Many women with congenital heart defects may safely bear children, although pregnancy is not advisable in some cases.*

6. *Peripartal cardiomyopathy, an infrequent complication of pregnancy, is a disease that produces a gradual softening, thickening, or enlargement of the heart muscle.*

7. *Pre-eclampsia, a disease of unknown origin that occurs in pregnancy, causes blood pressure to rise, fluid to accumulate, and protein to be lost in the urine. If untreated, it can lead to eclampsia, a toxemia that seriously threatens the lives of both mother and baby.*

8. *Pregnancy sometimes causes inflammation and clot formation in the veins. These blood clots may break off and enter the circulatory system, lodging in the pulmonary system or interfering with blood flow to the brain. Phlebitis, or clots in the veins of the leg, is more common in the weeks immediately after delivery.*

9. *The use of oral contraceptives seems related to a number of complaints, including gall bladder disease, benign liver tumors, high blood pressure, and blood clots. Women with hypertension should avoid these agents; all women taking them should have regular blood pressure readings.*

infection are vaginal spotting, uterine cramps, or heavy or prolonged menstrual flow. If infection occurs, the IUD should be removed and the infection treated with antibiotics.

Although the list of cardiovascular complications in pregnancy and after delivery is long and in many ways frightening, great advances have been made in the knowledge, diagnosis, and treatment of heart disease. As a result, many women who as recently as a decade ago could not risk pregnancy are now successfully raising families.

24

BEHAVIORAL RISK FACTORS

C. David Jenkins, Ph.D.

Epidemiology, the branch of medicine dealing with the rates of diseases and their distributions in particular places and among populations, has been effectively applied to the study of cardiovascular diseases. The challenge presented by epidemiology to the medical profession is not new. It can be found in the advice of Hippocrates, 2,400 years ago, that when studying disease the physician must also consider ". . . the mode in which the inhabitants live, and what are their pursuits, whether they are fond of drinking and eating to excess, and given to indolence, or are fond of exercise and labor."

It is now well established that the risk of cardiovascular disease is increased by such factors as diet, weight, serum cholesterol, and cigarette smoking (see chapter 1). All these are largely controllable by changing one's behavior. For all that is known about the precursors of coronary heart disease, however, perhaps an equal amount remains unknown. From epidemiological studies examining this unknown terrain, it appears probable that psychosocial and behavioral variables are also involved with the risk both of heart attack and of hypertension.

"TYPE A" BEHAVIOR The scientific literature published between 1955 and 1976 has identified a condition known as the "coronary-prone behavior pattern, Type A." This type is characterized by intensive striving for achievement, competitiveness, easily provoked impatience, a sense of urgency about time, abruptness of speech and gesture, overcommitment to profession or vocation, excessive drive, and hostility. "Type A" behavior occurs not only under stress but as a habitual manner, a deeply ingrained and enduring style of life. The enumerated traits may be found in various combinations, and may not all be present in the same individual. Of more than forty studies reviewed, all but a few supported the connection of such behavior with incidence or prevalence of coronary disease.

Behavior Type A can be measured by a structured interview originally used in the Western Collaborative Group Study (WCGS). Follow-up reports after intervals of four and one-half, six and one-half, and eight and one-half years showed an incidence of new coronary disease in Type A men varying from 1.7 to 4.5 times greater than for men characterized by a more relaxed, easy-going behavior ("Type B").

Support for the Type A hypothesis can be found in a study of 6,579 Swedish construction workers, and in another from the Soviet Union, where 76 percent of a group of coronary patients, as compared with 23 percent of a control group without symptoms of cardiovascular disease and holding the same kind of jobs, exhibited behavior remarkably like the Type A pattern.

The Jenkins Activity Survey, a self-administered, computer-scored questionnaire for determining coronary-prone behavior, has been used in many studies. In studies in California, Connecticut, Florida, North Carolina, and Texas, and in Poland, persons with coronary disease scored significantly higher on the Type A scale and usually also on the "hard-driving" scale than noncoronary individuals used as controls.

An industrial screening program of the Chicago Heart Association, which evaluated 1,208 middle-aged white men, including 56 having myocardial infarction, found that the Type A score from the Activity Survey, considered alone, was only weakly associated with the prevalence of coronary disease. When standard risk factors such as age, serum cholesterol, diastolic blood pressure, and cigarette smoking were taken into account, however, the Type A score had a significant connection with conorary disease. The presence of Type A behavior was about as strong a correlate, in fact, as the presence of elevated serum cholesterol or diastolic blood pressure.

Not all studies of Type A behavior have supported the hypothesis. One major study that found negative evidence was based on data from participants in the Kaiser-Permanente Health Plan. There is uncertainty about whether the items used (derived from a questionnaire having a different purpose) measured Type A adequately.

Four studies of pathological evidence support the theory of a coronary-prone behavior pattern. These were conducted in Boston, New York, North Carolina, and Argentina. At the Boston University School of Medicine, ninety-six men with various cardiovascular diseases were given coronary angiography, a procedure involving the injection of a liquid visible to X-ray photography into the major blood vessels of the heart, so that motion pictures taken with an X-ray camera reveal any obstruction of the arteries of the heart. The men who underwent angiography also completed self-administered questionnaires, including the Jenkins Activity Survey. Those who had a 50 percent or greater obstruction in two or more coronary vessels had significantly higher scores than those with relatively little obstruction on the four scales of the Activity Survey—Type A scale, speed and impatience, job involvement, and hard-driving. Although another study in Boston failed to support these findings, other angiographic studies have tended to do so.

The association of excessive overtime work with the risk of coronary disease has been borne out by studies over the past five years. Sixty-two myocardial-infarction patients in Stockholm, who were compared with 109 healthy employees of a municipal agency, were found to have been doing much more overtime work, although they had less supervisory responsibility. In Texas, thirteen of fifty infarction patients reported working more than seventy hours a week, a much higher percentage than the matched controls.

STRESS AND SUSTAINED PAINFUL EMOTIONS

Several retrospective studies of cardiac patients have suggested a connection between life changes and cardiovascular disease. Although the findings are provocative, other studies with stronger methods failed to demonstrate a connection. Further prospective research is needed to test the hypothesis before any conclusions can be drawn.

Recent investigations suggest a number of possible psycho-social precursors of angina pectoris (chest pains caused by an insufficient supply of blood to the heart). This research connects anxiety, depression, psychophysiological complaints, emotional drain, chronic feelings of dissatisfaction, and conflicts with other people with the development of angina pectoris and, in some studies, with sudden death. The relation of such factors to myocardial infarction is more doubtful. Although the data are still limited, the most consistent of these findings appears to be the relation of insomnia and disturbed sleep both to angina and to myocardial infarction.

The relation of socioeconomic status and occupation to the incidence of coronary disease and mortality has been often studied, but with conflicting results. The same is true of marital status and religious affiliation.

SOCIAL MOBILITY AND OTHER SOCIOLOGICAL FACTORS

Several studies of large populations have suggested that coronary disease may be related to social mobility, including both movement between generations and that within the lifetime of the group at risk. The evidence thus far, however, has once again been somewhat conflicting. Although a study by the Honolulu Heart Program showed that occupational mobility, when combined with a high Type A behavior pattern score on the Jenkins Activity Survey, has a positive association with coronary heart disease in the 45-to-54-year age range, inconsistency across age groups in the same population suggests a cautious interpretation.

HYPERTENSION

Although it has been well established that high blood pressure is a risk factor for many cardiovascular diseases, relatively little is known about the risk factors involved in hypertension itself. Once thought to be an inevitable consequence of aging, surveys of populations in non-industrial, agrarian areas show that average blood pressure does not necessarily increase with age. As has already been mentioned (See chapter 1) race is strongly associated with hypertensive heart disease in the United States. Black men have three times the rate of white men, and black women twice that of white women, for virtually all ages from 20 to 70 years. However, there are clear indicators in the research so far that hypertension in both blacks and whites may be related in larger measure to environmental than genetic factors. This was the conclusion drawn by the Public Health Service a decade ago from a summary of published studies. Published reviews of experimental research (in animals and humans) and of observational studies of human populations, conclude (1) that sustained hypertension can be created in animals by purely social interventions (e.g., crowding); (2) that conditions requiring continuous behavioral and physiological adjustments keep blood pressure high; and (3) that individuals in socially subordinate positions tend to have more extreme damage to their health.

The accumulated research data suggests that demographic, social, and psychological factors may possibly be important contributors to the epidemic of hypertension in some population subgroups in the United States and many other industrialized nations. Further experimental and community research is needed before our understanding of the disease can be applied in systematic programs of treatment and prevention.

SUMMARY

The role of the central nervous system in cardiovascular pathology has been recognized at least since the time of William Harvey, who wrote in his classic *De Motu Cordis*, published in 1628: "Every affection of the mind that is attended with either pain or pleasure, hope or fear, is the cause of an agitation whose influence extends to the heart." During the last half century there has been much laboratory documentation of this principle in both human and animal subjects. An array of findings showing a great intensity of emotional problems in coronary heart disease patients clearly suggests that physicians should pay greater attention to these problems, utilizing the skills of psychiatrists, psychologists, and other counselors in a comprehensive treatment program. More research is needed to determine whether continuing anxiety, depression, and disturbance of sleep increase the risk of recurrent myocardial infarction and sudden death. If so, there should be further research into whether psychotherapy or treatment with so-called tranquilizing drugs can reduce the threat. Such psychological

PRINCIPLES

1. The incidence of coronary heart disease differs greatly between the populations of different countries. Genetic, sociocultural, and geographic factors may be involved in as yet undetermined degrees. Education, social status, marital status, social mobility, and cultural

interventions can be explored as secondary preventive measures, in addition to being justifiable as psychiatric therapy.

All habitual behavior is hard to change. The deeply set, hard-driving, competitive Type A behavior is especially so because of its neurotic roots in the personality, and because in present-day society it is so often rewarded with money and prestige. From what is known of efforts to modify Type A behavior, group rather than individual therapy seems to be more effective. This is a matter calling for further study. Experimental field trials ought also to be made, I believe, to investigate the treatment of sustained and intense episodes of painful emotion as a preventive for angina pectoris, and treatment to reduce coronary-prone Type A behavior, for the possible prevention of both angina pectoris and myocardial infarction.

change have all been found associated with the risk of coronary heart disease, but the relationships are not consistent enough or strong enough to have practical implications as yet.

2. Anxiety, depression, and neuroticism have been found associated prospectively with the development of angina pectoris in several studies and with general mortality in a few. They do not appear prospectively associated with myocardial infarction. All these painful emotions are stronger after clinical coronary disease is present. The several studies of chronic life dissatisfaction and conflict show much the same patterns of association with coronary heart disease. Long-term interference with sleep appears associated with the risk of coronary disease, both prospectively and retrospectively.

3. A coronary-prone behavior pattern, known as Type A, is characterized by intensive striving for achievement, competitiveness, easily provoked impatience, urgent sense of time, abruptness of speech and gesture, overcommitment to vocation and profession, and excesses of drive and hostility. A large number of studies have found this behavior pattern associated prospectively and retrospectively with angina pectoris, myocardial infarction, and advanced coronary atherosclerosis. How such a pattern of behavior may relate to heart disease is presently under investigation.

4. Widespread hypertension in the United States and other industrialized nations may be at least in part a response to factors in the social environment, economic circumstances, and psychological responsiveness. These factors appear to interact with the biological determinants of elevated blood pressure.

GLOSSARY

A Glossary of heart terms was written to give clear definitions of technical terms in nontechnical language. It is meant for use in libraries, schools and colleges, hospitals, communities, and homes by individuals who need to read, write, teach or learn more easily about heart subjects.

The Glossary contains a selection of words and phrases commonly used in the heart field. They were chosen on the basis of frequency of use and the possibility of general unfamiliarity or ambiguity.

Included are words from medicine, anatomy, physiology, instrumentation and pharmacology and some special terms used by certain related professions in dealing with the subject of heart disease. The terms are in alphabetical order. Most are followed by a phonetic spelling to indicate the preferred pronunciation; several are illustrated when necessary for clarity.

A Note on Pronunciation: one accent mark (′) follows the primary accent, two (″) indicate the secondary accent and a hyphen (-) follows unstressed syllables, as in (ad′ren-er′jik).

ADRENAL GLANDS *(ah-dre′nal)*

A pair of endocrine (hormone-secreting) glands that sit atop the kidneys. The inner portion of each—the adrenal medulla—secretes norepinephrine and epinephrine. Epinephrine is a heart stimulant and norepinephrine is a powerful blood vessel constrictor. The outer shell—the adrenal cortex—secretes aldosterone, cortisone, and other steroid hormones that influence the body's handling of salt, water, carbohydrates and other aspects of metabolism.

ADRENALIN *(ah-dren′ah-lin)* *See Epinephrine.*

ADRENERGIC BLOCKING AGENTS *(ad″ren-er′jik)*

Drugs which block the normal response of an organ or tissue to nerve impulses transmitted by the adrenergic nervous system (more or less the same as the sympathetic nervous system). Blocking adrenergic nerves to the heart and blood vessels tends to decrease heart rate and the vigor of heart contraction and to suppress the constriction of blood vessels. Adrenergic blocking agents are often used to treat angina pectoris (since by reducing heart work they reduce its need for oxygen). Some are also used to treat arrhythmias and to control high blood pressure, especially when it is accompanied by a hyperactive heart.

There are two classes of these drugs, alpha- and beta-adrenergic blocking agents. Both can be used in cardiovascular disorders, although beta-adrenergic blocking agents are used more often; of these, propranolol is the most common.

ALDOSTERONE *(al-dos′ter-on* OR *al″do-ster′on)*

A hormone secreted by the adrenal cortex that promotes the retention of salt and water by the kidneys. Aldosteronism, or excessive secretion of this hormone, may cause an increase in blood pressure. In this case drugs known as aldosterone antagonists can be given; one example is spironolactone.

ALDOSTERONISM *(al″do-ster′on-izm″)* *See Aldosterone.*

AMINE *(ah-meen′* OR *am′in)*

An organic compound that may be derived from ammonia by the replacement of one or more of the hydrogen atoms by hydrocarbon fractions.

ANEURYSM *(an′u-rizm)*

A ballooning-out of the wall of a vein, an artery or the heart due to weakening of the wall by disease, traumatic injury or an abnormality present at birth.

ANGINA PECTORIS *(an-ji′nah* OR *an′ji-nah pek′tor-is)*

An episode of chest pain due to a temporary discrepancy between the supply and demand of oxygen to the heart. This may be due to low oxygen levels in the blood (from smoking or respiratory disease), to a restricted bloodflow to the heart (coronary insufficiency) or to an increase in heart work beyond normal levels. Most often, angina pectoris is a chronic condition caused by a blood supply restricted by hardening and narrowing of the coronary arteries supplying the heart muscle (coronary atherosclerosis).

An angina attack is not to be confused with a heart attack (myocardial infarction), which results from a severe and prolonged lack of oxygenated blood to a part of the heart.

ANGIOCARDIOGRAPHY *(an″je-o-kar″de-og′rah-fe)*

A diagnostic method involving injection of an x-ray dye into the bloodstream. Chest x-rays taken after the injection show the inside dimensions of the heart and great vessels outlined by the liquid. *See Cineangiography.*

ANOREXIA *(an″o-rek′se-ah)*

Lack or loss of appetite for food.

ANOXIA *(an-ok′se-ah)*

Literally, no oxygen. This condition most frequently occurs when the blood supply (and hence the oxygen supply) to a part of the body is completely cut off. This results in the death of the affected tissue. For example, a specific area of the heart muscle may die when the blood supply has been blocked, as by a clot in the artery supplying that area.

ANTIARRHYTHMIC DRUGS *(an″ti-ah-rith′mic)*

Drugs which are used to treat disorders of the heart rate and rhythm. The drugs lidocaine, procaine amide, quinidine, digitalis, and propranolol are often given to correct arrhythmias. Atropine and isoproterenol are used in cases of abnormally slow heart rates.

ANTICOAGULANT *(an″ti-ko-ag′u-lant)*

A drug which delays clotting of the blood (coagulation). When given in cases of a blood vessel plugged up by a clot, it tends to prevent new clots from forming, or the existing clots from enlarging, but does not dissolve an existing clot. Examples are heparin and coumarin derivatives.

ANTIHYPERTENSIVE DRUGS *(an″ti-hi″per-ten′siv)*

Drugs which can be used to control high blood pressure (hypertension). Those most often given are the diuretics (primarily the thiazides), which promote the natural elimination of excess fluids in the tissues and circulation. Some of the other major antihypertensive drugs lower blood pressure by their direct or indirect dilating effect on the arteries. Hydralazine, for example, directly relaxes the tiny muscles in the artery walls. Other drugs block or damper the nerves which signal the arteries to constrict. Some of these are reserpine, methyldopa and guanethidine. The drug propranolol slows the heartbeat, decreases the force of the heart's contraction and thus lowers the blood pressure.

ANXIETY *(ang-zi′e-te)*

A feeling of apprehension.

AORTA *(a-or′tah)*

The main trunk artery which receives blood from the left ventricle of the heart. It originates from the base of the heart, arches up over the heart like a cane handle, and passes down through the chest and abdomen in front of the spine. It gives off many lesser arteries which conduct blood to all parts of the body except the lungs.

AORTIC ARCH *(a-or′tik)*

The part of the aorta, or large artery leaving the heart, which curves up like the handle of a cane over the top of the heart.

AORTIC INSUFFICIENCY *(a-or′tik in″su-fish′en-se)*

An improper closing of the valve between the aorta and the left ventricle of the heart permitting a backflow of blood.

U.S. DEPARTMENT OF HEALTH, EDUCATION, AND WELFARE, **Public** *Health Service, National Institutes of Health. DHEW Publication No. (NIH) 78-131.*

AORTIC STENOSIS *(a-or'tik ste-nos'sis)*

A narrowing of the valve opening between the left ventricle of the heart and the large artery called the aorta. The narrowing may occur at the valve itself or slightly above or below the valve. Aortic stenosis may be the result of scar tissue forming after a rheumatic fever infection, or may have other causes.

AORTIC VALVE *(a-or'tik)*

Valve at the junction of the aorta, or large artery, and the left ventricle of the heart. Formed by three opposing cup-shaped membranes, it allows the blood to flow from the heart into the aorta and prevents a backflow. *See Valve.*

AORTOGRAPHY *(a"or-tog'rah-fe)*

X-ray examination of the aorta (main artery conducting blood from the left ventricle of the heart to the body) and its main branches. This is made possible by the injection of a dye which is opaque to x-rays.

APEX *(a'peks)*

The blunt rounded end of the heart, normally directed downward, forward, and to the left.

ARCUS *(ar'kus)*

A curved or bowlike structure. *See Corneal Arcus.*

ARRHYTHMIA *(ah-rith'me-ah)*

Any variation from the normal rhythm of the heartbeat.

ARTERIAL BLOOD *(ar-te're-al)*

Oxygenated blood. The blood is oxygenated in the lungs and passes from the lungs to the left side of the heart via the pulmonary veins. It is then pumped by the left side of the heart into the arteries which carry it to all parts of the body. *See Venous Blood.*

ARTERIOLES *(ar-te're-ols)*

The smallest arterial vessels (about 0.2 mm. or 1/125 inch in diameter) resulting from repeated branching of the arteries. They conduct the blood from the arteries to the capillaries.

ARTERIOSCLEROSIS *(ar-te"re-o-skle-ro'sis)*

A group of diseases characterized by thickening and loss of elasticity of artery walls. This may be due to an accumulation of fibrous tissue, fatty substances (lipids) and/or minerals. *See Atherosclerosis.*

ARTERITIS *(ar"te-ri'tis)*

A general term for inflammation of arteries. This may be secondary to some underlying condition (such as an infectious disease) or it may be the primary phenomenon. Primary arteritis includes polyarteritis nodosa (which is disseminated throughout the body), temporal arteritis (occurring at the temples) and aortitis (arteritis of the aorta and its major branches).

ARTERY *(ar'ter-e)*

Blood vessels which carry blood away from the heart to the various parts of the body. They usually carry oxygenated blood except for the pulmonary artery which carries unoxygenated blood from the heart to the lungs for oxygenation. *See Vein.*

ASCHOFF BODIES *(ash'of)*

Spindle-shaped nodules, occurring most frequently in the tissues of the heart, often formed during an attack of rheumatic fever. Named after Ludwig Aschoff (1866-1942), a German pathologist who described them.

ASSIST DEVICES

Special mechanical devices used to provide pumping assistance to a heart weakened by acute heart attack or heart failure.

ASYMMETRIC SEPTAL HYPERTROPHY (ASH) *(a"sim-met'rik sep'tal hi-per'tro-fe)*

Also called idiopathic hypertrophic subaortic stenosis (IHSS). A disease of the heart muscle (cardiomyopathy) in which there is an asymmetric enlargement (hypertrophy) of the walls of the left ventricle—the interventricular septum thickens more than the outer wall does. This makes the contraction of the left ventricle less

effective and obstructs bloodflow to the aorta (and therefore to all parts of the body including the heart muscle itself). This condition is fairly common, is sometimes hereditary, and can create such symptoms as chest pain and dizziness. Treatment, when necessary, includes surgery, drugs or reduced physical exertion.

ATHEROMA *(ath"er-o'mah)*

Also called plaque. A deposit of fatty (and other) substances in the inner lining of the artery wall, characteristic of atherosclerosis. Plural is ATHEROMATA *(ath"er-o-mah'ta)*. *See Atherosclerosis.*

ATHEROSCLEROSIS *(ath"er-o-"skle-ro'sis)*

A kind of arteriosclerosis in which the inner layer of the artery wall is made thick and irregular by deposits of a fatty substance. These deposits (called atheromata or plaques) project above the surface of the inner layer of the artery, and thus decrease the diameter of the internal channel of the vessel. *See Arteriosclerosis.*

ATRIAL FIBRILLATION *(a"tre-al fi-bri-la'shun)* *See Fibrillation.*

ATRIAL FLUTTER *(a'tre-al flut'er)*

An arrhythmia which occurs occasionally in healthy hearts, but more commonly in diseased hearts. It results in a rapid regular heartbeat. Drugs are often used to slow the rate.

ATRIAL SEPTUM *(a'tre-al sep'tum)*

Sometimes called interatrial septum. Muscular wall dividing left and right upper chambers of the heart which are called atria. *See Septum.*

ATRIOVENTRICULAR BUNDLE *(a"tre-o-ven-trik'u-lar)*
See Bundle of His.

ATRIOVENTRICULAR NODE *(a"tre-o-ven-trik'u-lar)*

A small mass of special muscular fibers at the base of the wall between the two upper chambers of the heart. It forms the beginning of the Bundle of His which is the only known normal direct muscular connection between the upper and the lower chambers of the heart. The electrical impulses controlling the rhythm of the heart are generated by the pacemaker, conducted through the muscle fibers of the right upper chamber of the heart to the atrioventricular node, and then conducted to the lower chambers of the heart by the Bundle of His. *See Bundle of His and Pacemaker.*

ATRIOVENTRICULAR VALVES *(a"tre-o-ven-trik'u-lar)*

The two valves, one in each side of the heart, between the upper and lower chambers. The one in the right side of the heart is called the tricuspid valve, and the one in the left side is called the mitral valve.

ATRIUM *(a'tre-um)*

Formerly "auricle." One of the two upper chambers of the heart. The right atrium receives unoxygenated blood from the body. The left atrium receives oxygenated blood from the lungs.

ATROPINE *(at'ro-peen)*

A drug used to treat, among other things, an abnormally slow heart rate; an anti-arrhythmic drug.

AUENBRUGGER, LEOPOLD JOSEPH
(1722-1809)

Austrian physician who invented the technique of tapping the surface of the body to determine the condition of organs beneath. The technique is called percussion.

AURICLE *(aw're-kl)*
Archaic term for atrium.

AUSCULTATION *(aws"kul-ta'shun)*

The act of listening to sounds within the body, usually with a stethoscope.

AUTONOMIC NERVOUS SYSTEM *(aw"to-nom'ik)*

Sometimes called the involuntary nervous system. The nerves of this system regulate tissues and functions not normally under conscious control (heartbeat, blood pressure, etc.). It consists of two divisions, the sympathetic and parasympathetic, which usually have opposing effects on the cardiovascular system: the sympathetic nerves, when stimulated, tend to increase heart rate, constrict blood vessels, and raise blood pressure; the parasympathetic tend to slow the heart rate, relax blood vessels, and lower blood pressure.

A-V BUNDLE

See Bundle of His.

BACTERIAL ENDOCARDITIS *(bak-te're-al en"do-kar-di'tis)*

An inflammation of the inner layer of the heart caused by bacteria; it may be a complication of another infectious disease, an operation or injury. The lining of the heart valves is most frequently affected, most commonly valves with previous damage from rheumatic disease or congenital abnormality.

BARLOW'S SYNDROME *(bar'loz)*

Also called floppy mitral valve syndrome as well as systolic click-murmur syndrome, billowing mitral leaflet syndrome, and prolapsed mitral valve leaflet syndrome (among other terms). A structural alteration of the mitral valve (which normally permits a one-way flow of blood from the left atrium down to the left ventricle of the heart) leading to stretching and weakness of the cusps or valve leaflets. Thus when the heart pumps, some of the blood leaks back into the left atrium instead of being pushed through the aorta to the body.

This syndrome is associated with unusual chest discomfort and arrhythmias.

BARORECEPTORS *(bar"o-re-sep'torz)*

Sensory nerve endings which respond to changes in pressure, as those in the walls of blood vessels.

BEHAVIOR, TYPE A AND TYPE B

Two kinds of behavior patterns, as recognized in medicine. Type A behavior is characterized by high degrees of competitiveness, aggressiveness and feelings of the pressure of time. This type of behavior is thought by some cardiologists to be a risk factor in the development of coronary heart disease. Individuals with the converse Type B behavior are more easygoing and contemplative and more easily satisfied.

BENZOTHIADIAZIDES
(ben"zo-thi"ah-di'ah-sidz)
See Thiazides.

BETA-BLOCKING AGENTS *(bay'tah)*

Also called beta-adrenergic blocking agents. *See Adrenergic Blocking Agents.*

BICUSPID VALVE *(bi-kus'pid)*

Usually called mitral valve. A valve of two cusps or triangular segments, located between the upper and lower chambers in the left side of the heart. However, in cardiology a "bicuspid valve" usually refers to the common congenital abnormality of the aortic valve's having two cusps instead of its usual three.

BIOFEEDBACK *(bi"o-feed'bak)*

A technique using instrumentation to provide moment-to-moment information about bodily processes which a person is not normally aware of, so that he or she can learn to control them. For example, one setup may include a blood pressure measuring device and colored lights to indicate whether the blood pressure is in the high or normal range. Evidence indicates that biofeedback may be used to teach a person to regulate his or her heart rate, blood pressure, bloodflow, skin temperature, and the activity of the gastrointestinal tract.

This term also refers to the normal and physiologic mechanisms the body uses to regulate myriad physiologic phenomena.

BLOOD PRESSURE

The force the flowing blood exerts against the artery walls. Two pressures are usually measured:

1. The upper, or *systolic*, pressure occurs each time the heart contracts (systole) and pumps blood into the aorta.
2. The lower, or *diastolic*, pressure occurs when the heart relaxes (diastole) and refills with blood flowing in from the large veins, the venae cavae.

The blood pressure is therefore expressed by two numbers, with the upper one over the lower one; for example, 120/80, which is spoken as "120 over 80."

BLUE BABIES

Babies having a blueness of skin (cyanosis) caused by insufficient oxygen in the arterial blood. This often indicates a heart defect, but may have other causes such as premature birth or impaired respiration.

BRADYCARDIA *(brad-e-kar'de-ah)*

Abnormally slow heart rate. Generally, anything below 60 beats per minute is considered bradycardia.

BRIGHT, RICHARD *(1789-1858)*

English physician who demonstrated the association of heart disease to kidney disease.

BUERGER'S DISEASE *(ber'gerz)*

A disease of the blood vessels which is more commonly called thromboangiitis obliterans. *See Thromboangiitis Obliterans.*

BUERGER'S SYMPTOM *(ber'gerz)*

In thromboangiitis obliterans (Buerger's disease), the pain in the affected leg when the patient is lying down is relieved only by letting the leg hang over the side of the bed. *See Thromboangiitis Obliterans.*

BUNDLE OF HIS *(hiss)*

Also called atrioventricular bundle or A-V bundle. A bundle of specialized muscle fibers running from a small mass of muscular fibers (atrioventricular node) between the atria of the heart down to the ventricles. It is the only known normal direct muscular connection between the atria and the ventricles, and serves to conduct impulses for the rhythmic heartbeat from the atrioventricular node to the heart muscle. Named after Wilhelm His, German anatomist.

CALORIE *(kal'o-re)*

Sometimes called large or kilocalorie. Unit used to express food energy. The amount of heat required to raise the temperature of 1 kilogram of water 1 degree Centigrade.

A high caloric diet has a prescribed caloric value above the total daily energy requirement. A low caloric diet has a prescribed caloric value below the total energy requirement.

CAPILLARIES *(kap'i-lar"ez)*

The tiniest blood vessels. Capillary networks connect the arterioles and venules. Capillary walls are composed of a single layer of cells through which oxygen and nutritive materials pass out to the tissues, and carbon dioxide and waste products are admitted from the tissues into the bloodstream.

CARBON DIOXIDE *(kar'bon di-ox'ide)*

A waste product of chemical reactions in the cells. It passes from the cells to the blood which eventually releases it in the lungs to be breathed out.

CARDIAC *(kar'de-ak)*

Pertaining to the heart. Sometimes refers to a person who has heart disease.

CARDIAC ARREST

Cessation of the heartbeat. As a result, blood pressure drops abruptly and the circulation of the blood ceases. Until recently, this was always fatal. Today, the heart can be stimulated to start beating again and death averted under certain circumstances. *See Cardiopulmonary Resuscitation.*

CARDIAC CYCLE

A cardiac cycle is the series of mechanical and electrical events associated with one heartbeat. One cycle or beat lasts about 0.9 seconds and includes contraction and pumping, relaxation and filling actions.

CARDIAC OUTPUT

The amount of blood pumped by the heart per minute.

CARDIAC RESERVE

The difference between the cardiac output at rest (about 5 quarts pumped by one ventricle per minute) and at the maximum physical effort (as much as 25 quarts per minute or more).

CARDIOLOGIST *(kar-de-ol'o-jist)*

A specialist in the diagnosis and treatment of heart disease.

CARDIOLOGY *(kar"de-ol'o-je)*

The study of the heart and its functions in health and disease.

CARDIOMYOPATHY *(kar"de-o-mi-op'ah-the)*

A general diagnostic term for diseases that involve mainly the myocardium (heart muscle) and not other heart structures (such as the valves, coronary vessels or pericardium). They may be caused by known toxic or infectious agents. For the majority of cases, however, the cause is not known.

CARDIOPULMONARY RESUSCITATION (CPR) *(kar"de-o-pul'mo-ner-e re-sus"i-ta'shun)*

Also called Basic Life Support. An emergency measure used by one or two people to artificially maintain another person's breathing and heartbeat in the event these functions suddenly stop. CPR consists of keeping the airway open and performing rescue breathing and external cardiac compression (heart massage) to keep oxygenated blood circulating through the body. *See Heart Massage.*

CARDIOVASCULAR *(kar"de-o-vas'ku-lar)*

Pertaining to the heart and blood vessels.

CARDIOVASCULAR-RENAL DISEASE
(kar"de-o-vas'ku-lar re'nal)

Disease involving the heart, blood vessels, and kidneys.

CARDIOVERSION *(kar'de-o-ver'zhun)*

The application of very brief discharges of direct-current electricity across the intact chest and into the heart muscle in order to stop a cardiac arrhythmia (rhythm disorder) and allow the normal heart rhythm to take over. This technique is most often used as an emergency measure, but can also be used to correct chronic conditions.

CARDIOVERTER *(kar'de-o-ver''ter)*

An instrument capable of delivering a brief direct-current electric shock. Used to terminate certain cardiac arrhythmias. *See Cardioversion.*

CARDITIS *(kar-di'tis)*

Inflammation of the heart.

CAROTID ARTERIES *(kah-rot'id)*

The left and right common carotid arteries are the principal arteries supplying the head and neck. Each has two main branches, the external carotid artery and the internal carotid artery.

CAROTID BODY *(kah-rot'id)*

A tiny (5 mm. or 1/5 inch) oval mass of cells located in each carotid sinus, that is, at the branching point in the arteries supplying the head and neck. The carotid bodies contain nerve endings known as chemoreceptors which are sensitive to oxygen and carbon dioxide content and to pH of the blood. For example, when the oxygen content of the blood is reduced, the carotid bodies cause an increase in respiration rate.

CAROTID SINUS *(kah-rot'd si'nus)*

On either side of the neck, a slight dilation at the point where the internal carotid artery branches from the common carotid artery. These arteries supply the head and neck with blood. The carotid sinus contains the carotid body and many baroreceptors, special nerve endings sensitive to changes in blood pressure to keep it relatively constant. For example, if blood pressure starts to rise, baroreceptors in the carotid sinuses are stimulated to reduce the rate and force of heart contraction and to dilate the arteries—thus lowering the blood pressure. *See Carotid Arteries and Carotid Body.*

CATHETER *(kath'e-ter)*

A thin, flexible tube which can be guided into body organs. A cardiac catheter is made of woven plastic, or other material to which blood will not adhere, and is inserted into a vein or artery (usually of an arm or a leg) and gently threaded into the heart. Its progress can be watched on a fluoroscope.

Cardiac catheters can be used for diagnosis (to take samples of blood or pressure readings in the chambers of the heart) or for treatment (to implant the electrodes of a pacemaker or to administer a drug).

CATHETERIZATION *(kath"e-ter-i-za'shun)*

In cardiology, the process of introducing a thin, flexible tube (a catheter) into a vein or artery and guiding it into the heart for purposes of examination or treatment.

CEREBRAL VASCULAR ACCIDENT *(ser'e-bral OR se-re'bral vas'ku-lar)*

Sometimes called cerebrovascular accident, apoplectic stroke, or simply stroke. An impeded blood supply to some part of the brain, generally caused by one of the following four conditions:

1. A blood clot forming in the vessel (cerebral thrombosis).
2. A rupture of the blood vessel wall (cerebral hemorrhage).
3. A piece of clot or other material from another part of the vascular system which

flows to the brain and obstructs a cerebral vessel (cerebral embolism).
4. Pressure on a blood vessel as by a tumor.

CEREBROVASCULAR *(ser"e-bro-vas'ku-lar)*

Pertaining to the blood vessels in the brain.

CHAGAS HEART DISEASE *(chag'as)*

A form of heart disease resulting from an infection by a microscopic parasite found in South America.

CHEMOTHERAPY *(ke"mo-ther'ah-pe)*

The treatment of disease by administering chemicals. Frequently used in the phrase "chemotherapy of hypertension," i.e., the treatment of high blood pressure by the use of drugs.

CHLOROTHIAZIDE *(klo"ro-thi'ah-zid)*

One of the thiazide diuretics (drugs which promote the excretion of urine). Sometimes used to treat high blood pressure and edema (waterlogged tissues).

CHOLESTEROL *(ko-les'ter-ol)*

A fat-like substance found in animal tissue. In blood tests the normal level for Americans is assumed to be between 180 and 230 milligrams per 100 cc. A higher level is often associated with high risk of coronary atherosclerosis.

CHOLESTYRAMINE *(ko"les-ti'rah-meen)*

A drug used to lower blood levels of the lipid cholesterol. *See Lipid-Lowering Drugs.*

CHORDAE TENDINEAE
(kor'di ten'dun-i)

Fibrous chords which serve as guy ropes to hold the valves between the upper and lower chambers. They stretch from the cusps of the valves to muscles called papillary muscles in the walls of the lower heart chambers.

CHOREA *(ko-re'ah)*

Involuntary, irregular twitching of the muscles, sometimes associated with rheumatic fever. Also called St. Vitus Dance, or Sydenham's Chorea.

CINEANGIOCARDIOGRAPHY
(sin"e-an"je-o-kar"de-og'rah-fe)

A diagnostic method similar to angiocardiography except that instead of still x-ray pictures, motion pictures of the heart are made by fluoroscopy, as an injected opaque liquid is carried through the heart and blood vessels. *See Angiocardiography.*

CIRCULATORY *(ser'ku-lah-to"re)*

Pertaining to the heart, blood vessels, and the circulation of the blood.

CLAUDICATION *(klaw"di-ka'shun)*

Pain and lameness or limping. Can be caused by defective circulation of the blood in the vessels of the limbs. *See Intermittent Claudication.*

CLOFIBRATE *(klo-fi'brat)*

A drug generally used to lower elevated levels of triglyceride lipids in the blood. *See Lipid-Lowering Drugs.*

CLUBBED FINGERS *(klubd)*

Fingers with a short broad tip and overhanging nail, somewhat resembling a drumstick. This condition is sometimes seen in children born with certain kinds of heart defects and in adults with heart, lung or gastrointestinal diseases. It may also be familial and insignificant.

COAGULATION *(ko-ag"u-la'shun)*

Process of changing from a liquid to a thickened or solid state. The formation of a clot.

COARCTATION OF THE AORTA
(ko"ark-ta'shun of the a-or'ta)

Literally a pressing together or narrowing of the aorta, the main trunk artery which conducts blood from the heart to the body. One of several types of congenital heart defects.

COLLATERAL CIRCULATION
(ko-lat'er-al ser"ku-la'shun)

Circulation of the blood through nearby smaller vessels when a main vessel has been blocked up.

COMMISSUROTOMY   *(kom"e-shur-ot'o-me)*

An operation to widen the opening in a heart valve which has become narrowed by scar tissue. The individual flaps of the valve are spread apart along the natural lines of their closure by a blunt instrument. This operation was developed to correct rheumatic heart disease. *See Mitral Valvulotomy.*

CONGENITAL ANOMALY   *(kon-jen'i-tal ah-nom'ah-le)*

An abnormality present at birth.

CONGESTIVE HEART FAILURE   *(kon-jes'tiv)*

"Heart failure" is a condition in which the heart is unable to pump its required amount of blood.

Heart failure is often congestive because loss of pumping power by the heart leads to congestion in the body tissues; fluid accumulates in the abdomen and legs and/or in the lungs (pulmonary edema). Congestive heart failure often develops gradually over several years, although it can be acute (short and severe). It can be treated by drugs or in some cases by surgery. *See Heart Failure.*

CONSTRICTIVE PERICARDITIS   *(kon-strik'tiv per"i-kar-di'tis)*

A thickening of the outer sac of the heart which prevents the heart muscle from expanding and filling normally.

CONTRACTILE PROTEINS   *(kon-trak'til pro'te-ins)*

Proteins which occur within all muscle fibers, including those of the heart muscle. Contractile proteins are responsible for shortening the muscle fibers and therefore causing the muscle to contract. There are several kinds of contractile proteins.

CORNEAL ARCUS   *(kor'ne-al ar'kus)*

A hazy ring around the edge of the cornea (the transparent covering over the front of the eye). It can have a variety of causes, including exposure to irritating chemicals, viral or bacterial infections, and old age. It can also be a normal finding in certain racial backgrounds.

In addition, corneal arcus can be a sign of Type II or Type IV hyperlipoproteinemia, blood-lipid disorders associated with premature development of atherosclerosis.

CORONARY ARTERIES   *(kor'o-na-re)*

Arteries, arising from the base of the aorta, which conduct blood to the heart muscle. These arteries, and the network of vessels branching off from them, come down over the top of the heart like a crown (corona).

CORONARY ARTHEROSCLEROSIS
(ath"er-o"skle-ro'sis)

Commonly called coronary heart disease. An irregular thickening of the inner layer of the walls of the arteries which conduct blood to the heart muscle. The internal channel of these arteries (the coronaries) becomes narrowed and the blood supply to the heart muscle is reduced. *See Atherosclerosis.*

CORONARY BYPASS SURGERY
(kor'o-na-re bi'pas)

Surgery to improve the blood supply to the heart muscle when narrowed coronary arteries reduce flow of the oxygen-containing blood which is vital to the pumping heart. This reduction in bloodflow causes chest pain and leads to increased risk of heart attack. Thus coronary bypass surgery involves constructing detours through which blood can bypass narrowed portions of coronary arteries to keep the heart muscle supplied. Veins or arteries taken from other parts of the body where they are not essential are grafted onto the heart to construct these detours.

CORONARY HEART DISEASE

Also called coronary artery disease and ischemic heart disease. Heart ailments caused by narrowing of the coronary arteries and therefore a decreased blood supply to the heart (ischemia).

CORONARY INSUFFICIENCY
(in"su-fish'en-se)

A condition which occurs whenever the coronary arteries (which supply the heart muscle with blood) do not provide oxygen adequate to the needs of the pumping heart. This may produce chest pain (angina pectoris) or a heart attack, or no pain may occur at all.

"*Acute* coronary insufficiency" is a term used to describe chest pain that is more severe than that of angina pectoris, but in which no heart muscle damage is done (as there would be in a heart attack).

CORONARY OCCLUSION   *(o-kloo'zhun)*

An obstruction in a branch of one of the coronary arteries which hinders the flow of blood to some part of the heart muscle. This part of the heart muscle then dies because of lack of oxygen supply. Sometimes called a coronary heart attack or simply a heart attack. *See Heart Attack.*

CORONARY THROMBOSIS   *(throm-bo'sis)*

Formation of a clot in a branch of one of the arteries which conduct blood to the heart muscle (coronary arteries). A form of coronary occlusion. *See Coronary Occlusion.*

COR PULMONALE   *(kor pul-mo-nal'e)*

Heart disease resulting from disease of the lungs or the blood vessels of the lungs. The lung problems cause high blood pressure in the pulmonary vessels (pulmonary hypertension). Thus the right ventricle enlarges because it must work harder to pump blood through the lungs.

CORVISART, JEAN NICOLAS   *1755-1821*

One of the earliest of the modern cardiologists, and the first person to call him or herself a "heart specialist." Favorite physician to Napoleon.

COUMARIN   *(koo'mah-rin)*

A class of chemical substances which delay clotting of the blood. An anticoagulant.

CPR   *See Cardiopulmonary Resuscitation.*

CRUDE DEATH RATE

Also called crude mortality rate. The ratio of total deaths to total population during a given period of time, such as a year. It is calculated by dividing the total number of deaths during the year by the mid-year population (estimated population on July 1) of the same year.

CYANOSIS   *(si"ah-no'sis)*

Blueness of skin caused by insufficient oxygen in the blood. Oxygen is carried in the blood by hemoglobin, which is bright red when saturated with oxygen. When hemoglobin is not carrying oxygen, it is dark burgundy and is called reduced hemoglobin. The blueness of the skin occurs when the amount of reduced hemoglobin exceeds 5 grams per 100 cc. of blood.

DECOMPENSATION   *(de"kom-pen-sa'shun)*

Inability of the heart to maintain adequate circulation, usually resulting in a waterlogging of tissues. A person whose heart is failing to maintain normal circulation is said to be "decompensated."

DEFIBRILLATION   *(de-fib"ri-la'shun)*

Termination of atrial or ventricular fibrillation. Usually refers to treatment by the application of electric shock (cardioversion). *See Fibrillation and Cardioversion.*

DEPRESSANT   *(de-pres'ant)*
Any drug which decreases functional activity.

DESCARTES, RENE   *(1596-1650)*

Author of the first physiology textbook which accepted the theory of the circulation of the blood as described by William Harvey.

DEXTROCARDIA   *(deks"tro-kar'de-ah)*

Two different types of congenital phenomena are often described as dextrocardia. The first is a condition more correctly termed "dextroversion" in which the heart is slightly rotated and lies almost entirely in the right (instead of the left) side of the chest. The second is a condition in which the left chambers of the heart are on the right side and the right chambers are on the left side, so that the heart and great vessels present a mirror image of the normal heart.

DIASTOLE   *(di-as'to-le)*

In each heartbeat, the period of the relaxation of the heart. Atrial diastole is the period of relaxation of the atria, or upper heart chambers. Ventricular diastole is the period of relaxation of the ventricles, or lower heart chambers. *See Cardiac Cycle.*

DIET   *(di'et)*

Daily allowance or intake of food and drink.

DIETETICS   *(di-e-tet'iks)*

The science and art dealing with the feeding of individuals or groups under different economic or health conditions.

DIETITIAN   *(di-e-tish'an)*
One skilled in the scientific use of diet in health and disease.

DIGITALIS *(dij"e-tal'is)*

A drug prepared from leaves of the foxglove plant. Its main effect is cardiotonic, that is, it causes the heart muscle to pump more forcefully and effectively, thereby improving the circulation of the blood and promoting the normal elimination of excess fluid. Digitalis is often used to treat heart failure because it can relieve one of the early effects of the condition—buildup of fluid in the body tissues.

Digitalis is the most frequently used cardiotonic drug; other examples are ouabain and strophanthidin.

DILATION *(di-la'shun)*

A stretching or enlargement of the heart or blood vessels beyond the norm.

DIURESIS *(di"u-re'sis)*

Increased excretion of urine.

DIURETIC *(di"u-ret'ik)*

A medicine which promotes the excretion of urine. These drugs are often used to treat conditions involving excess body fluid such as hypertension and congestive heart failure. One important class of diuretics is the thiazides.

DUCTUS ARTERIOSUS *(duk'tus ar-te"re-o'sis)*

A small duct in the heart of the fetus between the artery leaving the right side of the heart (pulmonary artery) and the artery leaving the left side of the heart (aorta). Normally this duct closes soon after birth. If it does not close, the condition is known as patent or open ductus arteriosus. *See Patent Ductus Arteriosus.*

DYSPNEA *(disp'ne-ah)*

The uncomfortable sensation or awareness of shortness of breath.

ECG

See Electrocardiogram.

ECHOCARDIOGRAPHY *(ek"o-kar"de-og'rah-fe)*

A diagnostic method by which pulses of sound (ultrasound) are transmitted into the body and the echoes returning from the surfaces of the heart and other structures are electronically plotted and recorded. Stop-action or real-time images of the heart can be made into a record of the heart's movements.

ECHOGRAM *(ek'o-gram)*

An image of the heart and great vessels, as would be produced by echocardiography.

ECTOMORPH *(ek'to-morf)*

Wiry body type.

EDEMA *(e-de'mah)*

Swelling due to abnormally large amounts of fluid in the tissues of the body.

EFFORT SYNDROME *(sin'drom)*

A group of symptoms (quick fatigue, rapid heartbeat, sighing breaths, dizziness) that do not result from disease of organs or tissues and that are out of proportion to the amount of exertion required. Often called functional heart disease.

EISENMENGER'S SYNDROME *(i'sen-meng"erz)*

A condition in which there is a large congenital shunting defect complicated by high blood pressure in the vessels of the lungs (pulmonary hypertension). A shunting defect is an abnormal opening between heart chambers (septal defect) or between the great vessels (such as patent ductus arteriosus) such that some oxygen-poor blood gets pumped to the body and some oxygen-rich blood gets pumped to the lungs.

The syndrome is also called Eisenmenger's Reaction. The term *Eisenmenger's Complex* is used only when the defect is in the ventricular septum.

EKG

See Electrocardiogram.

ELECTROCARDIOGRAM
(e-lek"tro-kar'de-o-gram")

Often referred to as ECG or EKG. A graphic record of the electric currents generated by the heart.

The word "electrocardiogram" most often refers to a resting electrocardiogram, that is, the patient is lying at rest while the recording is being made. The recording can also be made during exercise.

ELECTROLYTE *(e-lek'tro-lit)*

A substance which, when dissolved in a liquid, dissociates into ions (positively and negatively charged particles). A solution of electrolytes is capable of conducting an electrical current.

Electrolytes, especially sodium and potassium, occur naturally in the body fluids. Heart disease and medications to treat it can cause abnormal electrolyte concentrations in the body fluids. Physicians sometimes prescribe diet and medications to correct these disordered concentrations.

EMBOLISM *(em'bo-lizm)*

The blocking of a blood vessel by a clot or other substance carried in the bloodstream.

EMBOLUS *(em'bo-lus)*

A blood clot (or other substance such as an air bubble, fat or tumor) which drifts unattached in the bloodstream until it becomes lodged in a small vessel and obstructs circulation. *See Thrombus.*

ENDARTERECTOMY *(end"ar-ter-ek'to-me)*

Surgical removal of the innermost lining (intima) of an artery when it is thickened by fatty deposits (atheroma) and blood clots (thromboses).

ENDOCARDIAL FIBROELASTOSIS
(en"do-kar'de-al fi"bro-e"las-to'sis)

A heart disease of unknown cause occurring in adults, but mostly in infants. It involves thickening of the lining of the heart chambers (endocardium) with elastic tissue. The thickening is most pronounced in the left ventricle and greatly impairs cardiac function.

ENDOCARDITIS *(en"do-kar-di'tis)*

Inflammation of the inner lining of the heart (endocardium) usually associated with acute rheumatic fever or some infectious agents.

ENDOCARDIUM *(en"do-kar'de-um)*

A thin smooth membrane forming the inner surface of the heart.

ENDOMORPH *(en'do-morf)*

Short and thickset body type.

ENDOTHELIUM *(en"do-the'le-um)*

The thin lining of the blood vessels.

ENLARGED HEART

A state in which the heart is larger than normal. This may be due to heredity, a large amount of exercise over a period of time, or conditions which cause the heart to work harder—such as high blood pressure, obesity and defects of the heart or great vessels.

ENZYME *(en'zim)*

A complex organic substance which is capable of speeding up specific biochemical processes in the body. Enzymes are universally present in living organisms.

EPICARDIUM *(ep"e-kar'de-um)*

The outer layer of the heart wall. Also called the visceral pericardium.

EPIDEMIOLOGY *(ep'e-de"me-ol'o-je)*

The science dealing with the factors which determine the frequency and distribution of a disease in a human community.

EPINEPHRINE *(ep"e-nef'rin)*

One of the secretions of two small glands, called adrenal glands, located just above the kidneys. This secretion, also called adrenalin, and sometimes prepared synthetically, constricts the small blood vessels (arterioles), increases the heart rate, and raises blood pressure. It is a vasoconstrictor or vasopressor substance.

ERYTHROCYTE *(e-rith'ro-site)*

Red blood cell.

ESOPHAGEAL VARICES
(e-sof"ah-je'al var'i-seez)

Varicosed or swollen veins in the wall of the esophagus, the tube connecting the mouth and the stomach. These are dangerous because they may rupture and bleed profusely. Esophageal varices are often associated with cirrhosis of the liver. *See Varix.*

ESSENTIAL HYPERTENSION   (e-sen'shal hi"per-ten'shun)
Sometimes called primary hypertension, and commonly known as high blood pressure
An elevated blood pressure of unknown cause.

ETIOLOGY (e"te-ol'o-je)
The sum of knowledge about the causes of a disease.

EXERCISE ELECTROCARDIOGRAM   (e-lek"tro-kar'de-o-gram")
Often referred to as a "stress test." An electrocardiogram taken while the patient is
exercising—usually jogging on a treadmill, walking up and down a short set of stairs,
or pedaling on a stationary bicycle. See Electrocardiogram.

EXTRACORPOREAL CIRCULATION   (eks"trah-kor-po're-al)
The circulation of the blood outside the body as by a mechanical pump or pump-
oxygenator. This is often done while surgery is being performed on the heart.

EXTRASYSTOLE (eks"trah-sis'to-le)
A contraction of the heart which occurs prematurely and interrupts the normal rhythm.

EYEGROUND (i'ground)
The inside of the back part of the eye seen by looking through the pupil. Examining
the eyeground is one means of assessing changes in the blood vessels. Also called
fundus of the eye.

FABRICIUS AB AQUAPENDENTE,
HIERONYMUS (1560-1634)
Italian anatomist, a teacher of William Harvey at Padua. He studied the valves of
the veins. Harvey is reported to have credited the work of Fabricius with leading to
his own concept of the circulation of the blood.

FALLOT, ETIENNE LOUIS ARTHUR
(1850-1911)
French physician who gave an important description of a congenital heart defect
known as the Tetralogy of Fallot (more accurately, Tetrad of Fallot). See Tetralogy
of Fallot.

FEMORAL ARTERY (fem'or-al ar'ter-e)
Main blood vessel supplying blood to the leg.

FIBRILLATION (fi-bri-la'shun)
A kind of cardiac arrhythmia. Uncoordinated contraction of the heart muscle occurring
when the individual muscle fibers take up independent irregular contractions. ATRIAL
FIBRILLATION involves very rapid, irregular contractions of the atria, followed irregularly by contractions of the ventricles. This may occur suddenly and for a short time,
or, if there is an existing heart disease, can become chronic. Treatment is usually by
drugs and sometimes by cardioversion (brief electric shock). VENTRICULAR FIBRILLA-
TION involves contractions of the ventricles which are irregular, haphazard and ineffective, resulting in a rapid decline of blood circulation and death. Emergency
treatment may include external cardiac massage (cardiopulmonary resuscitation—
CPR), electrical defibrillation (cardioversion) or drugs. See Cardiopulmonary Resuscitation and Cardioversion.

FIBRIN (fi'brin)
An elastic, threadlike protein which forms the essential portion of a blood clot.

FIBRINOGEN (fi-brin'o-jen)
A protein dissolved in the blood which, by the action of certain enzymes, is converted
into the insoluble threadlike protein of a blood clot (fibrin).

FIBRINOLYSIN (fi"bri-no-li'sin)
An enzyme which can cause coagulated blood to return to a liquid state.

FIBRINOLYTIC AGENTS (fi"bri-no-lit'ik)
Also called thrombolytic agents. Substances which dissolve blood clots. Two examples
are streptokinase and urokinase.

FLUORESCENT ANTIBODY TEST   (floo"o-res'ent an'te-bod"e)
A rapid and sensitive laboratory test. Among other things, it can be used to detect the
disease-causing bacteria known as streptococci, especially those that cause rheumatic

fever and therefore rheumatic heart disease. The test consists of "tagging" with a
fluorescent dye the antibodies, i.e., substances in blood serum that have been built
up to defend the body against bacteria. This dyed antibody is then mixed with a smear
taken from the throat of the patient. If there are streptococci present in the smear,
the glowing antibodies will attach to them, and they can be clearly seen through a
microscope. See Rheumatic Fever and Rheumatic Heart Disease.

FLUOROSCOPE (floo'o-ro-skop)
An instrument for observing the internal body organs at work. X-rays are passed
through the body onto a fluorescent screen where the shadows of the beating heart
and other organs can be seen and studied.

FLUOROSCOPY (floo"or-os'ko-pe)
The examination of structures within the body by means of a fluoroscope.

FLUTTER
See Atrial Flutter.

FORAMEN OVALE (fo-ra'men o-va"le)
An oval hole between the left and right upper chambers of the heart which normally
closes shortly after birth. Its failure to close is one of the congenital defects of the
heart, called a patent (open) foramen ovale.

FUNDUS OF THE EYE (fun'dus)
The inside of the back part of the eye seen by looking through the pupil. Examining
the fundus of the eye is used as a means of assessing changes in the blood vessels.
Also called the eyeground.

GALEN (CLAUDIUS GALENUS)
(c. 130-200 A.D.)
Renowned Greek physician whose theory that life and health depended upon the
balance of four "humors" in the body dominated medical practice for 1500 years.
His concept of the ebb and flow of the blood (which transported the humors to various
parts of the body) was not refuted until William Harvey's discovery of the circulation of the blood in 1628.

GALLOP RHYTHM
An extra heart sound which, when the heart rate is rapid enough, resembles a horse's
gallop. It may or may not be significant.

GANGLION (gang'gle-on)
A mass of nerve cells which serves as a center of nervous influence.

GANGLIONIC BLOCKING AGENTS   (gang"gle-on'ik)
Drugs which block the transmission of a nerve impulse at the nerve centers (ganglia)
rather than at the nerve endings (as would adrenergic blocking agents). Some of
these drugs, such as hexamethonium and mecamylamine hydrochloride, may be used
in the treatment of high blood pressure.

GENETICS (je-net'iks)
The study of heredity.

GUANETHIDINE (gwa-ne'thi-deen)
One of the drugs used to control high blood pressure. See Antihypertensive Drugs.

HEART ATTACK
The death of a portion of heart muscle which may result in disability or death of the
individual, depending on how much of the heart is damaged. A heart attack occurs
when an obstruction in one of the coronary arteries prevents an adequate oxygen
supply to the heart. Symptoms may be none, mild or severe and may include chest
pain (sometimes radiating to the shoulder, arm, neck or jaw), nausea, cold sweat,
and shortness of breath.
    Doctors often refer to a heart attack in terms of the obstruction (i.e., coronary
occlusion, coronary thrombosis, or simply "coronary") or of the heart muscle damage
(myocardial infarction, "infarct," or "M.I."). In common usage, the term "heart
attack" often incorrectly refers to irregular heartbeats or attacks of angina pectoris.

HEART BLOCK
A condition in which the electrical impulse which travels through the heart's specialized conduction system to trigger the events of the heartbeat is slowed or blocked
along its pathway. This can result in a dissociation of the rhythms of the upper and
lower heart chambers and is the major disorder for which artificial pacemakers are
used. See Sinoatrial Node and Pacemaker.

HEART DISEASE

A general term used to mean ailments of the heart or blood vessels. Some of these are present at birth (congenital) and are either inherited or are the result of environmental influences on the embryo as it develops in the womb. The majority of cases of heart disease, however, are acquired later in life, for example, through the development of atherosclerosis.

HEART FAILURE

A condition in which the heart is unable to pump the amount of blood required to maintain a normal circulation. It can be isolated to either the left or the right side of the heart, or can involve the whole heart. Heart failure can develop from many heart and circulatory disorders, especially high blood pressure (an increased resistance to bloodflow in the arteries), heart attack, rheumatic heart disease and birth defects.

Heart failure often leads to congestion in the body tissues; fluid accumulates in the abdomen and legs and/or in the lungs (pulmonary edema). Congestive heart failure often develops gradually over several years, although it can be acute (short and severe). It can be treated by drugs or in some cases by surgery.

HEART-LUNG MACHINE

A machine through which the bloodstream is diverted for pumping and oxygenation, for example, during heart surgery. See Extracorporeal Circulation.

HEART MASSAGE

Also called cardiac massage. An emergency technique using compression of the heart to keep the blood pumping through the body in the event the heart stops pumping effectively. EXTERNAL HEART MASSAGE involves pressing on the chest to compress the heart between the breastbone and the spine. Also, raising the pressure inside the chest by external compression may aid the heart's emptying as well. INTERNAL CARDIAC MASSAGE is usually done in the operating room where the heart is directly compressed by the surgeon's hand through an incision in the chest.

HEMIPLEGIA (hem"e-ple'je-ah)

Paralysis of one side of the body caused by damage to the opposite side of the brain. Nerves cross in the brain, and one side of the brain controls the opposite side of the body. Such paralysis is sometimes caused by a blood clot or hemorrhage in a blood vessel in the brain. See Stroke.

HEMODYNAMICS (he"mo-di-nam'iks)

The study of the flow of blood and the forces involved.

HEMOGLOBIN (he"mo-glo'bin)

The oxygen-carrying red pigment of the red blood cells (corpuscles). When it has absorbed oxygen in the lungs, it is bright red and is called oxyhemoglobin. After it has given up some of its oxygen load in the tissues, it is dark burgundy in color and is called reduced hemoglobin.

HEMORRHAGE (hem'or-ij)

Loss of blood from a blood vessel. In external hemorrhage blood escapes from the body. In internal hemorrhage blood passes into tissues surrounding the ruptured blood vessel.

HEMORRHOIDS (hem'o-roidz)

Varices or excessively distended veins in the lower rectum and anus caused by a persistent increase in pressure within or against these veins. They are painful and often complicated by inflammation, bleeding, and clotting blood. See Varix.

HEPARIN (hep'ah-rin)

A naturally occurring substance which tends to prevent blood from clotting. Sometimes used in cases of an existing clot in an artery or vein to prevent enlargement of the clot or the formation of new clots. An anticoagulant.

HIGH BLOOD PRESSURE

An unstable or persistent elevation of blood pressure above the normal range. Uncontrolled, chronic high blood pressure strains the heart, damages arteries, and creates a greater risk of heart attack, stroke, and kidney problems. Also known as hypertension. See Primary Hypertension and Secondary Hypertension.

HIS, WILHELM (1831-1904)

German anatomist who discovered the bundle of specialized muscle fibers running from the upper to lower chambers of the heart. These fibers are known as the "Bundle of His."

HYDRALAZINE (hi-dral'ah-zeen)

One of the drugs used to control high blood pressure. See Antihypertensive Drugs.

HYDROGENATED (hi'dro-jen-a"tid)

Combined with more hydrogen; more saturated.

HYPERCHOLESTEREMIA (hi"per-ko-les"ter-e'me-ah)

An excess of a fatty substance called cholesterol in the blood. Sometimes called hypercholesterolemia or hypercholesterinemia. See Cholesterol.

HYPERLIPEMIA (hi"per-li-pe'me-ah)

An excess of fats or lipids in the blood. Also called hyperlipidemia.

HYPERLIPOPROTEINEMIA (hi"per-lip"o-pro"te-in-e'me-ah)

The name for several types of blood-lipid disorders involving high blood levels of lipoproteins (complexes of lipids—either cholesterol or triglycerides—and certain kinds of proteins). Some types of hyperlipoproteinemia (Type II and Type IV) are associated with the premature development of atherosclerosis (hardening of the arteries) and therefore with increased risk of heart attack and stroke.

HYPERTENSION (hi"per-ten'shun)

Commonly called high blood pressure. See High Blood Pressure, Primary Hypertension, and Secondary Hypertension.

HYPERTENSIVE (hi"per-ten'siv)

A person with high blood pressure (hypertension).

HYPERTHYROIDISM (hi"per-thi'roid-izm)

A condition in which the thyroid gland is overly active. This may eventually result in a speeded up rate of heartbeat.

HYPERTROPHY (hi-per'tro-fe)

The enlargement of a tissue or organ due to increase in the size of its constituent cells. This may result from a demand for increased work.

HYPOCHOLESTEREMIC DRUGS
(hi"po-ko-les"te-re'mik)
See Lipid-Lowering Drugs.

HYPOLIPEMIC DRUGS (hi"po-li-pe'mik)
Also called hypolipidemic drugs. See Lipid-Lowering Drugs.

HYPOTENSION (hi"po-ten'shun)

Commonly called low blood pressure. Blood pressure below the normal range. Most commonly used to describe an acute fall in blood pressure, as occurs in shock or syncope (fainting).

HYPOTHALAMUS (hi"po-thal'ah-mus)

A part of the brain which exerts control over activity of the abdominal organs, water balance, temperature, etc. Damage to the hypothalamus may cause abnormal gain in weight, among other things.

HYPOTHERMIA (hy"po-ther'me-ah)

Also called hypothermy. The state of low body temperature. Often induced (usually to 86-88 degrees F.) during heart surgery in order to slow the metabolic processes. In this cooled state body tissues require less oxygen, and are therefore less likely to be damaged by oxygen deprivation.

HYPOTHYROIDISM (hi"po-thi'roid-izm)

A condition in which the thyroid gland is underactive, resulting in the slowing down of many of the body processes including the heart rate.

HYPOXIA (hi-pok'se-ah)

Less than normal content of oxygen in the organs and tissues of the body. At very high altitudes a healthy person experiences hypoxia because of insufficient oxygen in the air.

IATROGENIC HEART DISEASE (i"at-ro-jen'ik)

Literally means "caused by the doctor." A heart ailment inadvertently caused by the doctor or simply by the patient's belief that he has heart disease inferred from the manner and actions of his physician or other member of the medical team.

IDIOPATHIC HYPERTROPHIC SUBAORTIC STENOSIS (IHSS) (id"e-o-path'ik hi"per-tro'fik sub"a-or'tik ste-no'sis) See Asymmetric Septal Hypertrophy.

ILIAC ARTERY *(il'e-ak ar'ter-e)*
A large artery which conducts blood to the pelvis and the legs.

INCIDENCE *(in'si-dens)*
The number of new cases of a disease developing in a given population during a specified period of time, such as a year.

INCOMPETENT VALVE *(in-kom'pe-tent)*
Any valve which does not close tight and leaks blood back in the wrong direction. Also called valvular insufficiency.

INFARCT *(in'farkt)*
The area of tissue which is damaged or dies as a result of receiving an insufficient blood supply. Frequently used in the phrase "myocardial infarct," referring to the area of heart muscle injury due to the interrupted flow of blood through the coronary artery which normally supplies it.

INFARCTION *(in-fark'shun)*
The occurrence of an infarct.

INNOMINATE ARTERY *(in-nom'i-nat)*
One of the largest branches of the aorta. It arises from the arch of the aorta and divides to form the right common carotid artery and the right subclavian artery.

INTERATRIAL SEPTUM
(in"ter-a'tre-al sep'tum)
Sometimes called atrial septum. Muscular wall dividing left and right upper chambers (the atria) of the heart.

INTERMITTENT CLAUDICATION
(in"ter-mit'ent klaw"di-ka'shun)
Pain in the muscles of a limb which, similar to angina pectoris, occurs intermittently—during stress but not at rest. This condition frequently accompanies diseases of the peripheral blood vessels, such as thromboangiitis obliterans. The resting muscle has an adequate blood supply, but when the need for blood increases (as during exercise), the disease impairs the circulation. An inadequate blood supply and the buildup of waste products of metabolism in the tissues cause pain. "Claudication" means lameness.

INTERVENTRICULAR SEPTUM
(in"ter-ven-trik'u-lar sep'tum)
Sometimes called ventricular septum. Muscular wall, thinner at the top, dividing the left and right lower chambers of the heart which are called ventricles.

INTIMA *(in'ti-mah)*
The innermost layer of a blood vessel (it includes the endothelium).

IN VITRO *(in vee'tro)*
Literally means "in glass," hence in a laboratory vessel. Describes a phenomenon studied outside a living body under laboratory conditions. *See In Vivo.*

IN VIVO *(in vee'vo)*
In a living organism. Describes a phenomenon studied in a living body. *See In Vitro.*

ISCHEMIA *(is-ke'me-ah)*
A local, usually temporary, deficiency of oxygen in some part of the body, often caused by a constriction or an obstruction in the blood vessel supplying that part.

ISCHEMIC HEART DISEASE *(is-kem'ik)*
Also called coronary artery disease and coronary heart disease. Heart ailments caused by narrowing of the coronary arteries and therefore a decreased blood supply to the heat (ischemia).

ISOPROTERENOL *(i"so-pro"te-re'nol)*
A drug which can be used as a cardiac stimulant to treat an abnormally slow heartbeat.

ISOTOPE *(i'so-top)*
Any of two or more species of a chemical element. The isotopes of one element are chemically identical, but differ by some physical property such as mass or radioactivity. Radioactive isotopes (radioisotopes) are often used in medicine to trace the fate of substances in the body. *See Radiosotopic Scanning.*

JUGULAR VEINS *(jug'u-lar)*
Veins which return blood from the head and neck to the heart.

LEUKOCYTES *(lu'ko-sitz)*
See White Blood Cells.

LIFESTYLE
An individual's typical way of life, including diet, kinds of recreation, job, home environment, location, temperament, and smoking, drinking and sleeping habits.

LINOLEIC ACID *(lin-o-lay'ik)*
An important component of many of the unsaturated fats. It is found widely in oils from plants. A diet with a high linoleic acid content tends to lower the amount of cholesterol in the blood.

LIPID *(lip'id)*
A fatty substance.

LIPID-LOWERING DRUGS
Drugs used to treat the various types of hyperlipoproteinemia, that is, abnormally high concentrations of lipids (fats) in the blood. Also called hypolipemic and hypolipidemic drugs; those drugs that lower blood levels of the lipid cholesterol are called hypocholesteremic.
    The most common lipid-lowering drugs used are cholestyramine, clofibrate and nicotinic acid.

LIPOPROTEIN *(lip"o-pro'te-in)*
A complex consisting of lipid (fat) and protein molecules bound together. Lipids do not dissolve in the blood, but must circulate in the form of lipoproteins.

LUMEN *(lu'men)*
The passageway inside a tubular organ. The vascular lumen is the passageway inside a blood vessel.

MALIGNANT HYPERTENSION
(mah-lig'nant hi"per-ten'shun)
Severe high blood pressure that may run a rapid course and cause damage to the blood vessel walls in the kidney, eye, and other organs. Its cardinal feature is central nervous system impairment, for example, coma, seizures, etc.

MESOMORPH *(mes'o-morf)*
Muscular body type.

METABOLISM *(me-tab'o-lizm)*
A general term designating all chemical changes which occur to substances within the body.

METHYLDOPA *(meth"il-do'pah)*
One of the drugs used to control high blood pressure. *See Antihypertensive Drugs.*

MITRAL INSUFFICIENCY *(mi'tral in"su-fish'en-se)*
An incomplete closing of the mitral valve between the upper and lower chamber in the left side of the heart which permits a backflow of blood in the wrong direction. Sometimes the result of scar tissue forming after a rheumatic fever infection.

MITRAL STENOSIS *(mi'tral ste-no'sis)*
A narrowing of the valve (called the mitral valve) opening between the upper and lower chamber in the left side of the heart. Sometimes the result of scar tissue forming after a rheumatic fever infection.

MITRAL VALVE *(mi'tral)*
A valve of two cusps or triangular segments, located between the upper and lower chamber in the left side of the heart. *See Valve.*

MITRAL VALVULOTOMY *(mi'tral val"vu-lot'o-me)*
An operation to widen the opening of the mitral valve by means of surgery with a knife. Usually performed when the valve opening is so narrowed as to obstruct bloodflow, which sometimes happens as a result of rheumatic fever. *See Commissurotomy.*

MONO-UNSATURATED FAT
(mon"o-un-sat'u-rat-ed)

A fat so constituted chemically that it is capable of absorbing additional hydrogen but not as much hydrogen as polyunsaturated fat. These fats in the diet have little effect on the amount of cholesterol in the blood. An example is olive oil. *See Poly-unsaturated Fat.*

MURMUR *(mur'mur)*

An extra heart sound, sounding like fluid passing an obstruction, heard between the normal heart sounds.

MYOCARDIAL INFARCTION
(mi"o-kar'de-al in-fark'shun)

The damaging and death of an area of heart muscle (myocardium) resulting from an interruption in the blood supply reaching that area. *See Heart Attack.*

MYOCARDITIS *(mi"o-kar-di'tis)*

Inflammation of the heart muscle (myocardium). It may be due to a variety of diseases, certain chemicals or durgs, trauma (e.g. electric shock or excessive x-ray treatment), or may be of unknown origin.

MYOCARDIUM *(mi"o-kar'de-um)*

The muscular wall of the heart. The thickest of the three layers of the heart wall, it lies between the inner layer (endocardium) and the outer layer (epicardium).

NEUROCIRCULATORY ASTHENIA
(nu"ro-cir'cu-lah-to"re as-the'na-ah)

Sometimes called soldier's heart, effort syndrome, or functional heart disease. A complex of nervous and circulatory symptoms, often involving a sense of fatigue, dizziness, shortness of breath, rapid heartbeat, and nervousness. *See Effort Syndrome.*

NEUROGENIC *(nu"ro-jen'k)*

Originating in the nervous system.

NICOTINIC ACID *(nik'o-tin"ik)*

A lipid-lowering drug which can be used to lower elevated levels of both cholesterol and triglycerides in the blood. *See Lipid-Lowering Drugs.*

NITRITES *(ni'trits)*

A group of chemical compounds, many of which cause dilation of the small blood vessels and thus lower blood pressure. Examples are amyl nitrite, sodium nitrite, nitroprusside and nitroglycerin.

NITROGLYCERIN *(ni-tro-glis'er-in)*

A drug (one of the nitrites) which relaxes the muscles in the blood vessels. Often used to relieve attacks of angina pectoris and spasm of coronary arteries. It is one of the vasodilators.

NORADRENALIN *(nor"ad-ren'ah-lin)* See *Norepinephrine.*

NOREPINEPHRINE *(nor"ep-e-nef'rin)*

An organic compound which produces a rise in blood pressure by constricting the small blood vessels. Sometimes used in the treatment of shock. Also called noradrenalin.

NORMOTENSIVE *(nor"mo-ten'siv)*

Characterized by normal blood pressure.

NUTRITIONIST *(nu-trish'un-ist)*

One professionally engaged in investigating and solving problems of nutrition.

OBESITY *(o-bees'i-te)*

An increase in body weight beyond physical and skeletal requirements due to an accumulation of excess fat. This puts a strain on the heart and increases the chance of developing two major heart attack risk factors—high blood pressure and diabetes.

OCCLUSIVE *(o-kloo'siv)*

Closing or shutting off. A coronary occlusion is a closing off of a coronary artery (which supplies the heart muscle with blood).

OPEN-HEART SURGERY

Surgery performed on the opened heart. This phrase is also often used to refer to all heart surgery—whether or not the heart itself is opened.

ORGANIC HEART DISEASE

Heart disease caused by some structural abnormality in the heart or circulatory system.

OXYGEN *(ok'si-jen)*

A gas which is the most important component of the air we breathe. It is vital to energy-producing chemical reactions in the living cells of the body. Breathed into the lungs, it enters the bloodstream and is carried by the blood to the body tissues.

PACEMAKER *(pas'mak-er)*

A small mass of specialized cells in the right atrium of the heart which gives rise to the electrical impulses that initiate contractions of the heart. Also called sinoatrial node or S-A node of Keith-Flack. Under abnormal circumstances, other cardiac tissues may assume the pacemaker role by initiating electrical impulses which stimulate contraction.

The term "artificial pacemaker" is applied to an electrical device which can substitute for a defective natural pacemaker and control the beating of the heart by a series of rhythmic electrical discharges. If the electrodes which deliver the discharges to the heart are placed on the outside of the chest, it is called an "external pacemaker." If they are placed within the chest wall, it is called an "internal pacemaker."

PALPITATION *(pal"pi-ta'shun)*

A sensation of fluttering of the heart or abnormal rate or rhythm of the heart as experienced by the person.

PAPILLARY MUSCLES *(pap'i-ler"e)*

Small, cone-shaped muscles projecting from the walls of the lower heart chambers (the ventricles) to which are attached fibrous cords (chordae tendineae) stretching up to the flaps of the valves between upper and lower chambers. When the ventricles fill with blood and contract, the papillary muscles also contract and tighten the cords, allowing the valves to be pressed shut, but preventing them from being pushed back and open into the upper chambers (the atria) by the surging blood.

PARASYMPATHETIC NERVOUS SYSTEM
(par"ah-sim"pah-thet'ik)

One of the two divisions of the autonomic nervous system. *See Autonomic Nervous System.*

PARIETAL PERICARDIUM
(pah-ri'e-tal per"e-kar'de-um)

A thickened protective membrane which is the outer wall of the pericardium, the double-walled sac surrounding the heart.

PAROXYSMAL TACHYCARDIA
(par"ok-siz'mal tak"e-kar'de-ah)

A period of rapid heartbeats which begins and ends suddenly.

PATENT DUCTUS ARTERIOSUS
(pa'tent duk'tus ar-te"re-o'sis)

A congenital heart defect in which a small duct between the artery leaving the left side of the heart (aorta) and the artery leaving the right side of the heart (pulmonary artery), which normally closes soon after birth, remains open. As a result of this duct's failure to close, blood from both sides of the heart is pumped into the pulmonary artery and into the lungs. This defect is sometimes called simply patent ductus. Patent means open.

PATENT FORAMEN OVALE
(pa'tent fo-ra'men o-va'le)

One type of congenital heart defect. An oval hole (the foramen ovale) between the left and right upper chambers of the heart, which normally closes shortly after birth, remains open.

PERCUSSION *(per-kush'un)*

Tapping the body as an aid in diagnosing the conditions of parts beneath by the sound obtained. A physician will often tap the chest to determine the state of the heart and lungs—for instance, whether there may be a fluid accumulation or an enlarged heart.

PERIARTERITIS NODOSA
(per"e-ar"te-ri'tis no-do'sa)

See *Polyarteritis Nodosa.*

PERICARDIAL TAMPONADE
(per"i-kar'de-al tam"pon-ad')

An accumulation of excess fluid between the two layers of the membrane sac surrounding the heart (the pericardium). This can happen rapidly or gradually and impairs the normal functioning of the heart. *See Pericardium.*

PERICARDITIS *(per"e-kar-di'tis)*

Inflammation of the membrane sac (pericardium) which surrounds the heart.

PERICARDIUM *(per"e-kar'de-um)*

A closed sac surrounding the heart and roots of the great vessels. The sac is formed by two walls:

The VISCERAL PERICARDIUM is on the inside, closely adhering to the heart. It forms the outermost layer of the heart wall and is also called the epicardium.
The PARIETAL PERICARDIUM is on the outer side of the sac and is anchored to other chest structures such as the breastbone. It is a protective membrane.
The space inside the sac (THE PERICARDIAL CAVITY), between the two walls, contains a fluid which provides for smooth movements of the heart as it beats.

PERIPHERAL RESISTANCE *(pe-rif'er-al)*

The resistance offered by the arterioles to the flow of blood. An increase in peripheral resistance causes a rise in blood pressure.

PERIPHERAL VASCULAR DISEASE
(pe-rif'er-al vas'cu-lar)

A term which, in its broadest sense, refers to diseases of any of the blood vessels outside of the heart and to diseases of the lymph vessels. These are circulation disorders caused by changes in the caliber of the vessels. FUNCTIONAL peripheral vascular diseases are not structural or organic in cause, but are transient and reversible. An example is Raynaud's disease, which can be triggered by cold temperatures, emotional stress, work with vibrating machinery or smoking. The term ORGANIC describes circulation disturbances which are caused by structural changes in the vessels (such as inflammation and tissue damage). An example is Buerger's disease (thromboangiitis obliterans).

PHEOCHROMOCYTOMA
(fe-o-kro"mo-si-to'mah)

A tumor which arises in the adrenal glands. It produces and releases into the bloodstream large quantities of norepinephrine and epinephrine. These powerful natural stimulants may then create such symptoms as high blood pressure, elevated heart rate, headaches, anxiety, and excessive sweating.

PHLEBITIS *(fle-bi'tis)*

Inflammation of a vein, often in the leg. Sometimes a blood clot is formed in the inflamed leg. *See also Thrombophlebitis.*

PHOSPHOLIPIDS *(fos"fo-lip'idz)*

One of the three major classes of lipids (fatty substances) in the blood. Unlike the other two classes—cholesterol and triglycerides—phospholipids are *not* known to be associated with atherosclerosis (hardening of the arteries).

PLAQUE *(plak) See Atheroma.*

PLASMA *(plaz'mah)*

The cell-free liquid portion of uncoagulated blood. It is different from serum which is the fluid portion of the blood obtained after coagulation.

PLATELETS *(plat'letz)*

One of the three kinds of formed elements found in the blood. Literally "little plates," they are small, colorless, disk-shaped bodies which are involved in the formation of blood clots. Also called thrombocytes. *See Red Blood Cells and White Blood Cells.*

POLYARTERITIS NODOSA
(pol"e-ar"te-ri'tis no-do'sa)

A disease of unknown cause characterized by inflammation and destruction along segments of small and medium-sized arteries, creating lumps or nodes of scar tissue. This leads to functional impairment of the tissues supplied by the affected vessels.

POLYCYTHEMIA *(pol"e-si-the'me-ah)*

An abnormal condition of the blood characterized by an excessive number of red blood cells.

POLYUNSATURATED FAT
(pol"e-un-sat'u-rat-ed)

A fat so constituted chemically that it is capable of absorbing additional hydrogen. These fats are usually liquid oils of vegetable origin, such as corn oil or safflower oil. A diet with a high polyunsaturated fat content tends to lower the amount of

cholesterol in the blood. These fats are sometimes substituted for saturated fat in a diet in an effort to lessen the hazard of fatty deposits in the blood vessels. *See Monounsaturated Fat.*

PRESSOR *(pres'or)*

Tending to increase blood pressure, as a pressor substance.

PREVALENCE *(prev'ah-lens)*

The number of cases of a given disease existing in a given population at a specified moment of time.

PRIMARY HYPERTENSION *(hi"per-ten'shun)*

Also called essential hypertension. High blood pressure of unknown origin (as opposed to secondary hypertension, which is caused by some primary disease, such as kidney disease). Most people who have high blood pressure have primary hypertension. *See Secondary Hypertension.*

PROCAINE AMIDE *(pro'kane am'id)*

A drug sometimes used to treat abnormal rhythms of the heartbeat; an antiarrhythmic drug.

PROPRANOLOL *(pro-pran'o-lol)*

A member of the group of drugs known as beta-blocking agents. Propranolol is used to treat angina pectoris, cardiac arrhythmias, high blood pressure, and other disorders of the cardiovascular system. *See Adrenergic Blocking Agents.*

PROSTAGLANDINS *(pros"tah-glan'dinz)*

Hormone-like substances made from fatty acids which are found throughout the body tissues. They are thought to have important roles in tissue metabolism and bloodflow, among other things.

PROSTHESIS *(pros-the'sis)*

An artificial substitute for a body part, such as a leg, tooth, heart valve or blood vessel. The plural form is *Prostheses.*

PSYCHOSOMATIC *(si"ko-so-mat'ik)*

Pertaining to the influence of the mind, emotions, fears, etc., upon the functions of the body, especially in relation to disease.

PULMONARY *(pul'mo-ner"e)*

Pertaining to the lungs.

PULMONARY ARTERY

The large artery which conveys unoxygenated (venous) blood from the lower right chamber of the heart to the lungs. This is the only artery in the body which normally carries unoxygenated blood, all others carrying oxygenated blood to the body.

PULMONARY CIRCULATION

The circulation of the blood through the lungs, the flow being from the right lower chamber of the heart (right ventricle) through the lungs, back to the left upper chamber of the heart (left atrium). *See Systemic Circulation.*

PULMONARY EDEMA
(pul'mo-ner"e e-de'mah)

A condition, usually acute (sudden and severe) but sometimes chronic, marked by an excess of fluid in the extravascular (outside the vessels) spaces in the lungs. It may be confined to the interstitial spaces or may appear in the alveoli (the millions of tiny air sacs in each lung). Pulmonary edema occurs most often as a complication of left ventricular failure due to ischemic heart disease, high blood pressure or disease of the aortic valve. *See Congestive Heart Failure and Heart Failure.*

PULMONARY EMBOLISM *(em'bo-lizm)*

A condition in which a blood clot (embolus), usually one formed in a vein of the leg or pelvis, breaks loose and becomes lodged in one of the arteries of the lungs. This may produce no symptoms at all or may create very serious impairment of pulmonary circulation.

PULMONARY HYPERTENSION
(hi'per-ten'shun)

High blood pressure (hypertension) in the blood vessels of the lungs. The two most common causes are chronic obstructive lung diseases (such as emphysema) and septal defects (holes in the wall which separates the left and right sides of the heart).

PULMONARY VALVE

Valve formed by three cup-shaped membranes at the junction of the pulmonary artery and the right lower chamber of the heart (right ventricle). When the right ventricle contracts, the pulmonary valve opens and the blood is forced into the artery leading to the lungs. When the chamber relaxes, the valve is closed and prevents a backflow of the blood. *See Valve.*

PULMONARY VEINS

The veins which conduct oxygenated blood from the lungs into the left upper chamber of the heart (left atrium).

PULSE *(puls)*

The expansion and contraction of an artery which may be felt with the finger.

PULSE PRESSURE

The difference between the blood pressure in the arteries when the heart is in contraction (systole) and when it is in relaxation (diastole).

PULSUS ALTERNANS *(pul'sus awl-ter'nanz)*

A pulse in which there is regular alternation of weak and strong beats.

PURKINJE FIBERS *(pur-kin'je)*

Specialized muscular fibers forming a network in the walls of the lower chambers of the heart and believed to be involved in conducting electrical impulses to the muscular walls of the two lower chambers (ventricles).

QUINIDINE *(kwin'i-deen)*

A drug sometimes used to treat abnormal rhythms of the heartbeat; an antiarrhythmic drug.

RADIOISOTOPE *(ray"de-o-i'so-top)*

A radioactive form ("isotope") of an element. *See Isotope.*

RADIOISOTOPIC SCANNING
(ray"de-o-i'so-top-ik skan'ning)

A diagnostic technique involving radioactive labelling of tissues and organs by the injection of radioisotopes into the bloodstream. The emitted radioactivity is detected by a scanner and a record or "scan" of the labelled area is made. Used by cardiologists to visualize the heart and great vessels, it can often reveal areas of heart damage. *See Isotope and Radioisotope.*

RAUWOLFIA *(raw-wol'fe-ah)*

A drug consisting of powdered whole root of a plant (Rauwolfia serpentina) which lowers blood pressure and slows the heart rate. Sometimes used in treatment of high blood pressure. An antihypertensive agent. *See Reserpine.*

RAYNAUD'S DISEASE *(ray-noz')*

Also called Primary Raynaud's Phenomenon. A disorder characterized by occurrences of Raynaud's Phenomenon, but not known to have an underlying cause.

RAYNAUD'S PHENOMENON *(ray-noz')*

Short episodes of pallor and numbness in the fingers, toes and, rarely, the nose and ears, due to temporary constriction of the arterioles in the skin. Pallor in the affected area is followed by blueness (due to insufficient oxygen supply), then occasionally by redness as oxygenated blood rushes in. These episodes may be triggered by cold temperatures, emotional stress, working with vibrating machinery or cigarettes.
PRIMARY RAYNAUD'S PHENOMENON is called RAYNAUD'S DISEASE, is generally benign, and has no known cause.
SECONDARY RAYNAUD'S PHENOMENON is a symptom of one of several serious disorders, which, if not detected and treated, may have serious consequences.

RED BLOOD CELLS (CORPUSCLES)

One of the three kinds of formed elements found in the blood. Their most important function is to carry oxygen by means of hemoglobin, the red pigment these cells contain. Also called erythrocytes. *See White Blood Cells and Platelets.*

REGURGITATION *(re-gur"ji-ta'shun)*

The backward flow of blood through a defective valve.

REHABILITATION *(re"hah-bil"i-ta'shun)*

The return of a person disabled by accident or disease to the maximum attainable physical, mental, emotional, social and economic usefulness, and, if employable, to an opportunity for gainful employment.

RENAL *(re'nal)*

Pertaining to the kidney.

RENAL CIRCULATION

The circulation of the blood through the kidneys. Important in heart disease because of its function in the elimination of water, certain chemical elements, and waste products from the body.

RENAL HYPERTENSION
(re'nal hi"per-ten'shun)

High blood pressure caused by damage to or disease of the kidneys or their blood vessels.

RESERPINE *(re'er-peen OR re-ser'peen)*

One of the organic substances found in the root of the Indian snake root plant (Rauwolfia serpentina) which lowers blood pressure, slows the heart rate, and has a sedative effect.

REVASCULARIZATION
(re-vas"ku-lar-i-za'shun)

Restoration of sufficient bloodflow to body tissues when supplying arteries are narrowed or blocked by injury or disease. Such surgery can be done on the legs, kidneys, brain, neck or (most commonly) the heart.
One procedure for cardiac revascularization is endarterectomy, removal of the thickened inner lining of a narrowed coronary artery. Other procedures may involve the use of additional blood vessels, either artificial ones or ones from elsewhere in the body. Vessels from other parts of the body may either be rerouted from nearby structures (for example, the internal mammary artery) or by grafting whole sections of vessels onto the heart (as is done with the saphenous vein in coronary bypass surgery). *See Endarterectomy and Coronary Bypass Surgery.*

RHEUMATIC FEVER *(roo-mat'ik)*

A disease, usually occurring in childhood, which may follow a few weeks after a streptococcal infection. It is sometimes characterized by one or more of the following: fever, sore swollen joints, a skin rash, occasionally by involuntary twitching of the muscles (called chorea or St. Vitus Dance) and small nodes under the skin. In some cases the infection affects the heart and may result in scarring the valves, weakening the heart muscle, or damaging the sac enclosing the heart. *See Rheumatic Heart Disease.*

RHEUMATIC HEART DISEASE *(roo-mat'ik)*

The damage done to the heart, particularly the heart valves, by one or more attacks of rheumatic fever. The valves are sometimes scarred so they do not open and close normally. *See Rheumatic Fever.*

RISK FACTORS

In cardiology, characteristics which are associated with an increased risk of developing coronary heart disease. These include high blood pressure (hypertension), elevated blood levels of cholesterol and other lipids (hyperlipoproteinemia), cigarette smoking, obesity, diabetes and a family history of heart disease. A competitive, aggressive lifestyle (Type A Behavior) is also thought to predispose a person to heart disease.

S-A NODE
See Sinoatrial Node.

SAPHENOUS VEIN *(sah-fe'nus)*

A large vein in the leg which can be removed and grafted onto the heart in coronary bypass surgery to provide adequate coronary circulation. *See Coronary Bypass Surgery.*

SATURATED FAT *(sat'u-rat"ed)*

A fat so constituted chemically that it is not capable of absorbing any more hydrogen. These are usually the solid fats of animal origin such as the fats in milk, butter, meat, etc. A diet high in saturated fat content tends to increase the amount of cholesterol in the blood. Sometimes these fats are restricted in the diet in an effort to lessen the hazard of fatty deposits in the blood vessels.

SCLEROSIS *(skle-ro'sis)*

Hardening, as in the term "arteriosclerosis," hardening of the arteries.

SECONDARY HYPERTENSION
(hi"per-ten'shun)

High blood pressure caused by (i.e. secondary to) certain specific diseases or infections. See *Pheochromocytoma* and *Renal Hypertension.*

SEMILUNAR VALVES *(sem"e-lu'nar)*

Cup-shaped valves. The aortic valve at the entrance to the aorta and the pulmonary valve at the entrance to the pulmonary artery are semilunar valves. They consist of three cup-shaped flaps which prevent the backflow of blood.

SEPTAL DEFECT *(sep'tal)*

An abnormal opening in the wall (septum) that normally divides the right and left sides of the heart. There are both atrial and ventricular septal defects, depending on whether the upper or lower heart chambers are involved.

SEPTUM *(sep'tum)*

A dividing wall.
1. Atrial or interatrial septum. Muscular wall dividing left and right upper chambers (atria) of the heart.
2. Ventricular or interventricular septum. Muscular wall, thinner at the top, dividing the left and right lower chambers (ventricles) of the heart.

SEROTONIN *(ser"o-to'nin)*

A naturally occurring compound, found mainly in the gastrointestinal tract and in lesser amounts in the blood, which has a stimulating effect on the circulatory system.

SERUM *(se'rum)*

The fluid portion of blood which remains after the cellular elements have been removed by coagulation. It is different from plasma which is the cell-free liquid portion of uncoagulated blood.

SERVETUS, MICHAEL *(1509-1553)*

Spanish physician who discovered the circulation of the blood through the lungs. Burned at the stake in Geneva for his religious doctrines.

SHOCK

The collection of symptoms resulting from an inadequate volume of fluid circulating through the body to maintain normal metabolism. This may be due to a large loss of blood or to some derangement of circulatory control. Shock is marked by hypotension (low blood pressure), pale, cold skin, usually tachycardia (weak, rapid pulse), and often anxiety. Cardiogenic shock is shock resulting from a greatly diminished cardiac output, such as may occur in a large heart attack.

SHUNT

A passage between two blood vessels or between the two sides of the heart, as in cases where an opening exists in the wall which normally separates them. In surgery, the operation of forming a passage between blood vessels to divert blood from one part of the body to another.

SIGN

Any objective evidence of a disease. See *Symptom.*

SINOATRIAL NODE *(si"no-a'tre-al)*

A small mass of specialized cells in the right upper chamber of the heart which give rise to the electrical impulses that initiate contractions of the heart. Also called S-A node or pacemaker.

SINUS RHYTHM *(si'nus rith'm)*

Normal heart rhythm as initiated by electrical impulses in the sinoatrial node or pacemaker. See *Pacemaker.*

SINUSES OF VALSALVA *(si'nus-sez of val-sal'vah)*

Three pouches in the wall of the aorta behind the three cup-shaped membranes of the aortic valve.

SODIUM *(so'de-um)*

A mineral essential to life, found in nearly all plant and animal tissue. Table salt (sodium chloride) is nearly half sodium. In some types of heart disease the body retains an excess of sodium and water, and therefore sodium intake is restricted.

SPHYGMOMANOMETER *(sfig"mo-mah-nom'e-ter)*

An instrument for measuring blood pressure in the arteries.

STARLING'S LAW OF THE HEART

A law which states that the more the heart muscle is stretched when an increased

amount of blood fills the ventricles, the more vigorous its contraction will be, resulting in a greater amount of blood pumped out of the heart.

STASIS *(sta'sis)*

A stoppage or lessening of the flow of blood or other body fluid in any part.

STENOSIS *(ste-no'sis)*

A narrowing or stricture of an opening. Mitral stenosis, aortic stenosis, etc., mean that the valve indicated has become so narrowed that it does not function normally.

STETHOSCOPE *(steth'o-skop)*

An instrument for listening to sounds within the body.

STRESS

Bodily or mental tension caused by physical, chemical or emotional factors. Stress can refer to physical exertion as well as mental anxiety.

STRESS TEST

A diagnostic method used to determine the body's response to physical exertion (stress). Usually involves taking an ECG and other physiological measurements (such as breathing rate and blood pressure) while the patient is exercising—usually jogging on a treadmill, walking up and down a short set of stairs, or pedaling on a stationary bicycle.

STROKE *(strok)*

Also called cerebral vascular accident. An impeded blood supply to some part of the brain, generally caused by:
1. A blood clot forming in the vessel (cerebral thrombosis).
2. A rupture of the blood vessel wall (cerebral hemorrhage).
3. A blood clot or other material from another part of the vascular system which flows to the brain and obstructs a cerebral vessel (cerebral embolism).
4. Pressure on a blood vessel, as by a tumor.

STROKE VOLUME *(strok)*

The amount of blood which is pumped out of the heart at each contraction of the heart.

SYMPATHECTOMY *(sim"pah-thek'to-me)*

An operation which interrupts some part of the sympathetic nervous system. The sympathetic nervous system is a part of the autonomic or involuntary nervous system which normally regulates tissues not under voluntary control, e.g., glands, heart, and smooth muscles. Sometimes the interruption is accomplished by drugs, in which case it is called a chemical sympathectomy.

SYMPATHETIC NERVOUS SYSTEM *(sim"pah-thet'ik)*

One of the two divisions of the autonomic nervous system. See *Autonomic Nervous System.*

SYMPTOM *(simp'tum)*

Any subjective evidence of a patient's condition. See *Sign.*

SYNCOPE *(sin'ko-pe)*

A faint. One cause for syncope can be an insufficient blood supply to the brain.

SYNDROME *(sin'drom)*

A set of symptoms which occur together and are therefore given a name to indicate that particular combination.

SYSTEMIC CIRCULATION *(sis-tem'ik)*

The circulation of the blood through all parts of the body except the lungs, the flow being from the left lower chamber of the heart (left ventricle) through the body, back to the right upper chamber of the heart (right atrium). See *Pulmonary Circulation.*

SYSTOLE *(sis'to-le)*

In each heartbeat, the period of contraction of the heart. Atrial systole is the period of the contraction of the upper chambers of the heart, called the atria.

Ventricular systole is the period of the contraction of the lower chambers of the heart, called the ventricles. See *Cardiac Cycle.*

TACHYCARDIA *(tak"e-kar'de-ah)*

Abnormally fast heart rate. Generally, anything over 100 beats per minute is considered a tachycardia.

TETRALOGY OF FALLOT   *(te-tral'o-je of fal-o')*

A congenital malformation of the heart involving four distinct defects (hence tetralogy). Named for Etienne Fallot, French physician who described the condition in 1888. The four defects are:

1. An abnormal opening in the wall between the lower chambers of the heart (ventricular septal defect).
2. Misplacement of the aorta, "overriding" the abnormal opening, so that it receives blood from both the right and left lower chambers instead of only the left.
3. Pulmonary outflow obstruction usually below or at the valve.
4. Enlargement of the right ventricle.

THIAZIDES   *(thi'a-sidz)*

Also called thiazide diuretics or benzothiadiazides. A class of diuretics (drugs which promote excretion of urine) which includes chlorothiazide. The thiazides are often used to treat high blood pressure and for the relief of edema, or waterlogged tissues. *See Antihypertensive Drugs.*

THORACIC   *(tho-ras'ik)*

Pertaining to the chest (thorax).

THROMBECTOMY   *(throm-bek'to-me)*

An operation to remove a blood clot from a blood vessel.

THROMBOANGIITIS OBLITERANS   *(throm"bo-an"je-i'tis ob-lit'er-anz)*

Also called Buerger's disease. A disease of the blood vessels of the extremities, primarily the legs, which occurs most commonly in men and is associated with tobacco use. It is characterized by inflammation of the veins, arteries and nerves and by thrombosis in the vessels (blood clot formation). This leads to poor circulation and gangrene. *See Buerger's Syndrome.*

THROMBOEMBOLISM   *(throm"bo-em'bo-lizm)*

Obstruction (embolism) of a blood vessel by a blood clot (thrombus) formed elsewhere in the circulatory system and carried along by the bloodstream to plug a smaller vessel.

THROMBOLYTIC AGENTS   *(throm"bo-lit'ik)*

Substances which dissolve blood clots. Also called fibrinolytic agents. Two examples are streptokinase and urokinase.

THROMBOPHLEBITIS   *(throm"bo-fle-bi'tis)*

Inflammation and blood clotting in a vein.

THROMBOSIS   *(throm-bo'sis)*

The formation or presence of a blood clot (thrombus) inside a blood vessel or cavity of the heart.

THROMBUS   *(throm'bus)*

A blood clot which forms inside a blood vessel or cavity of the heart. *See Embolus.*

TOXIC   *(tok'sik)*
Poisonous.

TRANSPLANTATION, HEART

The replacement of a healthy heart from a recently deceased donor into the chest of a person whose own heart can no longer function adequately. The donor's heart then replaces or assists the failing heart.

TRANSPOSITION OF THE GREAT VESSELS   *(trans"po-zish'un)*

A congenital heart defect in which the two largest arteries occur in the wrong places: the aorta arises from the right (rather than left) ventricle and the pulmonary artery arises from the left (rather than right) ventricle. Thus the right heart pumps used blood from the body through the aorta and back to the body, and the left heart pumps oxygenated blood from the lungs back to the lungs. Only if there is a sizeable hole between right and left chambers (a septal defect) or a channel between the aorta and pulmonary artery (patent ductus arteriosus) will enough oxygenated blood get pumped to the body to sustain life for the infant.

TRICUSPID VALVE   *(tri-kus'pid)*

A valve consisting of three cusps or triangular segments located between the upper and lower chamber in the right side of the heart. Its position corresponds to the mitral valve (which is bicuspid) in the left side of the heart. *See Valve.*

TRIGLYCERIDE   *(tri-glis'er-id)*

The main type of lipid (fatty substance) found in the adipose (fat) tissue of the body and also the main dietary lipid. High levels of triglycerides in the blood may be associated with a greater risk of coronary atherosclerosis.

TRUNCUS ARTERIOSUS   *(trun'kus ar-te"re-o'sus)*

An arterial trunk arising from the fetal heart which develops into the aorta and pulmonary artery. It is a congenital defect if it persists past the birth of the infant.

ULTRASOUND   *(ul'tra-sownd)*

High frequency sound vibrations, not audible to the human ear. In a sonar-like application, it can be used by cardiologists for diagnosis. *See Echocardiography.*

UNSATURATED FAT   *(un-sat'u-rat"ed)*

A fat whose molecules have one or more double bonds, so that it is capable of absorbing more hydrogen. MONOUNSATURATED FATS, such as olive oil, have only one double bond (the rest are single) and seem to have little effect on blood cholesterol. POLYUNSATURATED FATS, such as corn oil and safflower oil, have two or more double bonds per molecule and tend to lower blood cholesterol. *See Saturated Fat.*

VAGUS NERVES   *(va'gus)*

Two of the nerves of the parasympathetic nervous system which extends from the brain, through the neck and thorax into the abdomen. Known as the inhibitory nerves of the heart, they slow the heart rate when stimulated.

VALVE

A flap of tissue which prevents backflow of blood to keep it moving through the heart and circulatory system in the right direction. There are tiny valves along the inside of the veins and four large valves at the entrances and exits of the ventricles in the heart. *See Aortic, Mitral, Pulmonary, and Tricuspid Valves.*

VALVULAR INSUFFICIENCY   *(val'vu-lar)*

Valves which close improperly and permit a backflow of blood in the wrong direction. *See Incompetent Valve.*

VARICOSE VEINS   *(var'i-kos)*

Also called "varicosities" and "varices," they are swollen veins found most frequently on the legs, especially the calves. *See Varix.*

VARIX   *(var'iks)*

A varicosity or abnormally swollen vein, artery, or lymph vessel. The plural form is "varices." Varices can occur in such locations as the esophagus, the anus, or the legs (where they are more commonly called "varicose veins"). *See Esophageal Varices, Hemorrhoids, and Varicose Veins.*

VASCULAR   *(vas'ku-lar)*

Pertaining to the blood vessels.

VASO-   *(vas'o)*

A combining form meaning vessel or duct.

VASOCONSTRICTOR   *(vas"o-kon-strik'tor)*

Vasoconstrictor nerves are a part of the involuntary nervous system. When these nerves are stimulated, they cause the muscles of the arterioles to contract, narrowing the arteriole passage, increasing the resistance to bloodflow, and raising the blood pressure.

Vasoconstrictor agents (or vasopressors) are chemical substances which stimulate the muscles of the arterioles to contract. An example is norepinephrine (noradrenalin).

VASODILATOR   *(vas"o-di-lat'or)*

Vasodilator nerves are certain nerve fibers of the involuntary nervous system which cause the muscle of the arterioles to relax, thus enlarging the arteriole passage, reducing resistance to the flow of blood, and lowering blood pressure.

Vasodilator agents are chemical compounds which cause a relaxation of the muscles of the arterioles. Examples are nitroglycerin and other nitrites, hydralazine, and many others.

VASOINHIBITOR   *(vas"o-in-hib'i-tor)*

An agent which inhibits the action of the vasomotor nerves, that is, an agent which prevents the blood vessels from a normal response (constriction or dilation) to stimuli.

VASOMOTOR   *(vas"o-mo'tor)*

Any agent (nerve or substance) that affects the caliber of a vessel, especially of a blood vessel, that is, any agent that is either a vasoconstrictor or a vasodilator.

VASOPRESSOR *(vas"o-pres'or)*

A vasoconstrictor agent. *See Vasoconstrictor and also Pressor.*

VECTORCARDIOGRAPHY
(vek"tor-kar"de-og'rah-fe)

Determination of the direction and magnitude of the electrical forces of the heart by using electrocardiography in three dimensions.

VEIN *(vain)*

Any one of a series of vessels of the vascular system which carries blood from various parts of the body back to the heart. All veins in the body conduct unoxygenated blood except the pulmonary veins which conduct freshly oxygenated blood from the lungs back to the heart.

VENA CAVA *(ve'nah ka'vah)*

One of the two great veins which conduct unoxygenated blood from the body to the right atrium of the heart. The superior vena cava brings blood from the upper part of the body (head, neck and chest). The inferior vena cava brings blood from the lower part of the body (legs and abdomen). Plural form is *Venae Cavae (ve'ni ka'vi).*

VENOUS BLOOD *(ve'nus)*

Unoxygenated blood. The blood, with hemoglobin in the reduced state, is carried by the veins from all parts of the body back to the heart and then pumped by the right side of the heart through the pulmonary artery to the lungs where it is oxygenated.

VENTRICLE *(ven'tre-kl)*

One of the two main pumping chambers of the heart. The left ventricle pumps oxygenated blood through the arteries to the body. The right ventricle pumps unoxygenated blood through the pulmonary artery to the lungs. Capacity of each ventricle in an adult averages 85 cc. or about 3 ounces.

VISCERAL PERICARDIUM *(vis'er-al per"i-kar'de-um)*

The inner wall of the pericardium, the double-walled sac which surrounds the heart. The visceral pericardium closely adheres to the heart and forms the outermost layer of the heart wall and is also called the epicardium.

WHITE BLOOD CELLS

One of the three kinds of formed elements found in the blood. There are various types of white blood cells. Their best-known function is defense: they destroy foreign bodies, such as bacteria, in areas of infection. Also called leukocytes. *See Red Blood Cells and Platelets.*

XANTHINE *(zan'theen)*

A class of drugs used among other things to increase the excretion of urine. A diuretic.

XANTHOMA *(zan-tho'mah)*

A new growth of skin occurring as small flat or slightly raised patches or nodules which are yellowish-orange in color. The various types of xanthomas are due to blood lipid disorders (hyperlipoproteinemias).

INDEX

Abbott, Maude 248
Abdominal pain 226, 227, 237, 259, 261
Abortion
  spontaneous 39
  therapeutic 335
Acetylcholine 142
Acidosis 251, 317
Acrolein 31
Acrocyanosis 229, 230
Actinomyces 320
Acupuncture 37
Acyanotic heart disease 297, 298
Adenitis, cervical 261
Adenosine 137
Adrenal glands 144–45, 150, 316
  and fluid retention 203
  and hypertension 8, 170, 173
  smoking and 38
Adrenalin 196
Adriamycin 326
Advanced cardiac life support units 112
Aerobic effect. See Cardio-vascular training effect
Age and aging, as risk factors 2, 17. See also entries under Atherosclerosis; Blood pressure; Cardiac output; Coronary artery disease; Hypertension
Air pollution, smoking and 31–32
Airway, emergency opening of 105–106, 109, 111–12
Alcohol 44, 66
  following heart attack 91
  hypertension and 88
  and myocarditis 322
  as nutrient 42
  and obesity 15, 44, 66
  and premature heart-beat 192, 193

as risk factor 2, 13–14, 115
smoking and 22, 24, 39, 40
toxic effects 326–27, 328
and triglyceride levels 5
Alcoholic cardiomyopathy 327
Alcoholism 194, 327
  teenage, increase in 14
Aldosterone 145, 170–71, 172, 203, 207
Allergy and allergenic substances 31, 126, 221, 263, 308, 309–10
Alphamethyl-DOPA 308
Alveoli 140
Ambulatory electrocardiography 123
American Cancer Society 36
American Heart Association
  diet recommendations 8, 51, 52
  emergency identification cards 93, 238
  information available 51, 254
  Pooling Project 5
  smoking cessation programs 36
  training in life support techniques 104, 112
American Lung Association 36
Amicar R 286
Amino acids 44–45, 46, 51
Amino-caproic (Amicar R) 286
Amitryptyline 326
Amputation 215, 218, 219, 220, 221, 222, 226
Amyloidosis 325
Anasarca 205

Anastomoses 209, 210
Anemia 48, 229, 252, 317, 320, 327
  pernicious 49, 51
  in pregnancy 331
  symptoms 156, 162, 191
Aneurysm 226–27, 228, 229–30, 300
  aortic 23, 335
  arterial 213, 223, 224
  and hemorrhagic stroke 168, 285–86
  rupture of 23, 226, 284, 319
  surgical removal of 296
  syphilis and 319
Angina pectoris 89, 91, 95, 102, 152–53, 161, 177, 179–80, 183–86, 304–306
  and atherosclerosis 168, 178, 295
  and congestive heart failure 201
  exercise and 19
  forewarning of heart attack 153
  night attacks 186
  obesity and 15
  psychosocial precursors 341, 343
  unstable 179–80, 186
  and valve disease 268, 274
  in women 18. See also Chest pain; Drug therapy
Angiography 289, 341
  arterial 217, 229
  cardiac 125, 126, 323
  cerebral 281
  coronary 90, 125
  pulmonary 316
Angiotensin II 145
Ankles, swelling of 95, 115, 119, 125, 204, 237, 268, 334
Anorexia nervosa 65
Antibiotics 130, 252, 314, 315
  against endocarditis 320
  and pneumonia 315
  and rheumatic fever 94, 96, 261, 262, 263, 269, 270
  tetracycline 263
  and ulceration 218, 221
  and valvular surgery 274
Antibodies 45, 130, 259
Anticoagulant drugs 11,

96–97, 98, 192, 195, 224, 237, 238, 281, 282, 288, 290, 311–12
  in pregnancy 335
  and valve replacement 273, 295
  and vascular surgery 300
Antidepressant drugs 309, 326
Antinomy drugs 326
Anturane 312
Anxiety 13, 341, 342, 343
  effect on heartbeat 157, 191, 193–94, 198
  pain-causing 155, 161
  smoking and 28
  symptoms of 156, 160–61, 162
Aorta 132–37 passim, 142, 146, 148–49, 170, 213, 240
  abdominal 125, 215, 223, 226, 229–30
  aneurysm of 227, 319
  bypass surgery 185, 210
  coarctation of 171, 243–44, 251, 254, 320, 335
  thoracic 134, 226, 227. See also entries under Regurgitation; Stenosis; Valves
Aortic valve 131, 136, 213, 227, 266, 270, 294, 298, 319–30, 355
Aortography 217, 227
Aphasia 279–80
Apnea 204
Arrhythmia, cardiac 91, 95–96, 97, 160, 180, 188–98, 309, 322, 323, 325
  alcohol and 326–27
  treatment of 309–10, 312
Arterial embolism 222–24, 228–29
Arterial injury 224–25, 229
Arteries 131, 134–35, 136, 148
  blockage of 168, 310
  hypertension and 166–67, 170, 173, 174, 240
  narrowing of 214, 310
  peripheral, diseases of 213–30
  severing of 225